Recent Progress in Mitral Valve Disease

Recent Progress in Mitral Valve Disease

Carlos Duran, MD, PhD
Professor, Jefe, Centro Medico Nacional, 'Marques de Valdacilla',
Santander, Spain

William W. Angell, MD
Director, Cardiovascular Surgical Research,
Scripps Clinic and Research Foundation, La Jolla, California

Allen D. Johnson, MD
Head of Cardiovascular Disease,
Scripps Clinic and Research Foundation, La Jolla, California

James H. Oury, MD
Head, Division of Cardiac Surgery,
Scripps Clinic and Research Foundation, La Jolla, California

Butterworths
London Boston Durban Singapore Sydney Toronto Wellington

First published, 1984

© Butterworth & Co. (Publishers) Ltd, 1984

British Library Cataloguing in Publication Data

Recent progress in mitral valve disease.
  1. Mitral valve—Diseases
  I. Duran, Carlos
  616.1'25   RC685.V2

  ISBN 0-407-00294-4

Library of Congress Cataloging in Publication Data
Main entry under title:

Recent progress in mitral valve disease.
  Bibliography: p.
  Includes index.
  1. Mitral valve—Surgery. 2. Mitral valve—Diseases.
I. Duran, Carlos. [DNLM: 1. Heart valve diseases.
2. Mitral valve. WG 262 R295]
RD598.R37 1984   617'.412   84-1759
ISBN 0-407-00294-4

Photoset by Phoenix Photosetting, Chatham, Kent
Printed and bound by Robert Hartnoll Ltd, Bodmin, Cornwall

Preface

The International Symposium on the Mitral Valve and these Proceedings owe their genesis to Dr Daniel Kalmanson who in 1976 organized the first International Symposium on the Mitral Valve held in Paris, France. This meeting brought together authorities from many varying disciplines relating to the mitral valve in a unique 'pluridisciplinary' approach. The information at the Paris Symposium served not only as a cornerstone for our present knowledge but also provided a stimulus for continued research in this evolving area. Paris also provided me with the opportunity to meet several individuals who became instrumental in the organization of our Symposium. At the Paris meeting I had the opportunity of meeting Dr Carlos Duran, a man who greatly influenced my interest in the mitral valve and provided an opportunity for me to learn from him, in the operating suite, the surgical techniques of reconstruction. A few years later while in Santander, Spain, after a day in the operating room, an evening stroll in downtown Santander and a wonderful Spanish tradition known as 'the vino', provided the setting in which a 'pluridisciplinary' group of Spanish physicians and I formulated the plans for a second International Symposium on the Mitral Valve.

Many friends and colleagues are responsible for the growth of this early idea. Dr Alain Carpentier, the first surgeon to demonstrate to me the intracacies of the mitral valve, graciously consented to attend and contribute to the Symposium. My friend and partner, Dr William Angell, responded enthusiastically to the idea of a second symposium and collaborated in its formulation. Dr Allen Johnson, Head of the Division of Cardiovascular Diseases at Scripps Clinic and Research Foundation, shared the responsibility of Program Chairman with Dr Duran and myself and lent his expertise in the understanding of mitral valve function from a cardiologist's perspective. Dr Charles Edwards, President of Scripps Clinic and Research Foundation, eagerly supported our desire to provide a suitable setting to address again in a multidisciplinary way the fascinating subject of the mitral valve. To Catherine Williams, our Cardiovascular Nurse Clinician, goes my gratitude for her tireless efforts in planning and coordinating the many different aspects of the Symposium.

My hope is that the Proceedings of this second International Symposium will once again provide a suitable stepping stone for future symposia of this nature and will generate continued interest in pursuing an understanding of the Mitral Valve.

James H. Oury

Contributors

F. Alonso-Lej, MD
Chief of Thoracic and Cardiovascular Surgery, Ciudad Sanitaria; Chief of Cardiac and Thoracic Surgery, Nueva Clinica Quiron, Zaragoza, Spain

William W. Angell, MD
Director of Cardiovascular Surgical Research, Scripps Clinic and Research Foundation, La Jolla, California, USA

Rene A. Arcilla, MD
Director, Pediatric Cardiology; Professor of Pediatrics, University of Chicago, Chicago, Illinois, USA

David B. Arkin, MD
Division of Anesthesiology, Donald N. Sharp Memorial Community Hospital, San Diego, California, USA

Timothy Bateman, MD
Associate Cardiologist, Cedars-Sinai Medical Center, Los Angeles, California, USA

Saroja Bharati, MD
Chairperson, Department of Pathology, Congenital Heart and Conduction System Laboratory, Deborah Heart and Lung Center, Brown Mills, New Jersey, USA

V. Bilca, MD
Cardiovascular Surgeon, Research Assistant, Clinic for Cardiovascular Surgery, Tirgu-Mureş, Romania

V. O. Björk, MD
Professor of Thoracic and Cardiovascular Surgery, Karolinska Sjukhuset Thoracic Surgical Clinic, Stockholm, Sweden

Kim Böök, MD
Thoracic Surgical Clinic, Karolinska Hospital, Stockholm, Sweden

G. Bougkioukas
Department of Cardiac Surgery, University of Munich, West Germany

S. Bradisteanu, MD
Cardiovascular Surgeon, Research Assistant, Clinic for Cardiovascular Surgery, Tirgu-Mureş, Romania

D. Bratu, MD
Cardiologist, Clinical Assistant, Clinic for Cardiovascular Surgery, Tirgu-Mureş, Romania

Blase A. Carabello, MD
Associate Professor of Medicine Physiology, Temple University, School of Medicine; Director, Cardiac Diagnostic Laboratory, Temple University Hospital, Philadelphia, Pennsylvania, USA

Alain Carpentier, MD, PhD
Professor Agrege Chirurgie, Cardiaque, Universite Paris IV: Head, Laboratoire D'Etudes des Geffes et Prothese Cardiaques, Hopital Broussais, Clinique de Chirugio Cardio-Vasculaire, Paris, France

Kanu Chatterjee, MB, FRCP
Associate Chief, Cardiovascular Division, University of California, San Francisco, California, USA

Aurelio Chaux, MD
Senior Associate Surgeon, Cedars-Sinai Medical Center, Los Angeles, California, USA

Lawrence H. Cohn, MD
Professor of Surgery, Harvard Medical School, Brigham and Women's Hospital, Boston, Massachusetts, USA

Peirre L. Coulon, MD
House Officer, The General Infirmary, Leeds, UK

Lawrence Czer, MD
Associate Cardiologist, Cedars-Sinai Medical Center, Los Angeles, California, USA

Gordon K. Danielson, MD
Professor of Surgery, Mayo Medical School, Thoracic and Cardiovascular Surgery, Mayo Clinic, Rochester, Minnesota, USA

Keith Dawkins, MD
Cardiac Department, Brompton Hospital, London, UK

R. Deac, MD
Chief, Clinic for Cardiovascular Surgery, Tirgu-Mureş, Romania

Carlos Duran, MD, PhD
Professor, Jefe, Centro Medico Nacional, Marques de Valdacilla, Santander, Spain

E. Fargaraşanu, MD
Cardiovascular Surgeon, Clinical Assistant, Clinic for Cardiovascular Surgery, Tirgu-Mureş, Romania

Robert W. Frater, MD
Professor and Chief, Division of Cardiothoracic Surgery, Albert Einstein College of Medicine, Montefiore Hospital and Medical Center, Bronx, New York, USA

Richard Gray, MD
Associate Cardiologist, Cedars-Sinai Medical Center, Los Angeles, California, USA

William Grossman, MD
Professor of Medicine, Harvard Medical School; Chief, Cardiovascular Disease, Beth Israel Hospital, Boston, Massachusetts, USA

S. Hagl, MD
Department of Cardiovascular Surgery, Deutsches Herzzentrum, Muenchen, Munich, West Germany

Laurence A. Harker, MD
Director, Roon Research Center for Arteriosclerosis and Thrombosis, Scripps Clinic and Research Foundation, La Jolla, California, USA

Syed S. Hasan, MD, FRCS
Senior Registrar, The General Infirmary, Leeds, UK

Werner Heimisch, MSEE
Department of Cardiovascular Surgery, Deutsches Herzzentrum Muenchen, Munich, West Germany

A. Henze, MD
Associate Professor, Thoracic Surgical Clinic, Karolinska Hospital, Stockholm, Sweden

Marian I. Ionescu, MD
Cardiothoracic Surgeon, The General Infirmary, Leeds, UK

Stuart W. Jamieson, MD
Assistant Proffessor, Cardiovascular Surgery, Stanford University School of Medicine, Stanford, California, USA

W. D. Johnson, MD
3112 W. Highland Blvd., Milwaukee, Wisconsin, USA

Daniel Kalmanson, MD
Director of Clinical Teaching; Chief, Department of Cardiology, CV Research Center ARNTIC, Foundation A. de Rothschild, Paris, France

Chuichi Kawai, MD
Third Division Department of Internal Medicine, Kyoto University Hospital, Kyoto, Japan

Philip Kay, FRCS
Brompton Hospital, London, UK

Kenneth L. Kayser, MS
St Mary's Hospital, Milwaukee, Wisconsin, USA

J. Ward Kennedy, MD
Chief, Cardiovascular Disease Section, Veterans Administration Hospital, Seattle, Washington, USA

E. Kreuzer, MD
Professor of Cardiovascular Surgery, Herzchirurgische Klinik der Universität München, West Germany

Robert Leachman, MD
Senior Cardiologist, Texas Heart Institute; Professor of Medicine, Baylor College of Medicine, Baylor College of Medicine, Houston, Texas, USA

Maurice Lev, MD
Director of Laboratories, Department of Pathology, Congenital Heart and Conduction System Laboratory, Deborah Heart and Lung Center, Brown Mills, New Jersey, USA

M. Liebhart, MD
Cardiovascular Surgeon, Clinical Assistant, Clinic for Cardiovascular Surgery, Tirgu-Mureş, Romania

D. Lindblom, MD
Thoracic Surgical Clinic, Karolinska Hospital, Stockholm, Sweden

Jack Matloff, MD
Director, Thoracic and Cardiovascular Surgery, Cedars-Sinai Medical Center, Los Angeles, California, USA

Hans Meisner, MD
Department of Cardiovascular Surgery, Deutsches Herzzentrum Muenchen, Munich, West Germany

Nikolaus Mendler, MD
Department of Cardiovascular Surgery, Deutsches Herzzentrum Muenchen, Munich, West Germany

D. C. Miller, MD
Associate Professor of Cardiovascular Surgery, Stanford University School of Medicine, Stanford, California, USA

David Olivera, MRCP
Brompton Hospital, London, UK

James H. Oury, MD
Head, Division of Cardiac Surgery, Scripps Clinic and Research Foundatin, La Jolla, California, USA

Philip E. Oyer, MD
Assistant Professor of Cardiovascular Surgery, Stanford Medical Center, Stanford, California, USA

Matthias Paneth, FRCS
Brompton Hospital, London, UK

P. M. Pedraza, MD
St Mary's Hospital, Milwaukee, Wisconsin, USA

Kirk L. Peterson, MD
Director, Cardiac Catheterization Laboratory; Professor of Medicine, University of California, San Diego, California, USA

M. Poliac
Clinic for Cardiovascular Surgery, Tirgu Mures, Romania

B. Reichart
Department of Cardiac Surgery, University of Munich, Munich, West Germany

Robert Replogle, MD
Chief, Division of Cardiac Surgery, Michael Reese Hospital, Chicago, Illinois, USA

Donald N. Ross, DSC, FRCS
National Heart Hospital, London, UK

John Ross, Jr, MD
Professor of Medicine; Head, Division of Cardiology, University of California, San Diego, California, USA

Shigetake Sasayama, MD
Second Department of Internal Medicine, Toyama Medical and Pharmaceutical University, 2630 Sugitami, Toyama 930-01, Japan

N. Schad
Community Hospital, Passan, West Germany

Nelson B. Schiller, MD
Associate Professor of Medicine, University of California, San Francisco, California, USA

Fritz Sekening, MD
Department of Cardiovascular Surgery, Deutsches Herzzentrum Muenchen, Munich, West Germany

Pravin M. Shah, MD
Professor of Medicine, School of Medicine, School of Medicine, University of California of Los Angeles; Chief of Cardiology, Wadsworth Veterans Administration Hospital, Los Angeles, California, USA

Norman E. Shumway, MD
Chief of Cardiovascular Surgery, Stanford University School of Medicine, Stanford, California, USA

N. Paul Silverton, MD, MRCP
Lecturer in Cardiovascular Studies, Leeds University, Leeds, UK

Albert Starr, MD
Professor and Chief, Cardiopulmonary Surgery, The Oregon Health Science University, Portland, Oregon, USA

Edward B. Stinson
Department of Cardiovascular Surgery, Stanford University School of Medicine, Stanford, California, USA

Travis E. Stripling, PhD
Brown and Root, Inc., Houston, Texas, USA

Tsukasa Tajimi, MD
Visiting Research Fellow, University of California, USA

Anard P. Tandon, MD, MRCP
Consultant Physician, The Royal Infirmary, Halifax, UK

Frans Van de Werf, MD
Division of Cardiology, University Hospital St Rafael, Leuven, Belgium

Colette Veyrat
Chargé de Recherche au CNRS, Paris, France

David W. Wieting, MD
10846 Half Moon Pass, Littleton, Colorado, USA

Edward L. Yellin, PhD
Professor of Surgery; Associate Professor of Physiology and Biophysics, Department of Surgery and Physiology, Albert Einstein College of Medicine, Bronx, New York, USA

Chaim Yoran, MD
Director of Cardiology, Bronx-Lebanon Hospital Center; Associate Professor of Medicine, Albert Einstein College of Medicine, Bronx, New York, USA

Contents

Section 1

Introduction

James H. Oury and Carlos Duran

'There are more things in heaven and earth, Horatio, than are dreamt of in your philosophy'

(Hamlet, I.v. 166)

When faced with a new problem we search and probe its causes, mechanisms and possible solutions. A certain degree of understanding is reached, this knowledge is organized and conclusions for action are drawn. Once this plateau is achieved, we move on to more demanding situations and assumed the initial problem has been solved. Our understanding of the solution crystallizes to become 'established knowledge'. This 'established knowledge' will be taught to new generations who ignore the many unsuccessful attempts, side avenues, interrupted alternatives and negative experiences. Even some well-established facts are considered irrelevant to the solving of our daily problems.

New situations that challenge this 'established knowledge' and find it inadequate are necessary to force us to rethink our initial attitudes, deepen our search and reach a new level of cognition. This continuous process is essential to progress. The interruption or negative attitude towards the demands of change result in a closed and eventually sterile system. The assumption that a subject is closed, besides being an oversimplification, condemns the mind to ankylosis.

In the case of mitral valve surgery, advances in open-heart technology have displaced the simple solution of closed commissurotomy and opened the era of the valve prosthesis. The surgical simplicity of implantation coupled with the superb immediate results have overshadowed other possibilities often considered archaic, complex and even suspicious. However, the emergence of new techniques for valve repair have rekindled the interest in the mitral valve. It forced the development of improved diagnostic techniques which in turn facilitate the search for basic anatomic and physiologic facts. This situation led to the momentous symposium organized by Dr Daniel Kalmanson and held in Paris in 1975. Its pluridisciplinary approach covered most aspects of the mitral valve and stimulated as well as distributed knowledge across the specialty barriers.

Since then, a number of factors have continued to sustain or even accelerate the interest in the mitral valve. First was the reported data by many centers using the bioprosthesis for 5–10 years. Unfortunately, their findings show that the long-term results are far from perfect. Secondly, the new mechanical devices with improved hemodynamic performances have also come of age resulting in a new entity which could be term 'prosthetic disease'. Lastly, the conservative approach to valve repair has gained numerous adepts and offers a valid alterntive in some patient groups. Choosing the right surgical intervention encourages the need for better diagnostic correction for mitral stenosis. This suggestion brought down a flood of condemnation and controversial correspondence in that journal culminating finally in a leading article in which it was said that, 'the view was so potentially dangerous that the suggestion of surgical operation for the relief of mitral stenosis casts a grave responsibility upon Sir Launder Brunton'. Sir Thomas Lauder Brunton can rightly be claimed as the founding father of mitral valve surgeons which reserves him an honoured placed among the angels and surgical immortals.

On the other hand, the German surgeon Bilroth could be assigned to those warmer, nether regions for he said in 1883 that 'No man who wishes to retain the respect of his colleagues would dare to attempt a suturing of the heart'. With this generally hostile attitude of the medical profession there was no further discussion or work on the surgical management of valvular heart disease until about the First World War.

In 1914, Tuffier is cited by Cutler as having performed a successful finger dilatation of the *aortic* valve by invaginating the aortic wall; and in 1925, Sir Henry Souttar of the London Hospital did, in fact, perform the first successful finger dilatation of the mitral valve through the left atrium. The patient was a young girl and had a remission of her symptoms for some years—truly he was a man well ahead of his time. It is fair to point out, however, that the suggestion of finger fracture was made as early as 1910 by that cardiovascular genius Carrell, although he did not put his theory into practice.

It is also relevant to mention the extensive experimental work of Cutler of the Harvard Medical School, who carried out a series of experiments in cats and dogs with a view to excising part of the stenosed mitral valve. In 1923 he used a tenotome through the left ventricle of an 11-year-old girl who survived and died 4½ years later in left ventricular failure. Six subsequent patients treated with various punching instruments died. Without wishing to detract from Cutler's historically important work, it probably represented a 'wrong turning' in surgical progress for the mitral valve and largely ignored the dire effects of surgically induced regurgitation. Beck, one of Cutler's co-workers, was later to say that the use of such instruments probably delayed the advent of mitral valvotomy for 20 years. Another example of a wrong turning was exemplified by attempts to relieve the left atrial pressure by creating an atrial septal defect or by the more successful operation used by Sweet in the USA and d'Allain in France of a pulmonary vein to azygos anastomosis.

After these bold but sometimes misplaced pioneering efforts, the modern surgical era was introduced by Charles Bailey of Philadelphia. He, above all, deserves the credit for establishing the surgery of the mitral valve on a sound clinical basis; as a result of his work on dogs, he concluded that the approach through the left atrium was satisfactory and that the heart tolerated the exploring finger well. His first clinical attempt with this approach was in 1945, but the patient died of a torn left atrial appendage. His first success was not until 1948. At about the same time, four clinical surgeons working more or less independently achieved similar success—namely Bailey, Glover and Harken in the United States, and Brock in England. To Brock, however, belongs the credit for clarifying the surgical anatomy and pathology of the valve and for offering a logical explanation for the classically encountered typical mitral stenotic orifice.

The subsequent mitral valvotomy story is well known and the limited possibilities of finger fracture alone led to the use of a transatrial dilator by Du Bost in 1953 and to the subsequently more popular method of transventricular dilatation introduced by Logan of Edinburgh in 1955.

Mitral regurgitation posed another problem and serious attempts to correct this lesion were delayed by the general belief that the condition was well tolerated and did not impose a great burden on the heart. Early surgical maneuvers included a number of ingenious attempts to block the regurgitant jet with various pedicled grafts fixed within the left ventricle. The most important contribution, however, was one which has its modern counterpart in the various annuloplastic rings and repairs now performed, circumferential suture of the annulus was developed by Davila in the USA and Borrie in New Zealand. Davila and Glover were able to report 58 patients in 1938 with a 56% mortality in patients in failure and 17% mortality in the less severely ill.

Unlike mitral stenosis, closed methods of palliation for mitral regurgitation were largely unsatisfactory before the advent of open-heart surgery. Visual repair of the valve, like so many firsts, was achieved by Walt Lillehei of Minneapolis, in August 1956. A number of techniques were used like annuloplasty and the repair of ruptured chordae, but little lasting success resulted which underlined the need for a prosthetic replacement of the valve.

Initial attempts at valve replacement were with various flap-like devices of the toilet-seat variety. They were used particularly by surgeons like Ellis and Frater at the Mayo Clinic but culminated ultimately in the Starr–Edwards ball-valve prosthesis. Starr reported eight cases with six survivors in 1961. This undoubtedly represented the greatest major advance in the surgery of mitral valve disease with immediate and universal acceptance throughout the world. Development did not stop at that point, and we are literally still at the beginning of a series of advances in valve replacement. The mitral valve is still lagging behind our generally more satisfactory aortic valve substitutes.

Shortly after the introduction of the Starr valve, the encouraging results we were able to report with the aortic homograft led to a number of attempts to use homografts, usually mounted with some form of supporting ring as a mitral valve replacement. The first experimental work in this direction was carried out in dogs by that extraordinary pioneer Gordon Murray who incidentally was also responsible for the first aortic homograft in the descending aorta. Also, Lower working with Shumway did experimental work on the use of the autologous pulmonary valve as a mitral valve substitute. We subsequently adapted this work clinically for replacement both of the aortic and of the mitral valves.

Recognizing the logic of replacing the mitral valve with another anatomically perfect mitral valve, Berghuis and Rastelli in 1964 inserted homologous mitral valves in dogs complete with chordae and papillary muscles. This was followed by a number of clinical attempts by Senning, of Zurich, and ourselves using homologous mitral valves and a fully flexible ring mounting. We operated upon six patients and in two of them inserted a complete homologous aortic and mitral valve as a composite structure. All the mitral valves failed, the longest at 10 months, from rupture of the vulnerable chordae. Nevertheless, I believe the principle of using an anatomically perfect mitral valve is still valid, provided the chordae can be preserved and tensioned correctly.

After a further series of indifferent results with frame-mounted aortic and pulmonary homograft valves came the introduction of mounted porcine xenografts by Binet and Carpentier in France and Hancock in the USA. These and particularly the glutaraldehyde tanning technique revolutionized our current concept of biological valves for use in the mitral position. A number of basic problems remain unsolved and largely unchallenged.

To my mind, the fundamental defect in out thinking lies in the fact that we persist in regarding any inverted aortic valve, mechanical or biological, as a satisfactory and acceptable mitral valve replacement. Looking at the other side of the coin, I look upon the Bjork–Shiley valve as the nearest approach to the ideal mitral valve from a purely design point of view, and for this very reason regard it as totally unacceptable as an aortic valve replacement. The anatomic and haemodynamic conditions relating to the aortic and mitral areas are quite different and it makes no sense to regard the valves we use as automatically interchangeable.

For instance, there is a little anatomical resemblance between the small unsupported three-cusp aortic valve and the large bicuspid or multi-cusp, fully supported and fully flexible mitral valve apparatus. These naturally occuring valves represent the end result of millions of years of evolutionary development under the moulding effects of the blood flow and we cannot ignore this fundamental fact. Consequently, it is not surprising that aortic homograft valves last longer in the aortic area as compared with those in the mitral area.

An even more exacting comparison has been to assess the function of double homografts placed in the aortic and mitral area and in the same patient. They are then both in the same bilogical environment for the same length of time. In all cases the aortic homograft out performs the mitral homograft.

This suggests that the three-cusp aortic valve is not as effective long term in the mitral as in the aortic area. Similar results are related to the use of three-cusp fascial valves inserted in the mitral and aortic areas. In all cases the mitral valves failed first.

Not only does the three-cusp valve seem to be less satisfactory as a mitral valve substitute, but nature takes a hand in guiding us if we have the sense to heed her guiding hand. For instance, in many cases where we inserted a living autologous three-cusp fascial valve in the mitral area the moulding effects of the blood flow in that area made strenuous efforts to turn the valve into a more acceptable bicuspid structure. To my way of thinking this seems like a fairly obvious piece of friendly advice from the chief surgeon up there, but still we do not seem to get the message. Again, the use of a rigid ring, which is mandatory in all mechanical prostheses, immediately negates another basic principle on which the mitral valve functions. That is, an unrestricted sphinter-like mechanism embracing the posterior cusp and reducing the effective orifice by about one third in systole and enlarging that orifice by a similar amount in diastole. The use of a rigid ring is therefore going to have the effect of splinting the inflow portion of the ventricle and effectively immobilizes a significant segment of the contractile portion of the left ventricle.

Quite apart from the anatomical distortions from using a three-cusp rigid valve, the hemodynamic forces acting upon the mitral valve are also quite different from those acting at the aortic area where there is a relatively stable and predictably consistent diastolic closing pressure in the region of 80–100 mm Hg. The mitral valve, on the other hand, closes normally under a pressure of at least 120 mm Hg or more and with enormous sweeps and rises of pressure as the left ventricular systolic pressure varies throughout the day with varying stress and exercise. Consequently, the mitral valve is provided with an elaborate tensioning apparatus supported by papillary muscles, the whole resembling a parachute and being ideally adapted to withstand the vastly increased and rapidly changing closing pressures generated within the left ventricle. On the other hand, the opening pressures are extremely low so that there must also be a large orifice with no impedance to forward flow. Working along these guidelines we made various attempts to develop fully flexible mitral valve replacements. These certainly worked initially but failed eventually; not, I believe, through shortcomings in design but because of the unsuitability of the biological membrane—in this case autologous fascia lata.

How do we reconcile these ideals or ideals or design criteria with the sober facts? Logically we are driven to the conclusion that for an ideal mitral valve we have to provide a large, flexible bicuspid valve structure which will be non-obstructive, preserve flow patterns and not interfere with ventricular contractility.

But, to return to earth and the hurly-burly of surgical practice, we are still faced with only two options or lines of development—mechanical and biological. For me the less attractive and less interesting mechanical option represents a continuing adherence to the Bjork–Shiley family of flap valves which represent the nearest approach to the true mitral cusp mechanism. It also implies an acceptance of the recognized disadvantages of a rigid splinted mitral orifice and a significant incidence of embolism—all this in the interests of valve durability.

Alternatively, there is a biological option which offers a less stereotyped approach and should mean a flexible, bicuspid mechanism with an attachment either to a simple frame or to the papillary muscles. The perfect design is readily available and not too difficult to emulate. However, the most intractible problem lies not with design but with the durability of the biological membrane used in its manufacture. Here we are still in a primitive state of knowledge and significant developments have been few and far between. For instance, we have to protect our membrane from mechanical fatigue and from biological attack, both humoral and cellular. This may be achieved by rendering it non-antigenic or by the use of immunosuppressives or by preventing calcification by one means or another. Alternatively, we can try to maintain the viability of its collagen structure or promote an ingrowth of host cells. In this respect there is interesting recent evidence that dura mater preserved in glycerol retains the ability for its collagen to grow and adapt to changing stresses. This makes glycerol a potentially ideal preserving medium, certainly for homologous tissue, and much more work needs to be done with it.

On the other hand, if we are simply going to continue to turn all biological membranes into boot-like leather by the glutaraldehyde tanning process, and have no constructive thoughts beyond that, then Nancy Sinatra had some good advice for us when she sang 'these boots are made for walking'; and like boots, these valves are wearing out and are going to continue to do so.

Section 2

Flow dynamics in mitral valve disease

3

Dynamics and fluid dynamics of the mitral valve

David W. Wieting and Travis E. Stripling

Introduction

Anatomy of the mitral valve

The mitral valve (valvula bicuspidalis mitralis) is a undirectional flow device situated between the low-pressure left atrium and the high-pressure left ventricle of certain mammalian hearts. The proper anatomical regulation of blood flow across the valve depends on a complex interaction among four components: (1) the mitral annulus of fibrous ring; (2) the mitral valve leaflets; (3) the chordae tendineae; and (4) the papillary muscles (*see Figure 3.1*). The interaction of the anatomy, physiology and pathology of these four components in man is described clearly in reviews by Silverman[1] and Ranganathan[2]. In the healthy heart this delicate structure closes rapidly, allowing little, if any, blood to regurgitate into the left atrium. Conversely, it also opens rapidly, providing a large flow area with almost no resistance to blood flowing into the left ventricle from the left atrium. The pressure difference necessary to propel blood through the valve is almost neglible as long as all components are normal and unaffected by disease.

The mitral ring is not a static structure but has a very definite sphincter-like action, being smaller during systole than diastole [3–6]. In general, the mitral valve is composed of two leaflets of unequal size. The larger is known as the anterior (anteromedial, ventral, aortic, major, or septal) leaflet, and the smaller is known as the posterior leaflet. The junctions between the two leaflets, known as commissures, never extend entirely to the mitral annulus; therefore, the leaflet tissue surrounds the circumference of the mitral annulus, forming an asymmetrical, flattened funnel or nozzle, during diastole (*see Figure 3.2*). Brock[4] calculated the ratio of the area of the mitral valve annulus to the area of the mitral valve orifice, i.e. AMV:AMO, and found a range from 1.5:1 to 2.2:1.

The chordae tendineae are attached to the ventricular surface of the valve leaflets and the papillary muscles. They act as anchors which prevent the valve leaflets from proplapsing into the left atrium during ventricular systole.

Function of the mitral valve: Brief historical review

Historically, the vital function of the mitral valve as a check valve was not recognized or demonstrated until the seventeenth century. Most physicians and

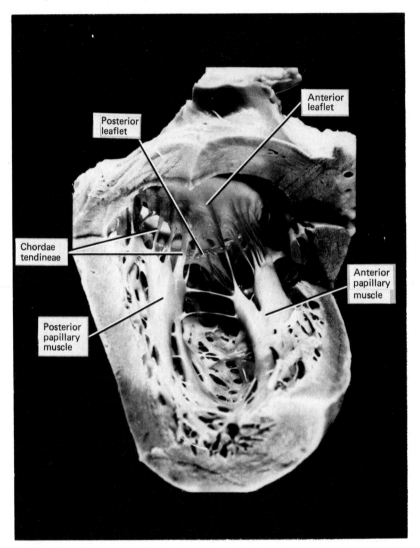

Figure 3.1 A human mitral valve, seen from the left ventricle with the septal wall of the left ventricle excised.

philosophers prior to the seventeenth century accepted the erroneous theory of Galen, a second century Graeco-Roman physician. According to Galen, the mitral valve served to prevent the escape of vital spirits from the left ventricle retrograde into the lung but had no significant function on the direction of blood flow. A detailed review of the historical understanding of the function of the mitral valve was presented in an earlier work[7]; therefore, only a brief summary will be presented here.

In 1628 William Harvey[8] finally put an end to the erroneous theory of Galen. In the words of Harvey, 'Good God! How do the mitral valves prevent escape of air and not of blood.' He conducted a series of experiments from which he concluded

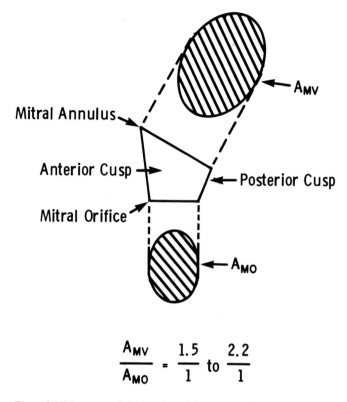

$$\frac{A_{MV}}{A_{MO}} = \frac{1.5}{1} \text{ to } \frac{2.2}{1}$$

Figure 3.2 Diagrammatic illustration of the asymmetric, flattened funnel shape of the mitral valve and the relative sizes and spatial orientation of the mitral annulus and mitral orifice. A_{mv} = Area of the mitral annulus; A_{mo} = area of mitral orifice.

that blood passed through the lungs and into the left ventricle via the mitral valve, which then prevented blood from going back into the lungs. Thus the true function of the mitral valve was finally established. The exact nature of the fluid mechanics of the left ventricle and the mitral valve, however, had not been clearly demonstrated.

A reasonably accurate theory of valve closure was proposed in 1891 by Krehl[9], who postulated that blood flowing through the ostia of the heart causes eddies (vortices) to form in the space in back of the valve leaflets. When flow ceases through the valves, these eddies open out like tightly wound clock springs and 'throw' the valve leaflets into approximation. The higher pressure which develops an instant later causes the leaflets to become tightly closed without regurgitation.

The first of the recent reports describing a vortex formation as an important mode of closure of the mitral valve leaflets was by Reid[10, 11] and Bellhouse[12–15, 31], both at Oxford. Reid based his conclusion on studies in human subjects using high-speed cineangiography with contrast medium injected into the right heart and observing its appearance in the left ventricle. The fluid entering the left ventricle was observed to recirculate behind the posterior and anterior leaflets, causing closure just prior to the onset of ventricular systole. Bellhouse based his conclusion of vortex formation upon fluid mechanics studies of a model mitral valve.

In-vivo studies of the influence of atrial contraction on mitral valve mechanics and ventricular filling were reported by Nolan[16] who concluded that the major contribution of atrial contraction was the augmentation of ventricular filling and not the prevention of mitral regurgitation. In 1966 Braunwald[17] reported effective closure of the mitral valve in the absence of left atrial contraction.

In 1972 Yellin, Frater and Peskin reported pulsatile flow studies across the mitral valve using hydraulic, electronic and computer simulation. Strong evidence was obtained from these studies to support the vortex formation theory and its importance as a mechanism of mitral valve closure[18].

The movements of the mitral valve are governed by the mechanical and fluid mechanical forces that act upon it. The rationale for this paper is to analyze the various forces which are responsible for the proper function of the mitral valve. Mitral valves were studied both *in vivo* and *in vitro* in order to correlate the results and draw definitive conclusions.

In-vitro studies

Methods and materials

For the *in-vitro* studies a series of healthy human hearts were procured from post-mortem examinations. The hearts with valves *in situ* were fixed by infusing formalin (10%) into the aortic roots and coronary arteries using physiologic pressures. The artria and ventricles were also filled with formalin and the entire hearts suspended in a container of formalin. After the hearts were fixed, the fibrous skeleton, including the aortic and mitral valves, was dissected from the surrounding myocardium (*see Figure 3.3*). Mitral valves with two distinct papillary muscles were selected. Most of the aortic root and myocardium were removed except for the region of the papillary muscles. When conducting studies of papillary muscle forces and chordae tendineae tension, the mitral valve was directed free from the aortic valve and studied as an isolated mitral valve. These studies have been reported previously[7, 19, 20]; therefore, the details of this method will not be presented here. Briefly, the isolated mitral valve was sutured to a Plexiglas disk and mounted in the mitral valve testing chamber of a pulse duplication system. Strain-gauge load cells were attached to each papillary muscle for measuring the dynamic force necessary for preventing mitral valve prolapse and regurgitation. The force applied to each papillary muscle was gradually increased until no regurgitation occurred. Flow patterns were photographed and analyzed to determine the velocity profiles proximal and distal to the isolated mitral valve under optimum conditions of papillary muscle forces and corresponding chordae tendineae tensions[19, 20]. The observations of these studies and a subsequent one[21] concerning the fluid mechanics of the isolated mitral valve led to the design of a left ventricular shaped chamber[7, 22, 23] which provides a method for studying the mitral and aortic valve in their normal or near normal anatomical geometrical configuration.

A detailed description of the design and fabrication of the left ventricular shaped (Model II) chamber has been given previously[7, 23]; therefore, only the critical aspects will be presented here. *Figure 3.4* presents a conceptual sketch of the Model II chamber. The reliability of any *in-vitro* study of fluid mechanics of heart valves depends upon the similarity between the valve testing chamber and the geometry of the human heart. It is impossible to duplicate all the properties of the healthy beating human heart; however, extreme care was taken in this study to duplicate as

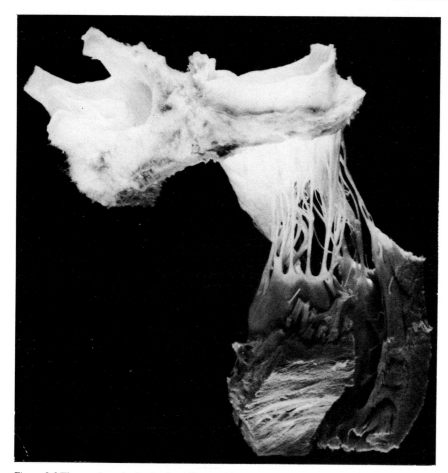

Figure 3.3 The aortic and mitral valves dissected from a normal adult heart at post mortem.

closely as possible the correct anatomical spatial relationship between the aortic and mitral valve as well as the left atrium, left ventricle and aorta.

The fabrication of the Model II chamber involved three steps: (1) making room temperature vulcanizing (RTV) silicone rubber castings of human hearts and aortas; (2) molding transparent plastic chambers around the silicone rubber castings; and (3) machining and hand sculpturing the various component parts in order to mount healthy human mitral and aortic valves as a single intact unit. The resulting chamber and a silicone rubber casting are shown in *Figure 3.5*.

An aortic and mitral valve specimen (*see Figure 3.3*) were selected so as to fit the size of the Model II chamber resulting from the silicone rubber casting. The two valves were sutured with a continuous 2–0 Ethiflex suture to the intermediate portion of the Model II chamber and sealed by means of Eastman 910 cement and medical grade Silastic adhesive. Each papillary muscle was trimmed and fitted with a nylon velour cuff or 'glove'. The lower portion of the velour was fashioned to form a loop for applying force to the papillary muscle and associated chordae tendineae. The entire papillary muscles and velour cuffs were then dipped three

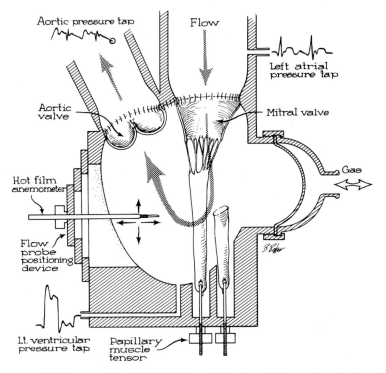

Aortic pressure tap

Flow

Left atrial
pressure tap

Aortic
valve

Mitral valve

Hot film
anemometer

Gas

Flow
probe
positioning
device

Lt. ventricular   Papillary
pressure tap   muscle
                         tensor

Figure 3.4 Conceptual sketch of the left ventricular shaped valve testing chamber, Model II.

times in polyurethane and four times in vinyl with sufficient time for curing between dipping. This procedure provided a tight-fitting polymeric 'glove' around each bundle of the papillary muscle and prevented tearing of the papillary muscles during the application of forces necessary to prevent prolapse and regurgitation of the mitral valve during simulated ventricular contraction.

Holes were drilled and papillary muscles inserted into the appropriate location of the left ventricular portion of the Model II chamber. Two threaded stainless steel rods with hooks were attached to the papillary muscles for independently adjusting the force applied to each papillary muscle.

A pneumatically driven diaphragm pump section was attached to the posterior wall of the left ventricular portion of the model II chamber as shown in *Figure 3.6(b)*. Left ventricular contraction was simulated by the diaphragm pump which was in turn powered by a Vitamek (Vitamek, Inc., Houston, Texas) pneumatic power unit. The Vitamek unit provides variable heart rates, systolic durations, systolic drive pressure and diastolic drive pressure.

The left atrium was simulated by a flexible silastic rubber tube attached to the upper left atrial section of the Model II chamber (*see Figure 3.6*)

A hot-film anemometer probe was inserted into the mid-plane of the Model II chamber for measuring fluid velocities. A special positioning device employing a series of 'O-ring' seals was designed to allow for moving the probe into any desired position along the mid-plane while the system was in operation. The assembled Model II chamber with the hot-film anemometer probe inserted is shown in *Figure*

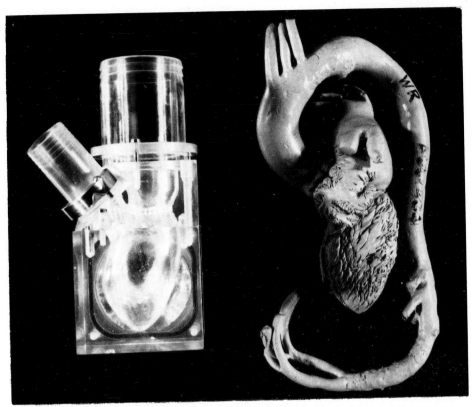

Figure 3.5 (Left) The Model II left ventricular shaped valve shaped valve testing chamber. (Right) silicone rubber injection corrosion casting of the left atrium, left ventricle and aorta of a human heart.

3.6. This chamber provides a geometrical shape approximating to the natural human left ventricle at end diastole.

The Model II chamber with the aortic and mitral valve was placed in the mock circulatory system of a pulse duplication system illustrated in *Figure 3.7* and described previously[24]. This system provides dynamic pressures and flows similar to those of the human heart. The Model II chamber is transparent, therefore valve dynamics as well as fluid flow patterns can be visualized and photographed with proper lighting and flow tracer particles by employing a transparent blood analog fluid. For the hot-film anemometry studies, a Cuno 5 μm filter and a heat-exchanger were employed in order to prevent contamination of the anemometer probe and to provide a stable temperature of blood analog fluid.

The blood analog fluid used in the study was an aqueous-glycerol solution composed of 46% glycerol by weight, which has a viscosity of 3.5 cP and a specific gravity of 1.25 at 30.5°C. The temperature of the blood analog fluid was monitored by means of a Curtin precision-grade thermometer Model 228-825.

Flow patterns associated with the mitral valve were obtained using a technique described previously[24]. It involves suspending small spherical-shaped plastic beads in the blood analog fluid and illuminating with a high-intensity slit-light source. This technique makes it possible to observe and photograph two-dimensional flow

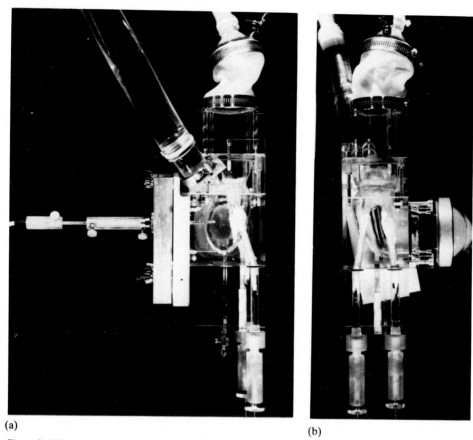

(a)   (b)

Figure 3.6 The assembled Model II valve testing chamber. (*a*) Front view. (*b*) Right-side view.

patterns at any desired plane in the three-dimensional flow field of the left ventricle of the Model II chamber.

Fluid velocity magnitudes within the left ventricle of the Model II chamber were measured with a Thermo-Systems, Inc., Model 1053B constant-temperature anemometer equipped with a TSI Model 1210–20W cylindrical probe. The direction of the velocity vector was determined from the still photographs of flow patterns in the left ventricle at the appropriate time during the cardiac cycle. The hot-film probes were calibrated by towing the probes through a temperature-controlled reservoir of the blood analog fluid at a known velocity. (The calibration curves are given in *Figure 3.A1* and *3.A2* in the appendix on p. 471.)

Statham physiological pressure transducers Model P23H and P23Db were used for simultaneous measurement of the aortic, left ventricular and left atrial pressures as well as the pressure drop across the mitral valve. Mean flow rates were measured with a Fischer Porter rotameter Model 10A 1027 whereas pulsatile flow rates were measured with a Carolina Square Wave Electromagnetic Flowmeter.

Flow patterns were photographed with three cameras as follows:

1.   A Leica M1 35 mm equipped with a Leitz Elmarit 1:2.9 90 mm lens;

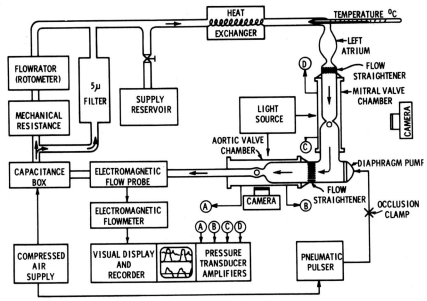

Figure 3.7 Schematic diagram of the pulse duplication system.

2. An Arriflex 16 mm movie camera; and
3. A Fastax High Speed Camera Model WF4.

The electrical signals from all transducers and sensors were routed through an Electronics for Medicine 12-channel recorder for monitoring, then post-conditioned by Honeywell Accudata Buffer Amplifiers, and recorded on magnetic tape in analog form using an Ampex Model FR 1300 eight-channel tape recorder. The data were later played back, recorded on a Bush Model 260 recorder and analyzed for the desired velocity, pressure and flow data.

The aortic and mitral valves mounted in the Model II chamber were placed in the mock circulatory system, the system primed with the blood analog fluid, and all residual air bled from the system. The Vitamek Pneumatic Power Unit was turned on the pulse duplication system tuned as follows: (1) pulse rate of 72 beats/minute; (2) mean flow rate of 5 l/min; (3) aortic pressure of 120/180 mm Hg; (4) left ventricular pressure of 120/0 mm Hg; (5) mean left atrial pressure between 5 and 10 mm Hg; and (6) a blood analog fluid temperature of 30.5°C. The static (resting) load applied to each papillary muscle was gradually increased while observing flow patterns with the slit-light source until the mitral valve was competent and little or no regurgitation was visible.

When the optimum condition for papillary muscle force was obtained, flow patterns in the left ventricle were photographed using the three camera systems. Still photographs of flow patterns were taken at various shutter speeds using Kodak Tri-X Pan film during peak diastolic flow and during peak systolic flow. High-speed 16 mm movies were taken at 500 frames per second using Kodak Tri-X Reversal film type 7278. A 16 mm color movie was also taken at 24 frames per second using Kodak Ektachrome E.F film type 7242.

After the flow patterns were photographed particles were filtered from the system by diverting the blood analog fluid through the 5 μm filter (*see Figure 3.7*), and the hot-film anemometer probe inserted for measurement of the velocity magnitudes at the 169 locations on the mid-plane and the left ventricle of the Model II chamber as illustrated in *Figure 3.8*. The system was again tuned and all data recorded on the Ampex magnetic tape system for one minute at each of the 169 data points. These data were later played back, recorded on a strip recorder and analyzed for 10 consecutive cycles.

A typical strip-chart recording of the various data is shown in *Figure 2.9*. For the purposes of analysis each of the individual 10 cardiac cycles at each of the 169 data points was divided into 10 equally spaced time increments, as illustrated in *Figure 2.10*. The linearized anemometer output voltage was measured at each of these discrete time increments and averaged over ten cardiac cycles. This average voltage was then converted to a velocity by using the calibration curve for the particular hot-film probe used. The results of these calculations have been tabulated and reported by Stripling[23]. It was assumed that the velocity component in the Y direction was negligible. The error introduced by this assumption is less than 3%

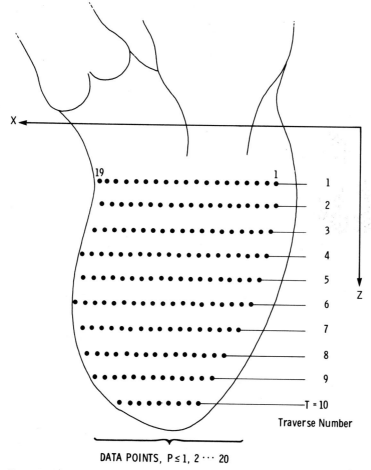

Figure 3.8 Data points at which blood analog fluid velocities were measured in the Model II chamber using hot-film anemometer.

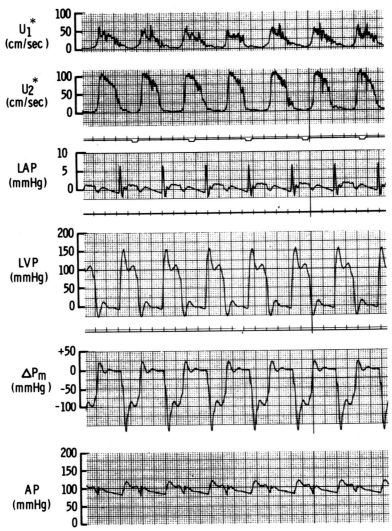

Figure 3.9 Typical control recording of data in the Model II chamber, at data point T = 5, P = 2. V = Linearized anemometer output voltage; AP = aortic pressure; LAP = left atrial pressure; LVP = left ventricular pressure; ΔP_m = LAP − LVP.

during peak diastolic flow[23] which was the primary concern of this work, i.e. during diastolic filling and closure of the mitral valve.

Results *in vitro*

The results for papillary muscle forces for an isolated mitral valve studied in the pulse duplication system are summarized in *Figures 3.11* and *3.12* and in greater detail in a previous publication[19]. The forces applied to the papillary muscles to prevent mitral valve prolapse and regurgitation were as follows. Posteromedial papillary muscle force ranged from a resting value during diastole of 2 N to a peak

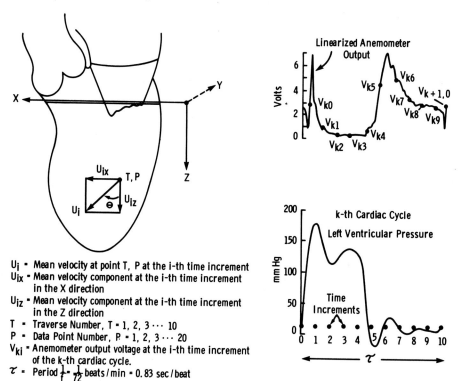

U_i = Mean velocity at point T, P at the i-th time increment
U_{ix} = Mean velocity component at the i-th time increment in the X direction
U_{iz} = Mean velocity component at the i-th time increment in the Z direction
T = Traverse Number, T = 1, 2, 3 ··· 10
P = Data Point Number, P = 1, 2, 3 ··· 20
V_{ki} = Anemometer output voltage at the i-th time increment of the k-th cardiac cycle.
τ = Period $\frac{1}{72}$ beats/min = 0.83 sec/beat

Figure 3.10 Coordinate system for measurement of velocity, U_i, in Model II chamber using the hot-film anemometer, at the *i*-th time increment of the K-th cardiac cycle.

value during systole of 4.36 N whereas the anterolateral papillary muscle force ranged from a resting value of 0.5 N during diastole to a peak value of 3.24 N during systole. A reduction of the (static loads applied to the) posteromedial papillary muscle force from the optimum value of 2.0–0.25 N and the anterolateral papillary muscle force from the optimum value of 0.5–0.15 N resulted in a reduction in mitral flow from 5 to 2.5 l/m due to regurgitation (*see Figure 3.11*). Conversely, if the papillary muscle force was increased above the optimum value, there was only a slight reduction in mean flow rate (*see Figure 3.11*). This reduction in flow is probably caused by the stiffening of the mitral valve leaflets caused by the greater than optimum force applied to the papillary muscles and the chordae tendineae, i.e. the valve leaflets are not free to move and open as widely as they do under optimum conditions. The flow patterns associated with the mitral valve during less than optimum papillary muscle forces are also grossly distorted due to the regurgitation as can be seen by comparing *Figures 3.12* and *3.13* as has been reported previously[19]. The vortices that are normally present behind the anterior and posterior leaflets are essentially obliterated by the regurgitation that occurs.

Velocity profiles proximal and distal to the isolated mitral valve as measured from flow patterns and hot-film anemometry mesurements compared favourably as illustrated in *Figures 3.13* and *3.14*. The peak velocity distal to the mitral valve was found to be approximately 100 cm/s at a plane 58 mm downstream from the mitral

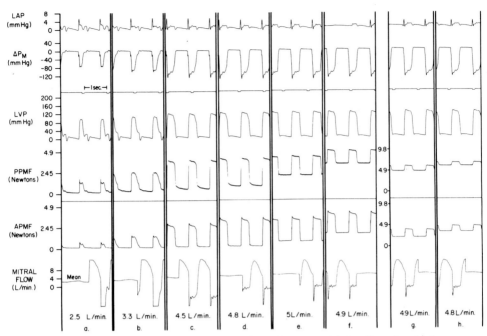

Figure 3.11 Plot of various parameters of left ventricular performance and the effect of gradually increasing papillary muscle force. Optimum force occurs in section e. Greater than optimum force (sections f–h) does not significantly affect mitral-valve function, but less than optimum force (sections a–d) results in considerable regurgitation. LAP = Left atrial pressure; P = pressure drop across mitral valve; LVP = left ventricular pressure; PPMF = posteromedial papillary muscle force; APMF = anterolateral papillary muscle force; mitral flow = electromagnetic flow signal for mitral flow rate.

valve annulus. A flow reversal associated with the large vortex immediately behind the anterior leaflet resulted in negative velocities of 25 cm/s at the same plane[7].

The results obtained in the Model II chamber are presented in *Figures 3.9* and *3.15–3.20*. The various pressure versus time tracings and the output voltage from the hot-film anemometer are presented in *Figure 3.9* for one data point (T=5, P=2 on *Figure 3.8*). Typical flow pattern photographs during diastole and systole are shown in *Figures 3.15* and *3.16*. The axial velocity profiles across 10 different planes or traverses (*see Figure 3.8*, Traverse 1–10) of the left ventricle at time increment $i = 6$, which occurs during peak diastolic filling of the left ventricle, are given in *Figure 3.17*. These represent the axial (i.e., base to apex) component of the velocity as measured with the hot-film anemometer probe in the Model II chamber. The direction of the velocity vector, U_i was determined by analysis of a series of flow pattern photographs and high-speed movies of flow tracer particle motion. Tracing paper was placed over flow pattern photographs and particle streak directions drawn. The resulting directions of the velocity vector during peak diastolic flow are illustrated by line segments and arrowheads in *Figure 3.18*. The angle, θ, was measured from the velocity directions of *Figure 3.18* using the coordinate system illustrated in *Figure 3.10*. These angles were then used to calculate the axial velocity component U_z at each of the 169 data points within the Model II chamber.

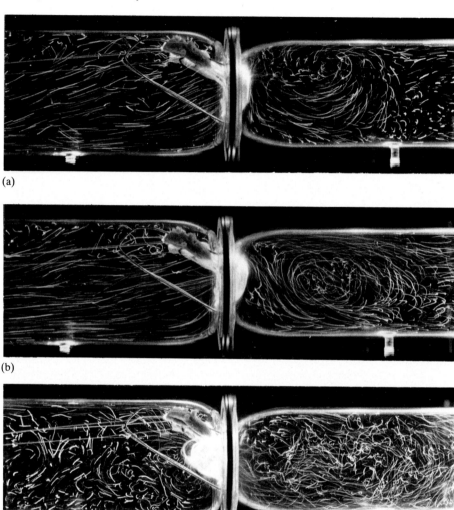

(a)

(b)

(c)

Figure 3.12 Flow patterns of a normal human mitral valve with less than optimum papillary muscle force. (*a*) During ventricular systole with about 50% optimum papillary force; (*b*) during ventricular systole with about 10% optimum papillary muscle force; (*c*) during ventricular diastole with about 10% optimum papillary force. (Note disturbance in flow when compared with optimum conditions of *Figure 3.13.*)

In like manner the axial velocity profile at each plane or traverse was calculated at time increment $i=1$ which occurred during peak ventricular systolic ejection. The resulting velocity profiles are given in *Figure 3.19*. The direction and magnitude of the velocity were determined as above; however, the directions of the velocity vectors could be accurately determined only in the left side of the flow pattern. Movement of the flow visualization particles on the right side of the flow patterns (*see Figure 3.16*) were not distinct enough or long enough to allow for determining

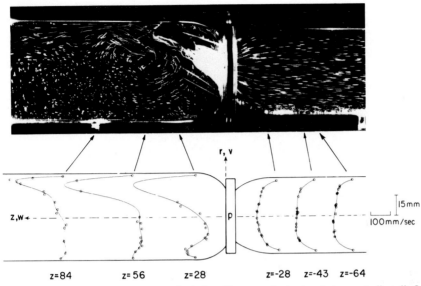

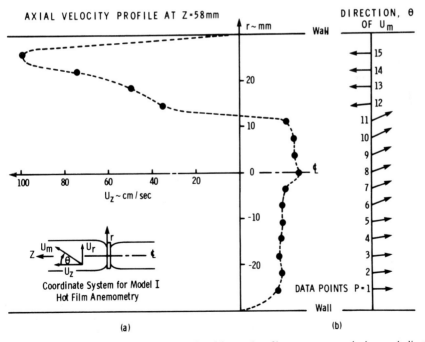

Figure 3.13 (Top) Flow pattern across the isolated human mitral valve during peak diastolic flow with optimum papillary muscle forces. (Bottom) Axial velocity profile calculated from a flow pattern during peak diastolic flow at six values of Z as indicated for a normal mitral valve in the isolated mitral valve Model I chamber.

Figure 3.14 (a) Axial velocity profile calculated from a hot-film anemometer during peak diastolic flow through a normal human mitral valve in the Model I chamber, at $Z = 58$ mm. *(b)* Direction, θ, of maximum velocity vector, U_m.

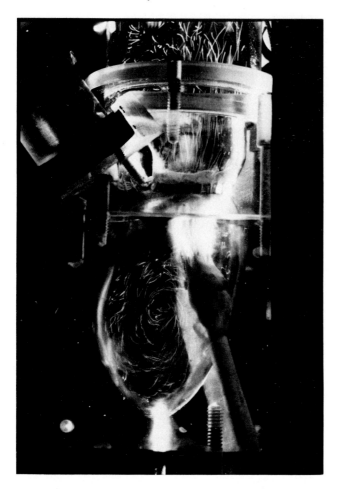

the angle θ; therefore, only one-half of the velocity profile is plotted in *Figure 3.19*. The directions that were determinable are indicated by the vectors drawn on *Figure 3.20*.

In-vivo studies

Methods and materials

In-vivo studies of fluid mechanics of the mitral valve were conducted in order to confirm the results of the *in-vitro* studies. Two different species of animals were used for the *in-vivo* studies, the dog and the calf. The dog was chosen as the primary experimental animal since the chest of the dog is small enough for definitive bi-plane angiography and large enough to allow measurements with the left ventricle using a catheter-tip hot-film anemometer probe without causing significant disturbance in blood flow patterns by the insertion of the catheter probe.

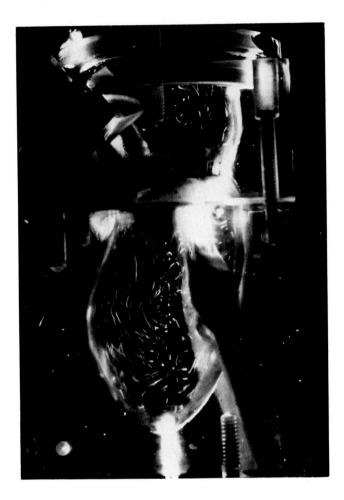

Figure 3.15 and 3.16 Typical flow pattern of a normal human mitral valve mounted in the left ventricular shaped Model II chamber, during peak diastolic flow (*left*) and peak systolic flow (*right*). Jacket No. 34400, Roll 72–004 No. 6 (*left*) Roll 72–009 No. 14A (*right*), 1/15th s.

Dogs weighing between 25 and 35 kg were anesthetized with initial doses of morphine sulphate (15–20 mg/kg) subcutaneously. Approximately 20 minutes later sodium pentobarbital (3–5 mg/kg) was administered intravenously. This combination of anesthetic agents was chosen in order to obtain a slow heart rate, since it was desired to obtain as many angiocardiograms as possible per cardiac cycle. The animals were reinforced with 50 mg of morphine either intramuscularly or subcutaneously at one hour intervals throughout the procedure. All animals were intubated and maintained by a Bird Mark 7 respirator throughout the lengthy procedure. Limb leads (Lead II) were attached for recording EKG. Body temperature was recorded throughout the procedure by use of a rectal thermometer probe.

Blood pressures were recorded in the following manner: (1) aortic via left femoral catheterization; (2) left ventricular via right femoral catheterization (using

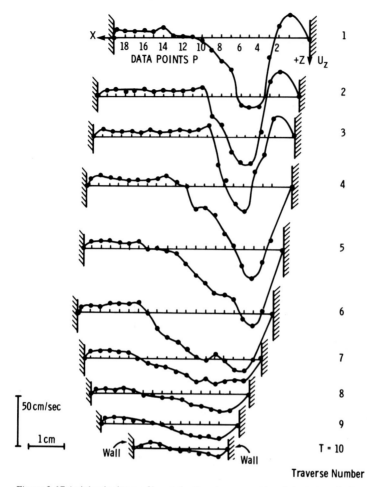

Figure 3.17 Axial velocity profiles at the time increment $i = 6$ during peak diastolic flow at 10 planes traversed (T = 1–10), measured with the hot-film anemometer for the human mitral valve in the Model II chamber.

a No. 7 French USCI 5440); and (3) left atrial (using a Brockenbrough Transseptal Catheter Model No. 7735 with a curved needle set No, 9152) via right femoral vein and transseptal puncture. A cardiac catheter was also inserted into the pulmonary artery via the left femoral vein for the purposes of injecting radiopaque dye. Blood velocity measurements were made in the aorta and the left ventricle by means of a DISA Model 55A87 Conical probe mounted on a No. 7 French USCI 5440 Cardiac Catheter in conjuction with the TSI Model 1053B Constant Temperature Anemometer. The sensors of this type probe are nickel film deposited circumferentially by sputtering on a cone-shaped quartz rod. The width of the film is 0.6 mm. Protection against mechanical and chemical degradation is provided by a quartz layer 2 μm thick. This type thin-film probe is most sensitive to fluid velocity 'head on' to the sensor, along the axis of the catheter. The effect of misalignment of the probe is a small decrease in the measured velocity. The directional characteristic measured in the free stream is parabolic, and rather flat. The

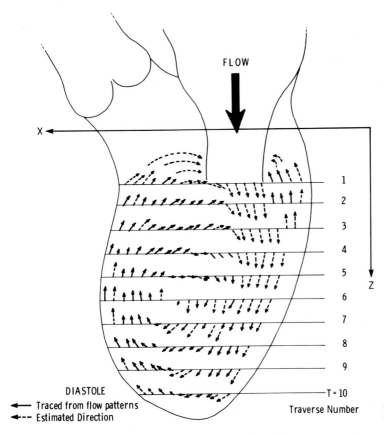

Figure 3.18 A sketch made by tracing the direction of particle movement on flow pattern photographs similar to *Figure 3.15* exposed during peak diastolic flow. Arrows indicate direction of velocity vector, U_i, at various points in the Model II chamber. Estimated directions were obtained from viewing high-speed movies of flow patterns.

apparent change of velocity with the angle of inclination is only 2% at 10 degrees[25]. The catheter-tip hot-film sensor was calibrated using the same tow-tank system used for the *in-vitro* studies except that bovine blood was employed at 37°C. A typical calibration curve for a DISA Model 55A87 Conical Probe is given in *Figure 3.A3* of the appendix on p. 472 and the linearized output voltage versus effective cooling velocity in bovine blood for the same probe is given in *Figure 3.A4* also on p. 472.

All EKG, blood pressures, and hot-film anemometer data were recorded and analyzed using the same equipment and techniques described for the *in-vitro* studies. The radiographic techniques used for determining the location of the hot-film anemometer velocity probe are described below.

Following control recording of EKG and blood pressures, the hot-film anemometer catheter-tip probe was inserted into the right carotid artery and a zero flow measurement of the anemometer output obtained by temporary ligation of the carotid artery. The hot-film anemometer catheter was advanced retrograde down the aorta and through the aortic valve into the left ventricle while observing the

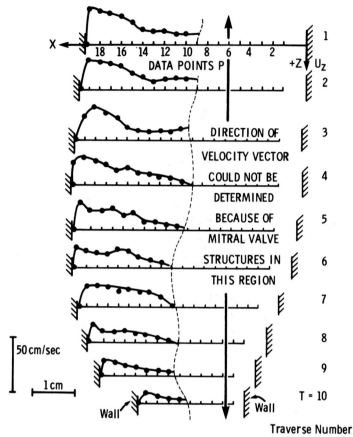

Figure 3.19 Axial velocity profiles at the time increment $i = 1$ during peak systolic flow, at 10 planes traversed (T = 1–10), measured with the hot-film anemometer for the human mitral valve in the Model II chamber.

output from the anemometer on the oscilloscope. The catheter-tip hot-film anemometer probe was positioned in the desired location in the left ventricle with the aid of fluoroscopy.

When the hot-film sensor was position in the desired location within the left ventricle, bi-plane angiograms of the entire heart and aorta were obtained by injecting Renovist radiopaque dye into the pulmonary artery by a Cordis angiography injector and cardiac programmer Model No. 64A–112. After allowing a few seconds for the dye to traverse the pulmonary system films were exposed by using two Odelca High-Speed Photofluorographic film changers and programmers Model No. RRS–100–3. Approximately 24 films were exposed during each run at 4 frames per second. Throughout this procedure all physiological data were recorded on magnetic tape similar to the *in-vitro* studies. When the desired data were recorded at this location the catheter-tip hot-film anemometer was repositioned in new locations and the same procedure repeated. Upon completion of data recording in the left ventricle the tape recording equipment was allowed to run continuously while the hot-film anemometer catheter was gradually withdrawn

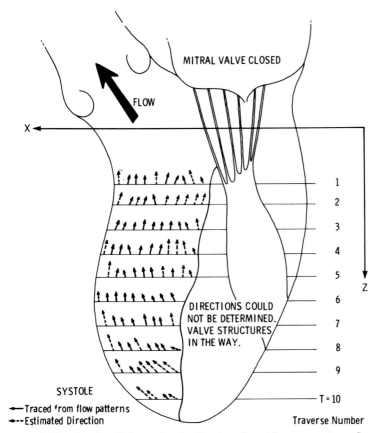

Figure 3.20 A sketch made by tracing the direction of particle movement on a flow pattern photograph similar to that in *Figure 3.16* exposed during peak ventricular ejection. Arrows indicate the direction of the velocity vector, U_i, at various points in the Model II chamber. Estimated directions were obtained from viewing high-speed movies of flow patterns.

from the heart and the cardiovascular system, a 'zero-flow' condition was again recorded to determine whether possible drift had occurred.

Velocity measurements were also made in the left ventricle of a calf weighing 100 kg (prior to prosthetic valve replacement). A similar protocol was followed for the calf. A transseptal catheter was not used since possible damage to the myocardium might have resulted from its use prior to the anticipated surgery. A cut down was made on only one carotid artery and one jugular vein to avoid possible sites of infection post-operatively. For this reason catheters were inserted only into the pulmonary artery for dye injection and into the aorta for monitoring arterial blood pressure. Other pressure catheters were omitted in this experiment. The hot-film anemometer catheter was inserted into the same cartoid artery as the arterial blood pressure catheter. In like manner, it was positioned in the desired locations within the left ventricle with the aid of a fluoroscopy. When the hot-film probe was positioned in the desired location, dye was injected via the pulmonary artery catheter and a series of cineangiograms obtained by using two Kodak 16 mm cine-cameras. The calf was too large to allow proper use of the Odelca cameras; in fact, only one plane of the cineangiogram was useful since the X-ray equipment was not large enough to penetrate sufficiently the large sternum of the calf.

The measurement of velocity with the hot-film anemometer in the left ventricle of the dog and the calf required careful coordination of the various types of angiography film and the signal from the hot-film anemometer. The magnitude of the velocity was readily obtained from the bridge or linearized output voltage of the anemometer and the known calibration curves (*see Figures 3.A3* and *3.A4*). Velocities were measured at 10 discrete points similar to those used for *in-vitro* studies (*see Figure 3.10*) in each of 10 successive cardiac cycles. The velocity measurements were conducted at two or three different locations in the left ventricle of the dog and the calf.

The location of the velocity measured was determined in two ways. In dogs it was possible to use the Odelca Bi-plane quick film changer. This camera provides approximately four films per second, each negative being four inch by four inch square. For each desired location, approximately 24 successive negatives were obtained from which the appropriate ones were selected and analyzed to determine the location of the catheter-tip transducer within the beating left ventricle. The negatives were projected on the ground-glass screen of a Helio 100 Constrastor. This technique provides a sharp image from which the cardiac silhouette and the ventricular chamber when opacified with radiopaque dye can easily be traced on acetate film. The hot-film anemometer catheter was also visible since weak dye injection was used intentionally in order not to obscure the images of the desired catheters. The biggest disadvantage of this technique is the fact that the Odelca camera exposed film at approximately four cycles per second and required approximately 150 ms for each exposure. Hence a very precise determination of velocity magnitude at an exact location in the left ventricle is not possible. It should be remembered, however, that the purpose of the *in-vivo* experiments in this work is merely to verify the validity of the *in-vitro* measurements which can be conducted at more precise locations within the plastic chambers.

The 16 mm cineangiograms obtained in the lateral position for the calf were analyzed with a Kodak Analyst 16 mm movie projector. This projector allowed frame-by-frame analysis (as well as projecting at normal 24 frames per second speed) for locating the hot-film anemometer catheter during the velocity measurements in the calf left ventricle.

Results (*in vivo*)

The results obtained in the left ventricle of the dog and the calf have been reported in detail[7]; therefore, only few examples in the calf will be given here to indicate the similarity between the *in-vivo* and *in-vitro* velocities measured in the left ventricle.

The results obtained in the calf are summarized in *Figures 3.21–3.24* and in *Table 3.1*. Each figure presents the electrocardiogram, the aortic pressure and the linearized output voltage from the conical anemometer probe at various locations in the left ventricle of the calf. The data in *Figure 3.21* were obtained during the first cineangiogram with the hot-film anemometer catheter located in the middle of the left ventricle. Note the interference signals on the baseline of the EKG during exposure of the cine cameras. *Figure 3.22* represents a recording made with the hot-film anemometer catheter probe near the posterior wall of the left ventricle. The hot-film anemometer catheter was then withdrawn until the tip was located in the mitral inflow tract of the left ventricle and the tracing of *Figure 3.23* obtained.

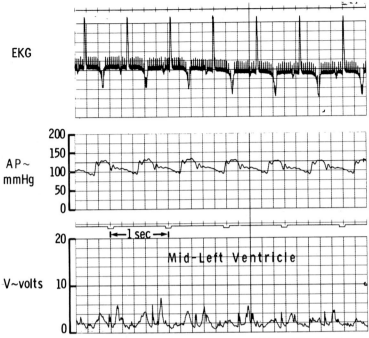

Figure 3.21 Strip chart records of EKG, aortic pressure (AP), and linearized anemometer voltage (V) with the anemometer probe position in the middle of the left ventricle of the calf heart.

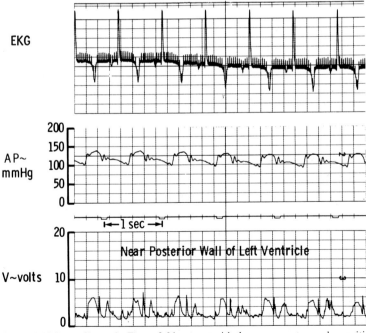

Figure 3.22 Same data as in *Figure 3.21*, except with the anemometer probe positioned off the posterior wall of the left ventricle.

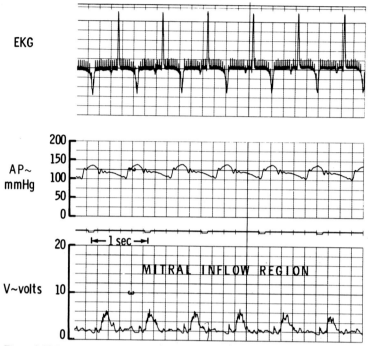

Figure 3.23 Same data as in *Figure 3.21*, except with the anemometer probe in the mitral inflow region of the left ventricle.

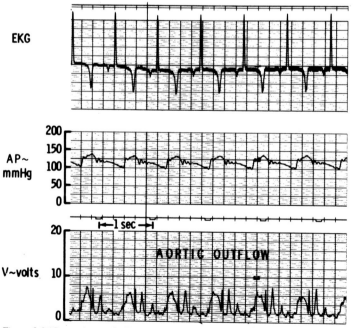

Figure 3.24 Same data as in *Figure 3.21* in the calf, except with the anemometer probe in the aortic outflow tract.

TABLE 3.1 Velocity measurements in the left ventricle and aorta of the calf at 10 equal time increments during the cardiac cycle averaged for 10 consecutive cardiac cycles.

				Velocity (U_i, cm/s)			
	Ascending aorta	Mid-left ventricle	Posterior left ventricle	Mitral inflow left ventricle	Aortic root	Apex left ventricle
0	11.7	15.7	23.6	24.3	13.3	25.8
1	97.5	27.9	58.6	29.3	116.7	25.0
2	105.8	36.4	60.0	29.3	126.7	28.3
3	76.7	24.3	41.4	22.9	123.3	24.2
4	27.5	29.3	22.1	32.9	66.7	30.0
5	30.0	22.1	55.0	25.8	39.2	30.0
6	25.8	52.5	39.2	55.0	27.5	31.7
7	21.7	36.7	30.0	65.8	21.7	25.0
8	16.7	25.0	23.3	48.3	17.5	25.8
9	12.5	16.7	28.3	32.5	17.5	25.0
10	12.0	17.5	25.0	25.8	19.2	25.8

The results obtained with the anemometer probe in the aortic outflow tract are presented in *Figure 3.24*.

Discussion

The mitral valve as referred to by Silverman[1] is not a simple valvular structure, but rather a structure called the 'mitral complex', consisting of the mitral annulus (or annulus fibrosus), the mitral leaflets, the chordae tendineae, and the papillary muscles. The first two components of the 'mitral complex', the mitral annulus and the mitral leaflets, are extremely critical; in fact, without the leaflets and the mitral annulus, there is no mitral valve. Assuming the presence of the mitral leaflets and an intact mitral annulus, the importance of functional papillary muscles and intact chordae tendineae for proper function of the mitral valve are well recognized.

The force on a single chordae tendineae has been reported by Salisbury *et al.*[26]. Bruch and De Pasquale[27] calculated the time course of tension in the papillary muscles by multiplying the left ventricular pressure at various points of interest in the cardiac cycle times the area of the atrioventricular orifice. Cronin and Associates[28] attached Walton–Brody strain gauge arches to the longitudinal surface of the papillary muscle of canine left ventricles and recorded the force of contraction simultaneously with that of an epicardial segment of the ventricle.

The results reported in this work compare favorably with those of Burch and Cronin. The theoretical considerations of Burch actually give the total force supported by the mitral valve. However, he suggests the following techniques for estimating the papillary muscle force. It was assumed that half of the force acting upon the mitral valve during systole is supported by the annulus of the mitral valve. Therefore, each papillary muscle supports approximately 25% of the total force acting upon the mitral valve. The peak force exerted by each papillary muscle, as calculated by Burch, for a normal size human heart with mitral circumference constant throughout systole is 3.25 N. This value compares favorably with the anterior papillary muscle peak systolic force of 3.24 N and the posterior papillary muscle peak systolic force of 4.36 N of this study. The mitral valve used in this portion of the study, however, had a larger posterior papillary muscle which apparently supported more of the chordae tendineae; therefore, it is not surprising that the two factors are unequal in magnitude.

It is not possible to make a direct comparison between the results of this study and those of Cronin[28], since the magnitude of the force was not given by Cronin; however, a qualitative comparison of the force versus time tracings, i.e. waveforms, can be made. The shape of these two tracings is similar. The results obtained in this study in the pulse duplication system have a sharper initial systolic spike probably caused by the inelastic nature of the valve testing chambers as compared with those measured in the elastic ventricles of dogs. The waveforms are also similar to those calculated and plotted by Burch and De Pasquale[27].

The importance of papillary muscle contraction has been studied by numerous investigators. Burch *et al.*[29] gave an excellent review of the literature concerning the syndrome of papillary muscle dysfunction and its clinical manifestations. Tsakaris *et al.*[30] reported studies of the effect of selective damage of one or both papillary muscles on mitral valve competence in the intact anesthetized dog. Papillary muscles were damaged by selective injection of 1–1.5 ml 10% formalin solution. Mitral regurgitation was measured with a Roentgen video-densitometer. Cronin[28] concluded that selective major damage of one or both papillary muscles of the left ventricle is compatible with competent mitral valve closure. These observations suggest that during ventricular systole the mitral valve leaflets can be restrained adequately by the chordae tendineae and underlying ventricular myocardium, and that the part played by the contracting papillary muscles is not essential for efficient closure of the mitral valve. The technique used by Cronin[28] preserved the papillary muscle in its normal length relationship or possibly even resulted in shrinkage with a decrease in length. An infarcted papillary muscle, however, can become elongated, and as a result regurgitation can occur. This condition was simulated by the reduced force applied to the papillary muscles (*see Figure 3.12*).

The function of the mitral valve with the damaged papillary muscles as reported by Cronin[28] is probably very similar to the isolated mitral valve studied in the pulse duplication system of this work. It was impossible in these studies to simulate the contraction of the papillary muscles and the mitral annulus. In all studies, however, sufficient force was applied to the chordae tendineae via the papillary muscles to prevent inversion of the leaflets into the left atrial chamber and the concomitant mitral regurgitation. Once the optimum magnitude was reached, no further increase in force supplied to the papillary muscles was needed to prevent regurgitation.

A comparison of the flow patterns obtained in the isolated mitral valve chamber for a normal human mitral valve with those of other investigators is difficult since, to the best of our knowledge, no one has previously reported two-dimensional flow patterns for the normal human mitral valve mounted in a pulse duplicator.

The flow-pattern studies of a model mitral valve and left ventricle were reported by Bellhouse[15, 31]. Flow patern photographs are not presented in the most recent publication, but sketches are drawn. Bellhouse described a 'ring vortex' in the model left ventricle. He observed that the incoming jet struck the apex of the ventricle and spread out to flow up the walls to the base of the ventricle and then turned back behind the leaflets toward the apex again to form a 'ring vortex'. The vortex in the model studies of Bellhouse was asymmetrical with the greatest strength concentrated in the outflow tract behind the anterior leaflet of the model mitral valve.

The data obtained in these studies (*see Figures 3.15 and 3.18*) during ventricular diastole confirmed the presence of vortices and the left ventricle of a pulse duplication system. In agreement with the findings of Bellhouse, the present studies indicate an asymmetry in the size of the vortices behind the anterior leaflet and the posterior leaflet of the mitral valve (*see Figure 3.15*).

Bellhouse[14] found that for a dilated left ventricular chamber, the vortex strength was negligible. The results reported in this study indicate that an increase in length of five times the average length of the left ventricle does not cause the strength of the vortex to become negligible. The strength of the vortex in the long cylindrical shaped chamber of the isolated mitral valve studies, however, does appear to be less than the strength of the vortex in the left ventricular shaped mitral valve chamber Model II. No studies were conducted in this investigation on the effect of the diameter of the left ventricular chamber. There is no doubt that the left ventricle of mammalian hearts can become dilated; however, the basic spatial relationships between a normal mitral valve annulus and the diameter of a dilated ventricle have a significant limit, namely less than the thorax; i.e., thoracic space minus lung volume space. It does not seem appropriate, therefore, to consider a large ventricle in which the vortex probably would not form. The studies of this work do indicate the importance of the apex to base length of the left ventricle and particularly the curvature of the apex for increasing the strength of the vortex which forms behind the anterior leaflet of the mitral valve. This vortex definitely does contribute to closure of the valve leaflets, as Bellhouse demonstrated by slow filling rates of the left ventricular chamber.

One additional, important function of the large vortex, which in our opinion fills the entire left ventricular chamber during end diastole, is the conservation of momentum. That is, the fluid entering the left ventricle through the mitral valve has considerable kinetic energy which is stored in the form of annular momentum in the large vortex. During the subsequent systolic contraction, the other high-velocity fluid exists from the periphery of the vortex through the open aortic valve. This represents a considerable energy-saving mechanism of the natural heart, which most artificial hearts do not duplicate.

The velocity profiles in the left ventricular chamber as measured from flow patterns (*see Figure 3.13*) compare favorably in shape to those measured with the hot-film anemometer (*see Figure 3.14*) in the same chamber. The magnitude of the velocity measured from the particle streaks and plotted by the least squares curve fitting technique is somewhat lower than that measured with hot-film anemometer. It was impossible, however, to measure accurately the streak length of particles in the very high velocity jet which enters the left ventricle during diastole; therefore, the magnitude of the velocity in both experiments is probably more nearly the same than the figures would indicate. The velocity profile obtained in the isolated mitral valve chamber Model I as shown in *Figure 3.14* compares favorably with the velocity profile as measured in the left ventricular shaped mitral valve chamber Model II with the hot-film anemometer and plotted with the assistance of flow patterns in *Figure 3.17*. The velocity profile at $Z = 58\,mm$ (*see Figure 3.14*) is equivalent to the velocity profile at traverse No. 4 in *Figure 3.17*.

A comparison with the data of other investigatiors is difficult since no velocity measurements *in vitro* of the normal human mitral valve have been conducted. Taylor[32, 33] reported measurements of velocity at different locations across the mitral valve orifice in man and dogs using an upstream and a downstream facing needle and found a peak flow velocity ranging from 90 to 120 cm/s. This valve compares favorably with the peak velocity measured in the left ventricular shaped mitral valve chamber Model II at traverse location No. 4 where the peak velocity was found to be 95 cm/s at time increment $i = 6$ (see Figure 3.10). This peak velocity is reached approximately 100 ms after the onset of diastole.

A significant difference was found in the investigations of this work when compared with those of Taylor regarding the shape of the velocity profile entering the left ventricle. Taylor[32] reported a flat profile except near the wall of the ventricle where measurements could not be made. The velocity profile found in this work was not flat, but had a very sharp spike immediately beneath the mitral orifice. The velocity profile through the valve leaflets probably is a flat profile, characteristic of undeveloped flow; however, when the fluid enters the left ventricular chamber surrounding fluid is brought into motion causing a profile which cannot be flat across the entire left ventricular chamber.

The peak velocity measured *in vivo* beneath the mitral valve orifice in the left ventricle of dogs was found to be approximately 100 cm/s which compares favorably with the measurements of Taylor[32, 33]. In this study, no attempt has been made to plot precisely the velocity versus time waveform throughout the entire beating left ventricle of the dog or the calf. This represents a very difficult, if not impossible task, since the geometry of the left ventricle changes continuously throughout the cardiac cycle. The *in-vivo* measurements in this study were conducted to verify the validity of the *in-vitro* studies of the human mitral valve. The shape of the waveforms obtained in the left ventricle of the calf compare favorably with those measured in the left ventricular shaped chamber Model II. Compare the velocity versus time tracing in *Figure 3.22* with that measured in the Model II chamber at the point, $T = 5$, and $P = 1$ (see Figure 3.25). In like manner comparing *Figures 3.21* and *3.26* indicates a similarity at two other locations in the left ventricle. The velocity immediately beneath the mitral valve orifice as measured in the calf (*see Figure 3.23*) is almost identical in shape and magnitude with the velocity measured in the left ventricular shaped mitral valve testing chamber Model II at the point, $T = 6$, $P = 1$, as shown in *Figure 3.27*.

The magnitude of the velocity measured in the aortic outflow tract in the Model II chamber is not as great as that measured in the aortic outflow tract of the calf; however, the character of the flow, i.e. the shape of the waveform is very similar in both instances (*see Figures 3.24 and 3.28*).

Unfortunately the direction of the velocity *in vivo* in the left ventricle of the dog and the calf could not be determined from the catheter-tip conical hot-film probe. The direction during diastolic inflow immediately beneath the mitral valve obviously must be directed from the base to the apex of the heart. In like manner the direction of flow along the septal portion of the ventricular wall near the aortic outflow tract during systolic contraction in the normal heart is probably from apex toward the aortic root. This fact combined with the shape of the waveform measured in the left ventricle of the dog and the calf indicate two spikes in the velocity versus time tracings (*see Figures 3.21, 3.22 and 3.24*). Apparently these two spikes in the velocity versus time tracings represent the acceleration of the vortex due to mitral inflow and the increased velocity of the vortex during systolic ejection. Additional credance to this theory is provided by the shape of the velocity tracings in the left ventricular shaped mitral valve testing chamber Model II beneath the mitral valve and also in the aortic outflow tract. Stated differently, the flow of fluid through the mitral orifice sets up the vortex formation in the left ventricle and creates one velocity peak. Then during systolic contraction the

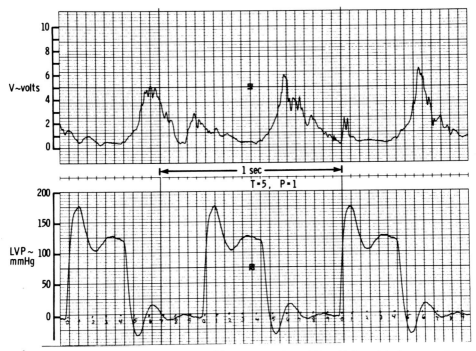

Figure 3.25 Typical linearized anemometer bridge output, voltage (V) and left ventricular pressure (LVP) versus time tracings in Model II chamber at T = 5, P = 1.

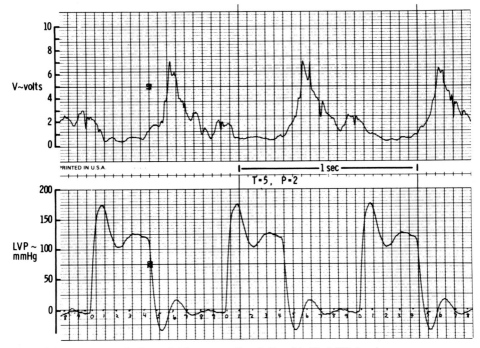

Figure 3.26 Same data as in *Figure 3.25*, except at T = 5, P = 2 in Model II chamber.

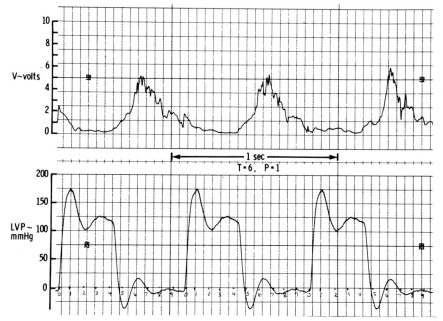

Figure 3.27 Same data as in *Figure 3.25* but at T = 6, P = 1 in Model II chamber.

velocity of this vortex is again increased as flow is accelerated out the aortic outflow tract as the vortex size decreases.

In-vivo observations of vortices observed during cineangiography in man have been reported by Reid[10, 11], and in the dog by Lynch and Bove[34] using the injection of radiopaque gelatin droplets in the left atrium and simultaneously recording cineangiograms. Each of these investigators report the presence of eddies forming in the left ventricle during diastolic filling. Lynch states, 'when the material (radiopaque) reaches the wall, larger eddies develop and a swirling motion in the lateral projection is easily seen.' Rushmer[35] described the concepts and mechanisms of mitral valve closure with the aid of several sketches showing flow currents behind the leaflets of the mitral valve. In our opinion this work represents the first attempt to correlate the measurement of velocity and flow patterns *in vitro* for a human mitral valve mounted in a left ventricular shaped valve testing chamber with measurements of velocity *in vivo*. There is of course no direct correlation of the results since the *in-vitro* measurements are made in a rigid non-flexing, non-contracting chamber whereas the *in-vivo* measurements are made in a pulsatile flow contracting left ventricular chamber of the dog and the calf. Nevertheless, striking similarly does occur at several points within the valve-testing chamber and the beating left ventricle.

Summary

Studies of the mechanical forces and fluid mechanical forces which interact with the mitral valve and left ventricle of certain mammalian hearts have been presented. Particular attention was given to the nature of these forces and the manner in which

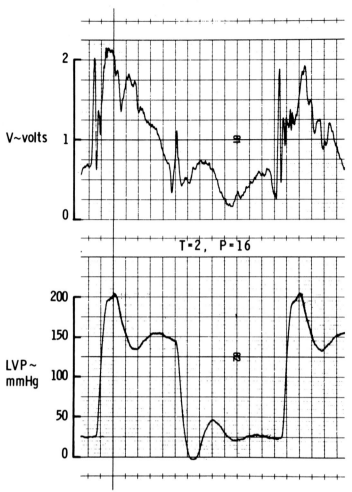

Figure 3.28 Linearized anemometer output voltage (V) and left ventricular pressure (LVP) in Model II chamber (T = 2, P = 16) in the aortic outflow tract.

they interact to form a precise, efficient, low-resistant, rapid-closing and durable check valve to regulate blood flow through the atrioventricular annulus of the heart. Both *in-vitro* and *in-vivo* studies were carried out.

The initial *in-vitro* studies were made by mounting an isolated human mitral valve in a cylindrical plastic chamber (Model I) with cross-sectional flow areas immediately proximal and distal to the valve analogous to those in the heart. Special load cells were fabricated and used to measure the magnitudes of posteromedial and anterolateral papillary muscle forces necessary to prevent regurgitation. The optimum magnitudes of the peak systolic forces were 3.25 N and 4.36 N for the anterolateral and posteromedial papillary muscles, respectively. Forces less than these values resulted in significant regurgitation; however, forces greater than the optimum values resulted in little or no regurgitation. No provision was made in the *in-vitro* studies for papillary muscle contraction.

Flow patterns associated with the isolated human mitral valve were observed and photographed with still, movie, and high-speed movie cameras. These flow patterns demonstrated that a large vortex forms behind the anterior leaflet, and a smaller vortex forms behind the posterior leaflet of the mitral valve during diastole at 72 pulses per minute and a mean flow rate of 5 l/min. These vortices tended to 'drift' downstream along the axis of the cylindrical chamber, since the apex of the left ventricle was not simulated. It appeared that the vortices do contribute to the approximation of the valve leaflets just prior to the onset of the subsequent systole. The rapid rise in ventricular pressure compeletes closure of the valve leaflets with essentially no visible regurgitation. The only reverse flow of blood analog fluid appeared to be associated with the movement of the leaflets in a dome-like shape into the mitral annulus.

The previously well-defined flow patterns both during systole and diastole were significantly altered when papillary muscle forces were reduced below the optimum levels. The vortices did not form; consequently the leaflets moved in a much move erratic manner and significant regurgitation occurred.

Axial and radial velocities proximal and distal to the isolated mitral valve under optimum conditions were calculated from flow pattern photographs and also measured with a two-channel hot-film anemometer. Velocity profiles obtained in this manner compared favorably.

The peak pressure drop accross the isolated human mitral valve was found to be approximately 3 mm Hg at 72 pulses per minute and a mean flow rate of 5 l/min.

A second series of *in-vitro* studies were carried out with the mitral and aortic valves dissected as a single unit from a human heart at autopsy and mounted in a plastic chamber (Model II) which was designed to simulate the geometry of the left atrium, aorta, and left ventricle at the end of diastole. The primary purpose of this chamber was to study the effect of 'capturing the vortex' within a simulated left ventricular shaped chamber.

Flow patterns in this chamber were photographed and analyzed in the same manner employed for the initial *in-vitro* studies in the Model I chamber. These flow patterns again demonstrated a large vortex behind the anterior leaflet and a smaller vortex behind the posterior leaflet; however, the large vortex expanded to fill almost the entire left ventricular chamber at the end of diastole. The stream of fluid entering the left ventricle from the mitral valve impinged on the apex, turned back up to the septal wall, and eventually merged with the small vortex which formed behind the anterior leaflet as a result of separation of the boundary layer. During the subsequent systole, the outer high-velocity fluid 'peeled off' from the vortex and was ejected through the aortic vestibule and aortic valve. The vortices behind the anterior and posterior leaflets again appeared to contribute to the efficient closure of the mitral valve by approximating the leaflets just prior to the onset of systole.

The vortex formation in the left ventricle also appears to serve as an energy-conserving mechanism. Fluid motion in the left ventricle probably remains in a constant state of rotation. As fluid enters during diastole the angular velocity increases. During systole the size of the rotating volume decreases but continues to rotate. This condition of flow can be compared to a flywheel which stores energy.

Blood analog velocity magnitudes were measured with the hot-film anemometer at 169 discrete data points in the Model II chamber. The direction of the velocity vector at each point was determined from flow pattern photographs during peak diastolic flow and during peak systolic flow. Axial velocity profiles were plotted at each of ten traverses in the x–z plane (bisecting the aortic valve annulus, the mitral valve annulus, and midway between the papillary muscles). The maximum velocity of 98.1 cm/s was measured during diastole immediately beneath the mitral valve at traverse $T = 2$ and data point $P = 4$ approximately 470 ms after the onset of systole.

Conclusions

An optimum force must be applied to each papillary muscle in order to prevent regurgitation through the mitral valve. Forces less than the optimum cause more regurgitation than forces greater than the optimum.

Regurgitation not only disturbs the flow pattern during diastole, but also during the subsequent systole.

Flow patterns made *in vitro* both in the isolated chamber (Mode I) and in the left ventricular shaped chamber (Model II) confirmed the existence of a large vortex behind the anterior leaflet and a smaller vortex behind the posterior leaflet of the mitral valve during diastole.

The vortices behind the mitral valve leaflets tend to approximate the margins of the leaflets just before the onset of systole and therefore prevent regurgitation during ventricular contraction.

Blood flow entering the left ventricle from the mitral valve strikes the apex and turns back up the septal wall of the left ventricle merging with the vortex behind the anterior leaflet. The result is one large vortex which essentially fills the entire left ventricle at the end of the diastole.

The large vortex that forms in the left ventricle probably serves as an energy-storing mechanism.

The fluid circulating in the outer part of the vortex 'peels off' and is ejected through the aortic valve during ventricular systole.

The vortex type flow pattern washes the entire left ventricle and tends to prevent thrombus formation as a result of stasis.

The peak pressure drop across the mitral valve during diastole is approximately 3 mm Hg. The mitral valve, therefore, represents a very minor resistance to blood flow.

Acknowledgement

This work was supported in part by USPHS Grants HL–13330, HE–05435 and GM 46009.

References

1. SILVERMAN, M.E. and HURST, J.W. (1968). The mitral complex. *American Heart Journal*, **75**, 399–418
2. RANGANATHAN, N., SILVER, M.D. and WIGLE, E.D. (1976). Recent advances in the knowledge of the anatomy of the mitral valve. In *The Mitral Valve, A Pluridisciplinary Approach* (Ed. D. Kalmanson), Chap. **1,** pp. 3–13. Acton, Ma.: Publishing Sciences Group
3. TSAKIRIS, A.G. (1976). The physiology of the mitral valve annulus. In *The Mitral Valve, A Pluridisciplinary Approach* (Ed. D. Kalmanson) Chap. **3**, pp. 21–60. Acton, Ma.: Publishing Sciences Group
4. BROCK, R.C. (1952). The surgical and pathological anatomy of the mitral valve. *British Heart Journal*, **14**, 489–513
5. SMITH, H.L., ESSEX, H.E. and BALDES, E.J. (1950). A study of the movements of heart valves and of heart sounds. *Annals of Internal Medicine*, **33**, 1357–9

6. VAN DER SPUY, J.C. (1958). The functional and clinical anatomy of the mitral valve. *British Heart Journal*, **20**, 471–8
7. WIETING, D.W. (1974). *Dynamics and Fluid Dynamics of the Mitral Valve*. Ph.D. Dissertation. Baylor College of Medicine, Houston, Texas
8. HARVEY, W. (1941). *Exercitatio Anatomica De Motu Cordis et Sanguinis in Animalibus*. (Translated and annotated by C.D. Leake.) Springfield: Charles C. Thomas.
9. KREHL, L. (1891). *Beiträge zur Kenntniss der Füllung and Entleerung des Herzens*. Leipzig: S. Hirzel.
10. REID, K.G. (1969). Mitral valve action and the mode of ventricular filling. *Nature (Lond.)*, **223**, 1383–4
11. REID, K.G. (1970). Design criteria for a prosthetic orthotopic heart and mitral valve. *Guys Hospital Reports*, **119**, 209–219
12. BELLHOUSE, B.J. (1960). Fluid mechanics of the mitral valve. *Nature (Lond.)*, **224**, 615–616
13. BELLHOUSE, B.J. (1970). Mechanism of closure of the mitral valve. *Clinical Science*, **39**, 13P–14P
14. BELLHOUSE, B.J. (1970). Fluid mechanics of a model mitral valve. *Journal of Physiology*, **207**, 72P–73P
15. BELLHOUSE, B.J. (1972). Fluid mechanics of a model mitral valve and left ventricle. *Cardiovascular Research*, **6**, 199–210
16. NOLAN, S.P., DIXON, S.H., FISHER, R.D. and MORROW, A.G. (1969). The influence of atrial contraction and mitral valve mechancis on ventricular filling. *American Heart Journal*, **77**, 784–791
17. BRAUNWALD, E., ROCKOFF, S.D., OLDHAM, H.N. and ROSS, J. JR. (1966). Effective closure of the mitral valve without atrial systole. *Circulation*, **33**, 404–409
18. YELLIN, E.L., PESKIN, C.S., and FRATER, R.W.M. (1972). Pulsatile flow across the mitral valve: hydraulic, electronic and digital computer simulation. A.S.M.E. Paper No. 72–WA/BHF–10
19. WIETING, D.W., HWANG, N.H.C., KENNEDY, J.H. and RUARK, B.S. (1971). Engineering evaluation of chordae tendineae tension and mitral valve function. ASME Paper No. 71/BHF–4
20. WIETING, D.W., KENNEDY, J.H., and HWANG, N.H.C. (1972). Testing of heart valve replacements. *Advances in Cardiology, 7: Long-Term Prognosis Following Valve Replacement*. Basel: S. Karger. pp. 2–11
21. WIETING, D.W., HWANG, N.H.C. and KENNEDY, J.H. (1971). Fluid mechanics of the human mitral valve. A.I.A.A. Paper No. 71–102
22. WIETING, D.W. (1972). An improved chamber for in vitro study of heart valves. *Proceed.* ACEMB **14**, 114
23. STRIPLING, T.E. (1972). *Left Ventricular Flow Characteristics of a Healthy Human Heart*. M.S. Thesis University of Houston, Houston, Texas
24. WEITING, D.W. (1969). *Dynamic Flow Characteristics of Heart Valves*. Dissertation. University of Texas, Austin, Texas
25. DISA Electronics (1970). *DISA Information*, No. 10. DISA Electronics, Franklin Lakes, New Jersey. October, p. 30
26. SALISBURY, P.F., CROSS, C.E. and RIEBEN, P.A. (1963). Chordae tendineae tension. *American Journal of Physiology*, **205**, 385–392
27. BURCH, G.E. and DE PASQUALE, N.P. (1965). Time course of tension in papillary muscles of the heart. *Journal of the American Medical Association*, **192**, 701–704
28. CRONIN, R., ARMOUR, J.A. and RANDALL, N.C. (1969). Function of the in situ papillary muscle in the canine left ventricle. *Circulatory Research*, **25**, 69–75
29. BURCH, G.E., DEPASQUALE, N.P. and PHILLIP, J.H. (1968). The syndrome of papillary muscle dysfunction. *American Heart Journal*, **75**, 399–415
30. TSAKIRIS, A.G., RASTELLI, G.C., AMORIM, D. DES., TITUS, J.L. and WOOD, E.H. (1970). Effect of experimental papillary muscle damage of mitral valve closure in intact anesthetized dogs. *Mayo Clinic Proceedings*, **45**, 275–285
31. BELLHOUSE, B.J. (1976). Fluid Mechanics of a Model Mitral Valve. *The Mitral Valve, A Pluridisciplinary Approach*. (Ed. D. Kalmanson), Chap. **9**, pp. 99–110. Acton, Ma.: Publishing Sciences Group
32. TAYLOR, D.E.M. and WADE, J.D. (1969). Flow through the mitral valve during diastolic filling of the left ventricle. *Journal of Physiology*, **200**, 75P–74P
33. TAYLOR, D.E.M. and WHAMOND, J.S. (1976). Velocity Profile and Impedance of the Healthy Mitral Valve. *The Mitral Valve, A Pluridisciplinary Approach*. (Ed. D. Kalmanson), Chap. **12**, pp. 127–136. Acton, Ma.: Publishing Sciences Group
34. LYNCH, P.R. and BOVE, A.A. (1969). Patterns of blood flow through the intact heart and its valves. *Prosthetic Heart Valves*. (Ed. L.A. Brewer), pp. 24–33. III, Springfield: Charles C. Thomas, Publisher
35. RUSHMER, R.F. (1970). *Cardiovascular Dynamics*, 3rd edn. Philadelphia; W.B. Saunders Company, pp. 293–299

4

Physiology of mitral valve flow

Edward L. Yellin, Chaim Yoran and Robert W.M. Frater

Introduction

Interestingly, although more than a decade has passed since publication of the first records of phasic mitral flow[1-3] the textbook illustrations of the cardiac cycle still do not include the mitral flow waveform. Perhaps this is due to a normal time delay between discovery and acceptance; perhaps this is due to an incomplete understanding of atrioventricular pressure-flow dynamics; or perhaps this is due to the fact that the time variations of diastolic filling are inherently more complex than those of systolic emptying. Whatever the reason, in this chapter we shall attempt to elucidate the physiology of mitral valve flow. We will offer a conceptual framework in which to analyze transmitral flow dynamics, review current knowledge and present some new data from conscious dogs. A model with a conceptual (i.e. analytical) approach is useful because it provides a framework into which the observed data must fit. Any deviation of the data from the accepted model must then be examined and explained so that the observation may be either questioned or rejected. Furthermore, the use of a model allows us to make predictions which can be tested by experiment.

Analysis

Soon after the first publication of electromagnetically measured aortic flow records, Spencer and Greiss[4] described the transaortic pressure–flow relations in terms of inertia and resistance. Nolan *et al.*[1] published the first records of phasic transmitral flow and recognized the importance of fluid inertia in explaining the delay between the timing of the atrioventricular pressure crossover and the cessation of mitral flow. Thus, aortic and mitral flow dynamics are governed by the same principles. Our understanding of these principles and their application to diastolic filling is helped considerably by the use of the model shown in *Figure 4.1*.

   The valve consists of a diode (middle path) which permits only unidirectional flow when the left atrial pressure (LAP) exceeds the left ventricular pressure (LVP). During that time the forward pressure difference consists of a component necessary for acceleration, *(A) dQ/dt*, and a component necessary to overcome viscous resistance, *(B)Q*. The upper path describes the viscoelastic properties of the valve, i.e. its ability to store energy by virtue of its compliance after the valve closes. Its properties partially determine the characteristics of the first heart sound. The lower path is included to describe the dynamics of mitral regurgitation (when the valve is competent the resistance is infinite). We have shown that in the equation of motion (*see Figure 4.1*): $n = 1$ when the valve is normal[5]; $n = 2$ when the valve is stenotic[6]; and $n = 2$ in the backflow path when the valve is incompetent[7–9]. The validity of this model can be tested by examining the experimental data for consistency with the following predictions which can be derived from the proposed conceptual approach.

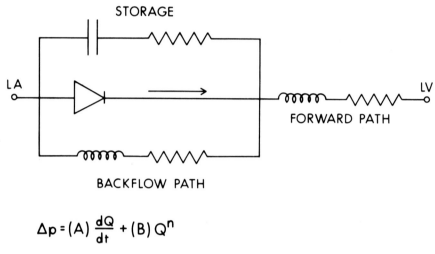

$$\Delta p = (A)\frac{dQ}{dt} + (B)Q^n$$

Figure 4.1 An electric analog of the mitral valve, with the equation of motion which describes the general pressure–flow relation across either the forward flow or backflow paths.

Let us measure flow at the level of the mitral annulus and start with the onset of isovolumic relaxation. As the LVP falls, the compliant valve, which has been stretched toward the atrium, will move toward the ventricle and although no flow will cross the leaflet free edges, there will be transport across the mitral annulus. This should appear as a small brief upstroke in mitral flow prior to the A-V pressure crossover. Forward flow should start at the pressure cross over, and as the LV rapidly relaxes a relatively large pressure gradient should develop to accelerate the blood during rapid early filling. To be consistent with the properties of an inertial system, the peak pressure gradient should precede the peak flow. The equation of motion also predicts that when the pressure difference goes to zero during diastasis there will be an exponential decay of flow toward zero:

If $\Delta P = (A)dQ/dt + (B)Q$, when $\Delta P = 0$, $dQ/Q = -B/A(dt)$
and $Q = Q_0 e^{-B/A(dt)}$, where Q_0 is the value of Q when ΔP first becomes zero.

Under normal conditions the exponential decay should end with an atrial contraction which once again accelerates mitral inflow. If the pressure difference during diastasis becomes negative rather than zero (i.e., LAP less than LVP) then mitral flow will decelerate more rapidly than the predicted exponential. Similarly, following an atrial contraction, when the atrium relaxes and/or the ventricle contracts, there will be a reversal of the pressure difference and flow will rapidly decelerate. Thus, mitral valve closure will of necessity be delayed with respect to the time of pressure crossover. As long as there is flow the valve must be open! Furthermore, we may conclude that the interrelation between flow and valve-closing motion will be highly dependent on the state of atrial contractility and on the duration of the PR interval.

The results presented below have been chosen to examine the predictions described above. In addition, the oscillographic records have also been selected to illustrate the application of the conceptual approach to our understanding of: the general diastolic interaction between valve motion and flow; the changes in flow patterns with heart rate; the atrial contribution to filling; the origin and determinants of the first heart sound; the influence of aortic regurgitation on mitral flow; and the control of ventricular filling during changes in contractility, preload, and vascular tone. Because our purpose is to elucidate the overall filling process, rather than its details, our emphasis will be primarily qualitative rather than quantitative.

Method

The experimental preparation has been described in previous publications from this laboratory[10–12] and is schematically illustrated in *Figure 4.2*. Briefly, in the acute studies, under pentobarbital anesthesia, micromanometers (Millar) were placed in the LV, LA and ascending aorta. An electromagnetic flow probe (Carolina Medical Electronics) was placed around the ascending aorta and during cardiopulmonary

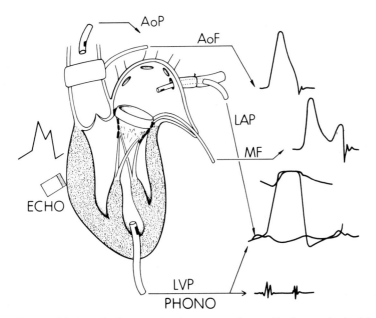

Figure 4.2 Schematic diagram of the instrumentation used in the anesthetized dog studies. Aortic pressure, aortic flow and the echo are not measured in the chronic dog preparation. AoP = Aortic pressure; AoF = aortic flow; LAP = Left atrial pressure; LVP = left ventricular pressure; and MF = mitral flow. (Re-drawn from *J. Applied Physiol.* (1975), **39**, 665, with kind permission of authors and publishers.)

bypass another flow probe was sutured to the mitral annulus. In some experiments radiopaque markers were implanted on the anterior and posterior mitral leaflets[10], and in others, echocardiography (Unirad) was used to record valve motion[11, 12]. The intracardiac phonogram and LV$dp/dt$ were obtained from the hi-fidelity LV pressure transducer. These hemodynamic parameters plus a standard limb lead ECG were recorded on an oscillographic recorder (Electronics for Medicine) at paper speeds of 100 mm/s.

Chronically instrumented dogs were studied in the resting state, lightly sedated with morphine sulphate (4–5 mg), 1 day to 4 weeks after operation, but without measuring aortic flow, aortic pressure and valve motion. In the chronic preparation we studied the responses to bolus injections of isoproterenol (2–20 μg) and nitroprusside (0.25–1.2 mg), and to volume loading (5% dextrose, 50 ml/min). Reflex bradycardia and AV block were created with bolus injections of norepinephrine (50 μg); and prolonged PR intervals were created with bolus injections of verapamil (4 mg).

Results and discussion

Since the purpose of this paper is to provide a didactic review rather than a scientific report, we have chosen a format that presents an original oscillographic record along with a simultaneous discussion of the data.

General description

Figure 4.3 is an oscillographic record taken from a conscious dog during a period of normal, but variable, rhythm (beats 2,4) and one junctional beat (No. 1), and has been selected because it illustrates many of the important results and concepts of mitral flow physiology. A characteristic mitral valve echogram had been superimposed on the record and is consistent with our other data[11, 12]. The A-V pressure gradient is established as the LV rapidly relaxes and its pressure falls below the LAP (diastolic suction). As the force on the valve decreases, the leaflets move toward the ventricle and open quickly and widely as blood is rapidly accelerated across the mitral annulus. Peak volume flow rate is 215 ml/s which translates into a velocity of 90 cm/s at the annulus, and which is produced by a peak pressure difference of 8 mm Hg. The peak pressure difference always precedes the peak flow by approximately 10 ms; this is consistent with the existence of fluid inertia. The mitral valve starts its diastolic closing motion while flow is still accelerating so that the E point precedes the flow peak by 27 ms; we postulate that this is due to a combination of vortices and chordal tension[12]. With atrial emptying and ventricular filling the A-V pressure decreases and equilibrates at zero. It is particularly important to note that flow then decelerates exponentially toward zero (beats 1,2,4). When the atrium contracts, flow accelerates and then decelerates entirely under the action of atrial relaxation since the ventricle has not yet contracted (beats 2–4). (See below for a further discussion of the P-R interval and filling.)

Contribution to filling of the atrial contraction

Having demonstrated that mitral flow would decay exponentially to zero in the presence of a long diastole and in the absence of an atrial contraction, we may now define the atrial systolic contribution to filling as follows: an atrial contraction contributes a filling volume equal to the flow *over and above* that which would have entered the ventricle if the atrium had not contracted and if *the duration of diastole were unchanged*. This is not the same as previous definitions which either measure the entire change in volume of the ventricle during the time of atrial systole[13, 14], or measure the change in volume when diastole has been shortened by a nodal beat that precedes the atrial contraction[1]. For example, the contribution of atrial systole in beats 2 and 3 (*see Figure 4.3*, shaded area) is 18% and 13%, respectively. The contribution which occurred during the period of atrial systole is 22% and 37%, respectively. Based on a large number of measurements taken during the resting state in conscious dogs, we find that the atrial contraction contributes 15±3% (mean ± SD) to the total filling volume.

Mitral flow, valve closure, and the first heart sound

The data of *Figure 4.3* (as well as others shown below) and our previous observations[10–12] lead us to support the concept that the first heart sound has its origin in the closure of the mitral valve and its subsequent vibrations. The energy level of the vibration is a function of the mass and elasticity of the cardiohemic system which is in oscillation[15] and of the impulsive force imparted to the system. Thus, S1 occurs after the pressure crossover when the valve has closed and flow

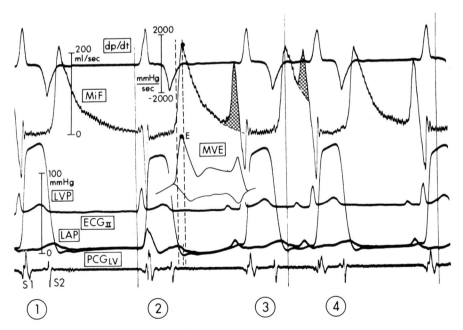

Figure 4.3 Original oscillographic record from a conscious dog with a typical mitral valve echogram (MVE) superimposed. The shaded areas denote the atrial contribution to filling. See text for discussion. Time lines are 1/s. dp/dt = LV$dp/dt$, ECG$_{11}$ = lead 11 of the electrocardiogram, PCG$_{LV}$ = intracardiac phonocardiogram, S1, S2 = first and second heart sounds. Filled circles denote peak mitral flow and the E point of the MVE. The broken vertical lines indicate the timing of the A-V pressure crossover, peak A-V pressure gradient and peak mitral flow rate.

ceased; its amplitude is strongly dependent on LV$dp/dt$ (compare beats 3 and 4); and flow deceleration is not necessary (beat 2, following the end of the long diastasis of beat 1). Note that S1 coincides with the flow oscillations at valve closure in all the beats.

Competence of valve closure in the absence of an atrial contraction

The first beat in *Figure 4.3* illustrates a normal competent valve closure in the absence of an appropriately timed atrial contraction. This is consistent with our previous observations[12, 16, 17], which have led us to conclude that an atrial contraction is not necessary for competent valve closure provided there is no unusual distortion of the mitral apparatus by, for example, an acute dilation of the ventricle. There is, however, considerable controversy over this question[18].

Role of left atrial reservoir pressure

Figure 4.4 illustrates the influence of the left atrial reservoir pressure (i.e., passive) ventricular filling. In this anesthetized dog study[16], a shunt from the subclavian artery to the left atrium was rapidly closed to measure the effect of changing the filling pressure before any reflex changes could occur. A sudden decrease in filling pressure at the crossover point from 11 mm Hg to 6 mm Hg led to 29% reduction in

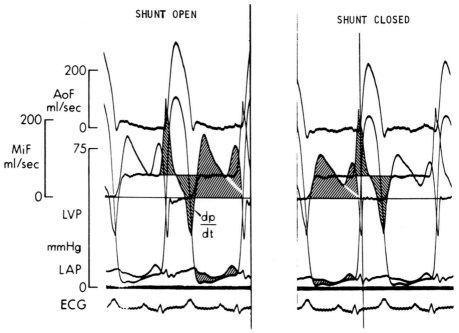

Figure 4.4 High-gain oscillographic records from an anesthetized dog illustrating the influence of left atrial reservoir pressure on phasic mitral flow. A shunt from the subclavian artery to the left atrium is open in the left panel. The record in the right panel was taken immediately after the shunt was closed. *dp/dt*, mitral flow, and the A-V pressure difference have been shaded for clarity. Shunt open: mean LAP = 8 mm Hg, filling volume = 26 ml. Shunt closed: mean LAP = 5 mm Hg, filling volume = 21 ml. (Reproduced from reference 16, with kind permission of authors and publishers.)

peak flow (rapid early filling) and a 25% reduction in total filling volume. The other hemodynamic parameters which influence filling—left ventricular relaxation and diastolic filling time—were unchanged. Thus, physiologically small increments in filling pressure produce large changes in filling volume.

Role of left ventricular relaxation

Figure 4.5 is another record from an anesthetized dog study[16] which illustrates the profound effect of left ventricular relaxation rate on early filling. This record was selected because in the post-extrasystolic beat there was a relatively small decrease in LAP at the pressure crossover, but there was a large decrease in LV relaxation rate. Following a 49% increase in the time constant of relaxation (and a 57% decrease in *dp/dt* min) there was a 25% decrease in peak flow and an 8% decrease in total filling volume, despite the 52% increase in diastolic filling time during the compensatory pause. We have previously reported that volume increases only 6% during the compensatory pause despite the 76% increase in filling time; primarily because of the slowed relaxation rate of the LV following the extrasystolic contraction[19].

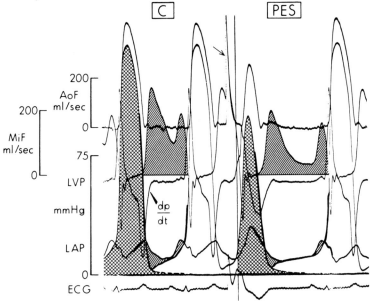

Figure 4.5 High-gain oscillographic record from an anesthetized dog illustrating the importance to filling of left ventricular relaxation rate. Shading and trace darkening have been added for clarity and emphasis. Note that the slowed rate of LV relaxation following the extrasystole has a profound influence on the peak flow and rate of increase of flow during the compensatory pause in postextrasystolic (PES) beat. The broken line on the LVP traces is an extrapolation of relaxation to zero pressure. Control: filling volume = 38 ml, diastolic filling time = 290 ms. PES: filling volume = 35 ml, diastolic filling time = 440 ms. (Re-drawn from reference 16, with kind permission of authors and publishers.)

Effect of P-R interval and atrial relaxation

In a conscious dog the P-R interval was prolonged by a bolus injection of verapamil (4 mg) and the results are shown in *Figure 4.6*. The early response (middle panel)

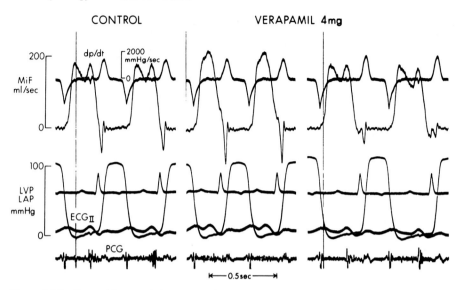

Figure 4.6 Oscillographic records from a conscious dog illustrating the effect on the mitral flow wave-form of prolonging the P-R interval with verapamil. Although there is a mixed effect due to the reflex changes in heart rate, atrial relaxation clearly may reverse the diastolic pressure gradient and decelerate mitral flow before the ventricular contraction. This is particularly evident in the right panel.

was a small increase in HR (128–140 beats/min) and a large increase in P-R interval (115–150 ms). Since the atrial contraction occurred early in diastole at the new HR, there was a significant amount of fluid momentum in the mitral flow, and the total filling volume decreased only 8% despite the early pressure crossover leading to a 25% reduction in the duration of the positive A-V pressure difference. The later response to verapamil is shown in the right panel where the HR has reflexly decreased to 110 beats/min and the P-R interval has increased further to 165 ms. This combination changes the waveform of mitral flow back to its control shape, but the mitral valve has clearly closed about 40 ms before the onset of ventricular contraction. Thus, although the filling volume is unchanged from control, the cardiac output has decreased 12%. The duration of systole is the same in the right panel as in the control so that 75 ms more was available for diastolic filling, but only 30 ms were actually used because the relaxing left atrium reversed the pressure difference 60 ms before the ventricle contracted.

An additional consequence of atrial relaxation is shown in *Figure 4.7*, a record from a conscious dog soon after receiving a bolus injection of norepinephrine (50 μg) which produced a reflex A-V block. It illustrates the phenomenon of mitral valve 'locking'[20]. Each atrial contraction resulted in a reversal of the pressure difference and an apparent closure of the valve, since the pressure gradient stayed negative and flow ceased in the intervals between atrial contractions. This phenomenon has been demonstrated by echocardiography[20].

Effect of aortic regurgitation on mitral flow

An interesting clinical correlate of the ideas discussed above is illustrated in the oscillographic record (*see Figure 4.8*) taken from a conscious dog who suddenly

A-V Block and Mitral Valve "Locking"

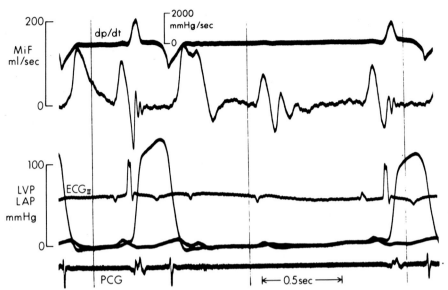

Figure 4.7 An oscillographic record from a conscious dog illustrating the ability of an atrial relaxation to reverse the pressure difference and to result in mid-diastolic valve closure. Transient A-V nodal block was produced by a reflex response to 50 μg norepinephrine.

AORTIC REGURGITATION

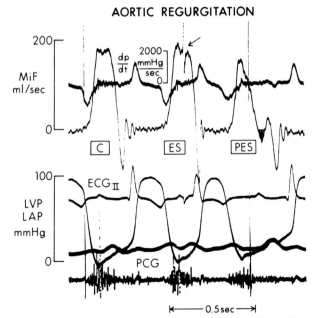

Figure 4.8 Oscillographic record from a conscious dog illustrating the effect on mitral flow of aortic regurgitation. In particular, note the shortening diastole with an extrasystole (ES) did not change the filling volume because in the control (C) beat there was an early pressure crossover. Note also that the slowed relaxation of the ES beat led to a decrease in filling during the compensatory pause of the post-extrasystolic (PES) beat. C and ES filling volume = 23 ml. PES = 15 ml.

developed aortic regurgitation on the 20th day following the surgery described above. In the control beat the combination of a rapidly rising LVP (due to retrograde aortic flow) and a long P-R interval resulted in an early pressure crossover and a reduced diastolic filling time. Thus, shortening the P-R interval by 20% with an extrasystole produced no change in filling volume. In contrast, the filling volume during the compensatory pause preceding the post-extrasystolic beat decreased by 34%, and there was a small amount of mid-diastolic and closing retrograde flow across the mitral valve. This decreased filling was due to a combination of a slowed relaxation rate, an enlarged stiff ventricle, a long P-R interval, and the consequent early pressure gradient reversal. We have shown in a previous study that aortic regurgitation reduces the actual diastolic filling time and shifts the bulk of mitral flow to the rapid filling phase so that increasing the heart rate in a patient with aortic regurgitation is beneficial because it reduces the minute volume of retrograde aortic flow and increases the forward cardiac output[21].

Effect of isoproterenol on filling

Figure 4.9 illustrates a typical response of the conscious dog to a bolus injection of isoproterenol (2 μg). Early filling is augmented by an increase in the A-V pressure difference due solely to a decrease in LVP_{min} which reflects the decreased end systolic volume. The force of atrial contraction and its contribution to filling clearly increase (middle and right panels), and this increase is maintained even after the early filling peak returns to control levels. We may conclude that isoproterenol

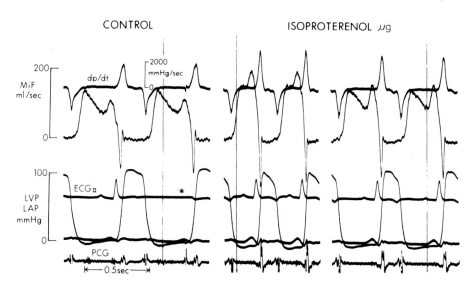

Figure 4.9 Oscillographic records from a conscious dog illustrating the hemodynamic response to isoproterenol. * Indicates that the QRS complex was blanked by a computational signal. Note the direct relationship between the amplitudes of S1 and *dp/dt*. Control: HR = 105 beats/min; filling volume = 30 ml; atrial contribution = 11%. Early response: HR = 168 beats/min; filling volume = 26 ml; atrial contribution = 14%. Later response: HR = 124 beats/min; filling volume = 33 ml; atrial contribution = 15%.

enhances ventricular filling by increasing elastic recoil (diastolic suction) without requiring an increased left atrial filling pressure. In this and the following records (*see Figures 4.9–4.11*), note the direct relation between the amplitude of S1 and $LVdp/dt_{max}$.

Effect of nitroprusside on filling

The typical response of the conscious dog to a bolus injection of nitroprusside (0.5 mg) is shown in *Figure 4.10*. The initial vasodilatation leads to a reduction of systemic pressure which, in turn, leads to a reflex increase in heart rate and contractility. The result is similar to that of isoproterenol: an increased A-V pressure difference due to a decreased end systolic volume and LVP_{min}, with no change in LAP, leads to an increase in peak flow; and an increased force of atrial systole leads to an augmented atrial contribution to filling.

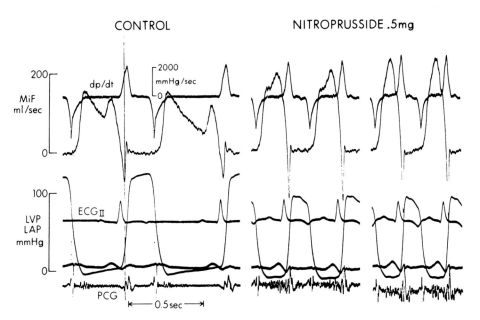

Figure 4.10 Oscillographic records from a conscious dog illustrating the hemodynamic response to nitro-prusside. Control (2 beats): HR = 105, 86 beats/min; filling volume = 32, 38 ml; atrial contribution = 12, 14%. Early response: HR = 161 beats/min; filling volume = 27 ml; atrial contribution = 15%. Later response: HR = 190 beats/min; filling volume = 23 ml; atrial contribution = 20%.

Effect of increasing preload by volume infusion

In contrast to the preceding two conditions, moderate increases in blood volume (100–200 ml) in the conscious dog increase the A-V pressure difference by increasing the filling pressure (LAP) rather than by decreasing LVP_{min}. This is illustrated in *Figure 4.11*.

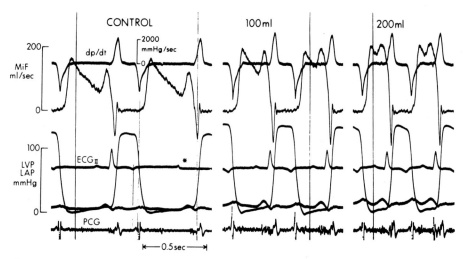

Figure 4.11 Oscillographic records from a conscious dog illustrating the hemodynamic response to increasing the preload by volume expansion. * Indicates that the QRS was blanked by a computerational signal. Control: HR = 89 beats/min; filling volume = 36 ml; atrial contribution = 14%. 100 ml: HR = 118 beats/min; filling volume = 37 ml; atrial contribution = 13%. 200 ml: HR = 151 beats/min; filling volume = 30 ml; atrial contribution = 11%.

Conclusions

We have employed highly invasive methods to study the physiology of mitral valve flow. We think the results are accurate and informative, and we hope this review will serve to clarify ventricular filling dynamics. Equally important, we hope that the data and the analysis presented will improve our ability to interpret and to elucidate the often ambiguous results obtained from high-technology, non-invasive methods. We hope thereby to stimulate the use and development of non-invasive techniques.

Acknowledgements

We thank all the Residents and Fellows who have been past collaborators with us in the Department of Surgery Cardiovascular Research Laboratory. Their names appear in the References. We thank Dr David and his co-authors[20] for sharing their ideas on mitral valve 'locking' with us before their publication. This work could not have been done without the technical skills of messrs A. Leon, P. Bon and F. Rivera. We thank Ms M. Olivera for typing the manuscript. This work was supported in part by USPHS Grants HL–19391 and HL–24638.

References

1. NOLAN, S.P., DIXON, S.H., FISHER, R.D. and MORROW, A.G. (1969). The influence of atrial contraction and mitral valve mechanics on ventricular filling. A study of instantaneous mitral valve flow *in vivo*. *American Heart Journal*, **77**, 784–91
2. FOLTS, J.D., YOUNG, W.P. and ROWE, G.G. (1971). Phasic flow through normal and prosthetic mitral valves in unanesthetized dogs. *J. Thoracic and Cardiovascular Surgery*, **61**, 235–41

3. KALMANSON, D., TOUTAIN, G., NOVIKOFF, N. and DERAE, C. (1972). Retrograde catheterization of left heart cavities in dogs by means of an orientable directional Doppler catheter-tip flowmeter: A preliminary report. *Cardiovascular Research*, **6**, 309–18

4. SPENCER, M.P. and GREISS, F.C. (1962). Dynamics of ventricular ejection. *Circulation Research*, **10**, 274–279

5. YELLIN, E.L., LANIADO, S., PESKIN, C.S. and FRATER, R.W.M. (1976). Analysis and interpretation of the normal mitral valve flow curve. In *The Mitral Valve: A Pluridisciplinary Approach* (ed. D. Kalmanson), pp. 163–172. Acton, Ma.: Publishing Sciences Group Inc.

6. YELLING, E.L., FRATER, R.W.M. and PESKIN, C.S. (1975). The application of the Gorlin equation to the stenotic mitral valve. In *Advances in Bioengineering* (eds. A.C. Bell and R.M. Nerem), pp. 45–47. ASME, N.Y.

7. YORAN, C., YELLIN, E.L., BECKER, R.M., GABBAY, S., FRATER, R.W.M. and SONNENBLICK, E.H. (1979). Mechanism for reduction of mitral regurgitation with vasodilator therapy. *Am. J. Cardiology*, **43**, 773–777

8. YORAN, C., YELLIN, E.L., BECKER, R.M., GABBAY, S., FRATER, R.W.M. and SONNENBLICK, E.H. (1979). Dynamic aspects of mitral regurgitation: Effects of ventricular volume, pressure and contractility on the effective regurgitant orifice area. *Circulation*, **60**, 170–176

9. YELLIN, E.L., YORAN, C., SONNENBLICK, E.H., GABBAY, S. and FRATER, R.W.M. (1979). Dynamic changes in the canine mitral regurgitant orifice area during ventricular ejection. *Circulation Research*, **45**, 677–683

10. LANIADO, S., YELLIN, E.L., MILLER, H. and FRATER, R.W.M (1973). Temporal relation of the first heart sound to closure of the mitral valve. *Circulation*, **47**, 1006–1014

11. LANIADO, S., YELLIN, E.L., KOTLER, M., LEVY, L., STADLER, J. and TERDIMAN, R. (1975). A study of the dynamic relations between the mitral valve echogram and phasic mitral flow. *Circulation*, **51**, 104–113

12. YELLIN, E.L., PESKIN, C., YORAN, C. *et al.* (1981). Mechanisms of mitral valve motion during diastole. *Am. J. Physiol.*, **241** (Heart Circ Physiol 10), H389–H400

13. HENDERSON, Y. (1906). The volume curve of the ventricles of the mammalian heart, and the significance of this curve in respect to the mechanics of the heart-beat and the filling of the ventricles. *Am. J. Physiol.*, **16**, 325–367

14. WIGGERS, C.J. and KATZ, L.N. (1921–22). The contour of the ventricular volume curves under different conditions. *Am. J. Physiol.*, **58**, 439–475

15. RUSHMER, R.F. (1976). *Cardiovascular Dynamics*, 4th ed. W.B. Saunders Co. Philadelphia, p. 423

16. YELLIN, E.L., SONNENBLICK, E.H. and FRATER, R.W.M. (1980) Dynamic determinants of left ventricular filling. In *Cardiac Dynamics* (eds. Baan, Artzenius and Yellin, Martin Nijhoff), pp. 145–158. B.V., The Hague.

17. YELLIN, E.L. and FRATER, R.W.M. (1981). Mitral regurgitation in ventricular premature contractors. *Chest*, **79**, 371

18. LITTLE, R.C. (1979). The mechanism of closure of the mitral valve: A continuing controversy. *Circulation*, **59**, 615–618

19. YELLIN, E.L., KENNISH, A., YORAN, C., LANIADO, S., BUCKLEY, N.M. and FRATER, R.W.M. (1979). The influence of left ventricular filling on post-extra-systolic potentiation in the dog heart. *Circulation Research*, **44**, 712–722

20. DAVID, D., MICHELSON, E.L., NAITO, M. *et al.* (1983). Diastolic 'locking' of the mitral valve: The importance of atrial systole and intraventricular volume. *Circulation*, **67**, 640–645

21. LANIADO, S., YELLIN, E.L., YORAN, C. *et al.* (1982). Physiologic mechanisms in aortic insufficiency. *Circulation*, **66**, 226–235

5

A new approach to mitral valve exploration using a two-dimensional echo–Doppler technique

Daniel Kalmanson and Colette Veyrat

Non-invasive diagnosis and evaluation of mitral valve disease has been substantially enhanced by the advent of one- and two-dimensional echocardiography. However, the role of the latter is mostly limited to mitral stenosis (MS). On the other hand, pulsed Doppler (PD) combined with two-dimensional echocardiography[1] has considerably improved the contribution of echocardiography, especially in the field of mitral regurgitation.

Materials and methods

The present study was performed on 135 subjects, 77 females and 58 males, ranging in age from 29 to 70 years.

The diagnosis was confirmed in all cases by invasive procedures (cardiac catheterization, angiography and whenever appropriate surgical findings).

Classification of the patients with mitral valve disease—The assessment of the severity of the lesions was made on a three-grade scale: (1) mild; (2) moderate; and (3) severe. It was based *for stenoses* on the catheterization results with determination of the mitral valve area using the Gorlin formula. The ranges were defined as : (1) above $1.8\,cm^2$; (2) between 1.3 and $1.8\,cm^2$; and (3) equal to and under $1.3\,cm^2$, with correction for any mitral regurgitation proven by angiography. The stenosis was exclusively assessed as moderate by surgery in one patient in whom left ventricular catheterization was unsuccessful.

For regurgitation the classification was based on the angiographic data, according to a scaled qualitative estimation of three grades. The 135 studied subjects included:

1. 25 patients with pure or predominant rheumatic mitral stenosis: three mild lesions, 11 moderate and 11 severe.
2. 44 patients had pure mitral regurgitation (MR) (with 46 lesions since two occurred on patients after operation on the mitral valve). Aetiology was rheumatic in 27 cases, prosthetic leaks in two cases, mitral valve prolapse in 10 cases, cardiomyopathy in three cases, congenital malformation in one case and undetermined in one case.
3. A control group of 66 subjects, including 50 patients without mitral valve disease and 18 normals.

Recording technique

Apparatus

We used an ATL 851 recorder, (ATL, Bellevue, Washington, USA), associating a pulsed Doppler (3 MHz) velocimeter and a two-dimensional 90 degree wide-angle mechanical sector using a single transducer for both techniques. The diameter of the transducer was 2.5 cm. According to the Doppler principle, the range gating system makes it possible to record the velocity of a small blood sample (2×4 mm) at any given location along the ultrasonic beam from 3 to 17 cm from the chest wall.

The output consisted of an audiosignal of the Doppler shift and of a graphic display of the frequency spectrum; in addition to the use of a time interval histogram with a demodulated analog flow velocity trace, using the zero crossing detector method, the apparatus was connected to a fast Fourier transform device (Angioscan/Uniscan, Unigon, Mount Vernon, New York, USA) in order to obtain a real-time spectral analysis. Analysis speed was 6.5 ms for one 128–point frequency spectrum. Other characteristics of this analyzer have been described previously[3]. We also used two video-monitors, one for the real-time scanning and the other for the Doppler display. Recordings were made on a Sony videotape recorder. Hard copies or real-time imaging were obtained on a 4633 Tektronix recorder. Doppler analog flow velocity traces, TM echocardiographic tracings, Doppler spectral displays as well as simultaneous electrocardiogram lead II and frequency selective phonocardiograms were recorded on an Irex I (Irex, Mahweh, New Jersey, USA) fibreoptics recording system.

Recording method

Subjects were generally studied in the supine left lateral position. The method used for two-dimensional echo-Doppler examination of the heart has been already reported. Briefly, it requires in succession: (1) dynamic visualization of the structure or chamber under investigation; (2) location of the Doppler beam, seen as a continuous white line, in order to transsect the area of interest; and (3) adjustment of the Doppler gate, seen as a bright spot, to control the depth of the sample volume along that beam. The image is then frozen while the apparatus is automatically switched to the Doppler system. When the characteristic Doppler sound is heard, the recording may be performed. We recorded several samples at the annulus, at least one at the centre and one at the commissures, using various approaches of the mitral valve (long and short axis and 4-chamber views)[4]. The Doppler study included, both for diagnosis and assessment of the lesions, the qualitative analysis of the recordings as previously described for invasive [5] and non-invasive[4, 6, 7] (references 4 and 7 for two-dimensional echo) procedures.

It comprised the detection of systolic or diastolic pattern anomalies of the flow velocity recordings if present. We studied for all lesions their spread over the annular area and the regurgitation within the atrium[7]. For the time interval histogram (TIH), the spectrum was considered as abnormally broadened when the dispersion of the dots was present according to the following criteria:

(1) Use of the minimal Doppler gain compatible with the recommended signal-to-noise ratio judged on the monitor from the bottom trace, called 'signal amplitude'.

(2) Amplitude of the dispersion at least twice as wide as that seen on the spectrum for laminar flow in segments of the same cardiac cycle.
(3) Duration of the disturbance equal to or longer than 0.1 s.
(4) Absence of interference with any cardiac structure motion.

The conclusion of both invasive and non-invasive data were made independently by separate teams.

Mitral regurgitation

A new method was devised, as follows, to determine quantitative parameters in order to enhance the accuracy of the assessment of regurgitation.

The procedure of examination used PD data derived from two complementary scan planes (*see Figure 5.1*).

1. Parasternal long axis visualization of the mitral valve and left atrium (LA), and PD mapping of the LA to detect or rule out the presence of an abnormal systolic Doppler signal related to the regurgitant jet; if present, measurement of its length and height in centimeters (cm) with calculation of the long axis regurgitant index (LARI) = 1/2 length × height.
2. Parasternal short axis visualization of the mitral annulus, and PD mapping of the annulus to detect or rule out the pressence of an abnormal systolic Doppler signal; if present, measurement of its width in cm corresponding to the short axis regurgitant index (SARI)
3. Calculation of the total regurgitant index (TRI) = LARI × SARI.
4. Correlative study of the evaluation of MR derived from these new PD indexes with left ventricular cineangiographic (LVCA) data.

Results

Mitral stenosis

Detailed results have been extensively published in a previous paper[8]. We shall here only briefly recall the following findings: sensitivity was 100%, specificity 96%, assessment of severity 88% and correct determination of the anatomic sites of the lesions 88%. Advantages of the Doppler technique will be discussed below (*Figures 5.2–5.4*).

Mitral regurgitation

Detailed results have been published elsewhere[9]. PD-positive diagnosis of MR was obtained in 90% of the cases, with an equal specificity. The regurgitant jet was measured in 87% of patients. The best result for the evaluation of the importance of MR was obtained from calculation of the TRI which was in agreement with LVCA classification in 88% of the cases with significantly ($p < 0.01$) increased values of each grade of severity (mild, 1.05 ± 0.55; moderate, 4.44 ± 2.08; severe, 10.92 ± 6.52). Isolated single-plane indexes (LARI and SARI) were less reliable than the TRI in differentiating moderate from severe MR. The identification of the involved regurgitant leaflet(s) predicted by PD from analysis of the LA direction of the jet and the annular site of the lesion (internal, central, and/or external) were further confirmed by LVCA and surgery when available (*see Figures 5.5 and 5.12*).

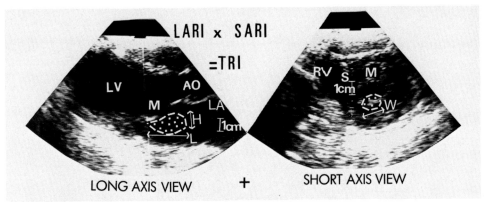

Figure 5.1 Measurement of regurgitant indices (during systole).
(*a*) Long axis view. LV = Left ventricle; AO = aorta; MV = mitral valve; LA = left atrium;
L = value of length; H = value of height; LARI = long axis regurgitant index; SARI = short axis reg-
urtitant index; TRI = total regurgitant index. (*b*) Short axis view along plane B. W = Value of width.
Note that plane B transsects the left cavities at the site of the mitral annulus.

Comments

One- and two-dimensional echocardiography have considerably enhanced our
diagnostic capacities for non-invasively exploring mitral valve disease. Their roles
have been particularly stressed for assessing mitral stenosis and mitral valve prolapse
and vegetations[10–15].

However, the role of one–, and even two-dimensional echocardiography has
turned out to be limited in the case of mitral regurgitation[14, 15]. In contrast, pulsed
Doppler is endowed with the unique ability to provide direct information on
transvalvular and intra-atrial blood flow disturbances, and therefore is particularly
suitable for diagnosing and assessing mitral regurgitation.

Mitral stenosis

Two-dimensional echocardiography remains the tool of choice for diagnosing and
evaluating mitral stenosis[11–13] and pulsed Doppler adds only limited help, although
it is sometimes very valuable.

Although two-dimensional echo is widely accepted for providing reliable results
in assessing the degree of severity of stenosis, it has been recognized that the
determination of the mitral valve area may run into some shortcomings[15] due in
particular to such factors as gain setting, and particularly subjective criteria for
delimiting the mitral orifice. It furthermore often overlooks concomitant mitral
regurgitation, for which a combined echo–Doppler technique may offer some
valuable advantages[4, 6, 7, 9, 16].

1. First, it can explore and detect the haemodynamic disturbances at all points of
    the mitral orifice, and thus detect turbulence at a commissure where the sole
    two-dimensional echo proved to be normal, or at best inconclusive (*see Figures 5.2
    and 5.3*).
2. It may help to delineate more correctly some parts of the orifice that are
    inapparent on the echo imaging, and thus enhance the accuracy of the
    calculation of the mitral valve area (*see Figure 5.4*).

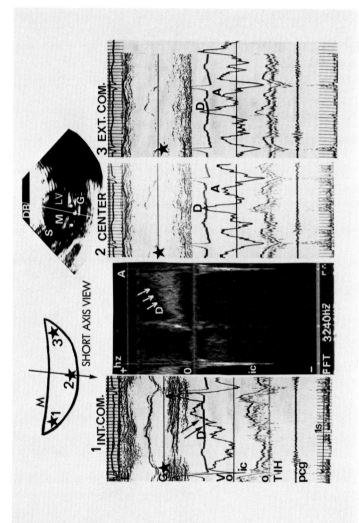

Figure 5.2 Detection of mild stenosis inapparent on two-dimensional imaging. M = Mitral valve; DB = Doppler beam; IC = isometric contraction; TIH = time interval histogram; PCG = phonocardiogram. Upper row. *Left:* schema of the mitral valve: stars 1, 2 and 3 are locations of Doppler gate. *Right:* two-dimensional imaging of the mitral valve. Lower row: 1, 2 and 3 correspond to the Doppler recordings at sites 1, 2 and 3. Left recording: real-time spectrum analysis. The mitral valve on the two-dimensional imaging appears normal. Only the Doppler can record turbulence at the internal commissure (1) whereas flow elsewhere is normal. These findings were confirmed on surgery.

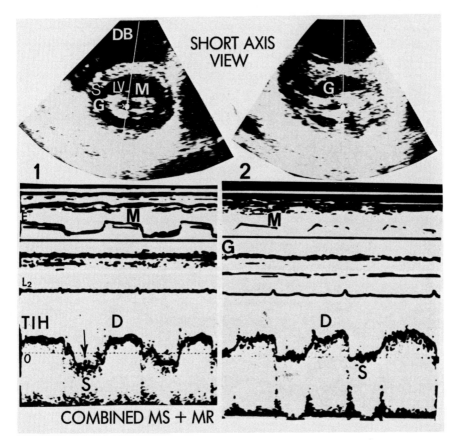

Figure 5.3 Detection of mild mitral regurgitation in mitral stenosis. S = Systolic wave; D = diastolic wave. The Doppler recording (lower left) corresponding to the positioning of the gate near the internal commissure (upper left) reveals a negative flow wave (S), whereas at the external commissure no negative wave can be detected (right).

3. In the same way, it offers a useful tool to study the postoperative benefits on transvalvular blood flow in a non-invasive way, which completes the information obtained by echo imaging alone.

Mitral regurgitation

Mitral regurgitation is precisely the lesion that highlights the supremacy of Doppler over echo.

1. First, it allows the direct detection of regurgitation either in the form of a negative blood flow velocity curve or that of a broadening of the spectral display.
2. Above all, it can provide information that can be particularly used by the

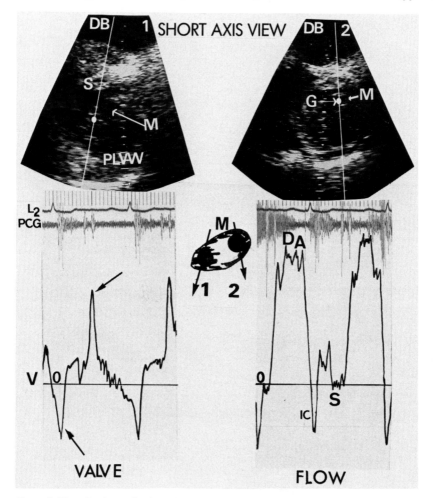

Figure 5.4 Doppler determination of the limits of mitral valve contour. *Left:* The Doppler gate 'hits' the structure of the mitral valve and can ascertain its limits. The corresponding recording (below) is specific of a Doppler 'structure sound'. *Right:* The gate is still within the contour since it records a typical flow of mitral stenosis (below). M = Mitral valve; PLVW = posterior wall on the left ventricle.

surgeon, by non-invasively refining the diagnosis of mitral lesions and regurgitation. It can, step by step, track the site of origin, the direction, the length and ending of the regurgitant jet throughout the left atrium, starting at the mitral annulus into the roof of the atrium or the branching of the pulmonary veins (*see Figures 5.5–5.8*).

3. The preceding information can provide the clue to the localization of the anatomical site of a lesion. For example, the singling out of one or more prolapsed scallops of the posterior mitral valve (*see Figure 5.10* and *5.11*). In case of mitral valve prolapse, the jet is directed anteriorly into and extends to the posterior wall of the aorta in case of posterior valve leaflet prolapse, and

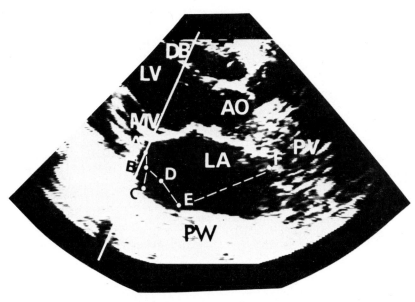

Figure 5.5 Two-dimensional scan/Doppler image of the mitral valve and of the left atrium. Long axis view. A–F are points of maximum turbulence. DB = Doppler beam; AO = aorta; MV = mitral valve; LA = left atrium; G = Doppler gate).

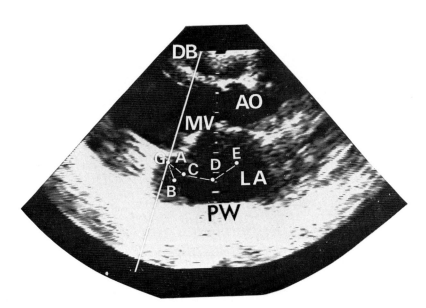

Figure 5.6 Two-dimensional scan/Doppler image of the mitral valve and of the left atrium. Long axis view. Same patient as in *Figure 5.5*. A–E = Points in the left atrium where a negative wave was recorded, but with minimal turbulence. DB = Doppler beam; AO = aorta; MV = mitral valve; LA = left atrium; G = Doppler gate.

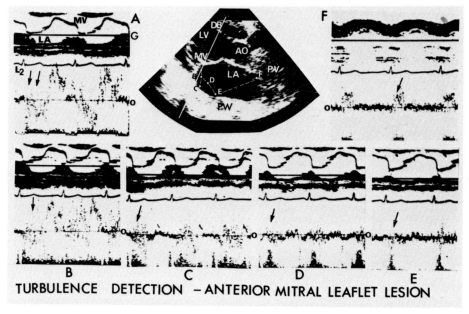

Figure 5.7 Detection of turbulence in mitral regurgitation due to anterior valve prolapse. Doppler scan of the mitral valve and left antrium. Display of turbulent flow (arrows) recorded at points A–F.

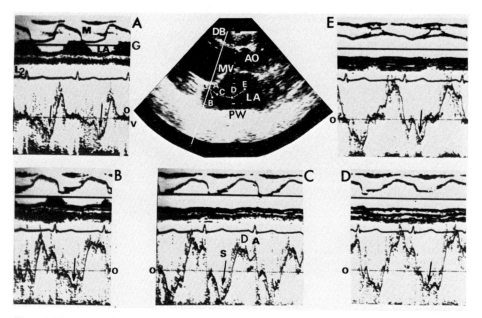

Figure 5.8 Detection of negative waves in mitral regurgitation due to anterior valve prolapse. Same patient as in *Figure 5.7*. Compare with the angiogram in *Figure 5.9*.

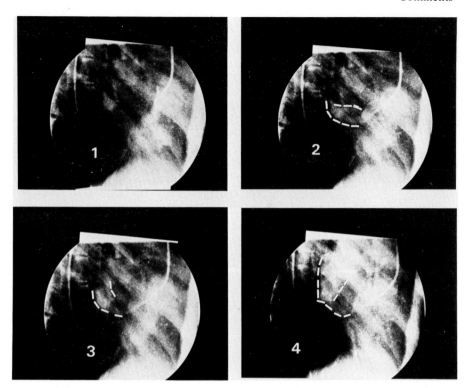

Figure 5.9 Angiogram of the left atrium in mitral regurgitation due to anterior mitral valve prolapse. (Same patient as in *Figures 5.5–5.8.* Note the right anterior oblique view, which gives a symmetrical image of the jet in contrast to the views in *Figures 5.7* and *5.8.*

posteriorly towards the floor of the left atrium in case of anterior valve prolapse (*see Figures 5.9* and *5.12*); it is mostly axial in rheumatic regurgitation. Aside from an anatomical prolapse, the jet may be found to be directed posteriorly in case of rheumatic retraction of the posterior leaflet, giving birth to a 'functional' prolapse[9].

4. One of the most advantageous and promising features of Doppler is to provide useful information on the severity of the regurgitation on a semi-quantitative basis using three grades of increasing severity[9]. The three-dimensional approach[9] is the first clue to a semi-quantitative assessment of MR using the above-mentioned indices (long axis, short axis and above all the most reliable total regurgitant index).

5. More recently, the detection of turbulence at specific points of the left cavities may provide the clue to the probability of ruptured or elongated chordae tendineae[9].

In conclusion, it may be stated that while Doppler studies provide complementary information in the case of mitral stenosis which may be of appreciable help to the physician and especially the surgeon, its main advantages consist in diagnosing and assessing reliably mitral regurgitation and also in offering a non-invasive procedure for studying the pathophysiology of both lesions.

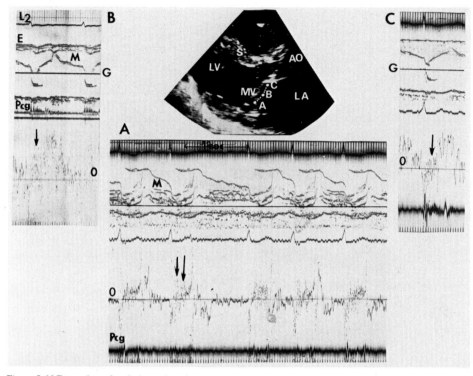

Figure 5.10 Detection of turbulence in mitral regurgitation due to posterior value prolapse. Note the ascending direction of the jet and compare with the jet of the aniogram in *Figure 5.12*.

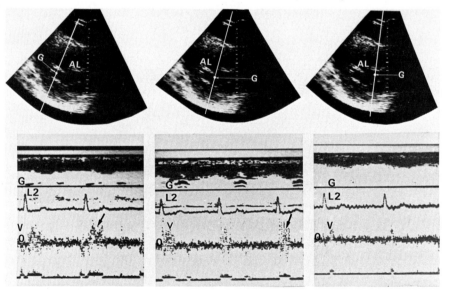

Figure 5.11 Doppler scan of the mitral valve. Short axis view. *Left:* Posterior commissure. *Middle:* Centre of the valve. *Right:* Anterior commissure. Turbulence is indicated by the spectral broadening. These recordings demonstrate that the prolapse involves the internal and central scallops. G = Doppler gate; AL = anterior leaflet of the mitral valve.

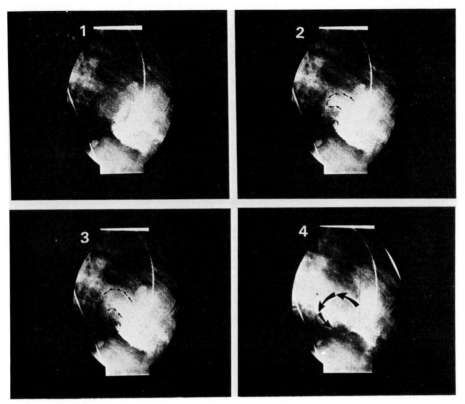

Figure 5.12 Left atrium angiogram. Mitral regurgitation due to posterior valve prolapse. Same patient as in *Figure 5.10*. Note the counter-clockwise direction of the jet, which is symmetrical like the jet in *Figure 5.10*, due to the right anterior oblique view.

References

1. BAKER, D.W., RUBENSTEIN, S. and LORCH, G. (1977). Pulsed doppler echocardiography. Principles and applications. *Am. J. Med.*, **63**, 69–80
2. GORLIN, R. and GORLIN, S.G. (1951). Hydraulic formula for calculation of the area of the stenotic mitral valve, other cardiac valves, and central circulatory shunts. *Am. Heart J.*, **41**, 1–29
3. MAC PHERSON P.C., MELDRUM S.J., TUNSTALLPEDOE D.S. (1981). Angioscan: a spectrum analyser for use with ultrasonic Doppler velocimeters. *J. Med. Engin. Tech.*, **5**, 84–85
4. KALMANSON, D., VEYRAT, C. and ABITBOL, G. (1979). Two-dimensional Echo Doppler velocimetry in mitral and tricuspid valve disease. In *Recent Advances in Ultrasound Diagnosis* (ed. A. Kurjak), pp. 335–48. Amsterdam: Excerpta Medica
5. KALMANSON, D., VEYRAT, C., BERNIER., A., SAVIER, CH., CHICHE, P. and WITCHITZ, S. (1975). Diagnosis and evaluation of mitral valve disease using transseptal Doppler ultrasound catheterization, *Br. Heart J.*, **37**, 257–271
6. KALMASON, D., VEYRAT, C., BOUCHAREINE, F. and DEGROOJE, A. (1977). Non-invasive recording of mitral valve flow velocity patterns using Doppler echocardiography. *Br. Heart J.*, **39**, 517–528
7. KALMANSON, D., VEYRAT, C., ABITBOL, G. and SAINTE-BEUVE D. (1981). Doppler echocardiography and valvular regurgitation with special emphasis on mitral insufficiency. Interest of real-time spectral analysis. In: *Echocardiography* (ed. Rijsterborgh), pp. 290–299. The Hague, The Netherlands: Martinus Nijhoff
8. VEYRAT, C., MANIN, J.P., VILLEMOT, J.P., CABROL, C. and KALMANSON, D. (1983). Anatomic and functional evaluation of pure and associated mitral stenosis using the scan- Doppler technique. *Ultrasound Medic and Biol.*, **9**, 7–17

9. VEYRAT, C., KALMANSON, D., BAS, S., ABITBOL, G. and MANIN, J.P. (1983). New indices for assessing the severity of mitral regurgitation. *Br. Heart J.*, **51**, 130–138

10. FEIGENBAUM, H. (1976). *Echocardiography*. Ed. 2 Philadelphia; Lea and Feibiger

11. HENRY, W.L., GRIFFITH, J.M., MICHAELIS, L.L., MCINTOSH, C.L., MORROW, A.G. and EPSTEIN, S.E. (1975). Measurement of mitral orifice are in patients with mitral valve disease by real-time, two-dimensional echocardiography. *Circulation*, **51**, 827–831

12. NICHOL, P.M., GILBERT, B.W. and KISSLO J.A. (1977). Two dimensional echocardiographic assessment of mitral stenosis. *Circulation*, **55**, 120–128

13. MARTIN, R.P., RAKOWSKI, H., KLEIMAN, J.H., BEAVER, W., LONDON, E. and POPP R.L. (1979). Reliability and reproducibility of two dimensional echocardiography measurement of the stenotic mitral valve orifice area. *Am. J. Cardiol.*, **43**, 560–568

14. POPP, R.L. (1979). Reliability of M-Mode and cross-sectional echocardiographic criteria for the diagnosis of mitral valve disorders. In *Echocardiology* (ed. Lancee C.T.), pp. 203–213. The Hague, Netherlands: Martinus Nijhoff

15. WANN L.S., FEIGENBAUM, H., WEYMAN, A.E. and DILLION, J.C. (1978). Cross-sectional echocardiographic detection of rheumatic mitral regurgitation. *Am. J. Cardiol.*, **41**, 1258–1263

16. MATSUO, H., KITABATAKE, A., HAYASHI, T., *et al.* (1977). Intracardiac flow dynamics with bidirectional ultrasonic pulsed Doppler technique. *Jap. Circ. J.*, **41**, 1258–1263.

17. VEYRAT, C., KALMANSON, D., FARJON, M., GUICHARD, J.P., SAINTE-BEUVE, D. and ABITOL, G. (1981). Combined pulsed Doppler echocardiography for the investigation of valvular heart diseases: 1-dimensional versus 2-dimensional approach. In: *Echocardiology* (ed. H Rijsterborgh), pp. 291–298. The Hague, Netherlands: Martinus Nijhoff

The integrated function of the mitral apparatus, left atrium, mitral annulus and papillary muscles

6

Functional anatomy of the mitral valve and annulus in man: lessons from echocardiographic observations

Pravin M. Shah and Chuwa Tei

Introduction

Although selective angiocardiography has been used to assess mitral valve function in man, it has not been possible to study anatomic components of functioning mitral valve complex prior to advent of echocardiography. This chapter will, therefore, review the detailed anatomic structure and function of the mitral valve in health and in diseased states as viewed by ultrasound imaging. An integrated approach using both m-mode and two-dimensional techniques will be utilized in this presentation. The complex anatomy of the mitral valve has been extensively illustrated in reports by Roberts. No attempt will be made to re-state anatomic substrates of the mitral valve complex, but rather to present their roles in mitral valve function.

Functional anatomy of the mitral complex will be described under the following major headings:

1. Normal functioning, structurally normal.
2. Abnormally functioning but structurally normal.
3. Abnormally functioning and structurally abnormal.
4. Structurally abnormal but normally functioning.

Functional anatomy of normal functioning, structurally normal valves

The cyclical motion of the mitral valve leaflets

M-mode echocardiography, with its high resolution and rapid pulse repetition rate, permits accurate analysis of rapidly moving structures such as the mitral valve leaflets. As shown in *Figure 6.1*, the two leaflets move synchronously but in opposite directions during phases of the cardiac cycle; however, excursions of the anterior leaflet far exceed those of the posterior. Left atrial contraction following the P wave of the EKG results in further opening of the mitral orifice by separating the two leaflets. Subsequent to atrial relaxation the leaflets execute a closing motion. Approximately 30–40 ms after onset of the QRS and with anticipated initiation of mechanical systole of the left ventricle, the mitral leaflets appose to a closed position. The two leaflets remain apposed throughout ventricular systole and open in early diastole some 80–100 ms after the aortic component of the second

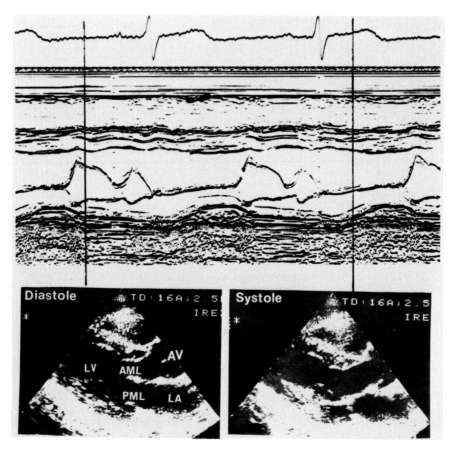

Figure 6.1 Normal mitral valve opening and closing motion as seen by M-Mode echo (upper panel) and two-dimensional echo obtained from the parasternal long axis views in diastole and in systole (lower panels). The cyclical motion of the two leaflets are observed as described in the text.

heart sound, an event that marks the termination of left ventricular systole. The leaflets attain a maximum opened position, which is maintained momentarily. During the rapid filling phase the two leaflets move rapidly toward a partially closed position. During diastasis, the leaflets remain in a partially open position and are opened further with the next atrial contraction. Major determinants of mitral leaflet motion are instantaneous pressure differences between left atrium and left ventricle; and transmitral flow into the left ventricle. Inertia of the normal leaflets results in coaptation occurring about 10 ms after left-ventricular–left-atrial pressure cross-over. The rapid mitral component of the first heart sound coincides with the early point of closure or coaptation, and opening snap times coincide precisely with the apex of the early diastolic opened position. There are, as a rule, no distinctive correlates of third or fourth heart sound on the mitral valve motion pattern.

Two-dimensional echocardiography additionally demonstrates, in parasternal or apical cross-sections, the disparity in lengths of the two leaflets. The anterior leaflet is a long, curtain-like structure which in its fully open position comes in close proximity to the interventricular septum and in its fully closed position covers a larger fraction of the mitral orifice in cross-section. The posterior leaflet is strikingly shorter, moves less and covers a smaller fraction of the orifice in cross-section. The two leaflets coapt at or near their free margins and maintain a closed position through systole slightly tented toward the left ventricle, inferoapical to the mitral annular plane.

The cyclical motion of the mitral annulus

Two-dimensional echocardiography has been used to reconstruct the mitral annulus as delineated by basal attachment of the mitral leaflets at the atrioventricular junction. This has provided a unique opportunity to measure cyclical changes in mitral annular size in man (*see Figure 6.2*). Briefly, the mitral annulus reaches a maximum size in late diastole around peak or end of the P wave on the EKG. A presystolic narrowing is then observed, and this continues into early to mid systole, which denotes the timing of smallest annular size. The annular size begins to increase in the latter half of ventricular systole and continues through the isovolumic relaxation phase. There is then a slower but progressive enlargement of the annulus to its maximum size following the P wave in late diastole. The mechanisms of these cyclical changes in the mitral annular size may be best explained by recalling a dual interplay of instantaneous changes in the left atrial and the left ventricular sizes.

The mitral annular area corrected for body surface area in normal subjects was to be $3.8 \pm 0.7\,cm^2/M^2$ in late diastole. The mean reduction in area through early to mid systole was $26 \pm 3\%$.

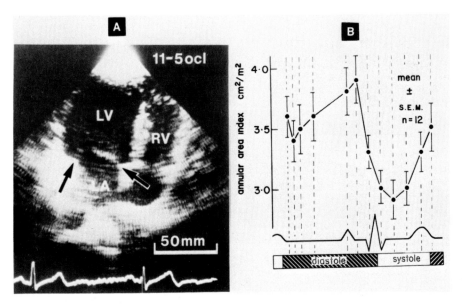

Figure 6.2 Apical two-dimensional echocardiography shows the mitral leaflets at their annular attachments as shown by arrows in left panel. The reconstructed mitral annular area at selected intervals during a cardiac cycle are plotted for a group of normal subjects. The areas are normalized for body surface area.

The 'submitral' apparatus

Although chordal structures may be visualized by two-dimensional echocardiography, identification of normal individual chordae tendineae is generally not obtained.

The two papillary muscles are commonly visualized in short axis cross-sections of the left ventricle. Their number, size and location may be assessed in this view. A modified long axis view to evaluate the papillary muscles along their long axes have been developed in our laboratory (*Figure 6.3*). These views are cross-sections in the

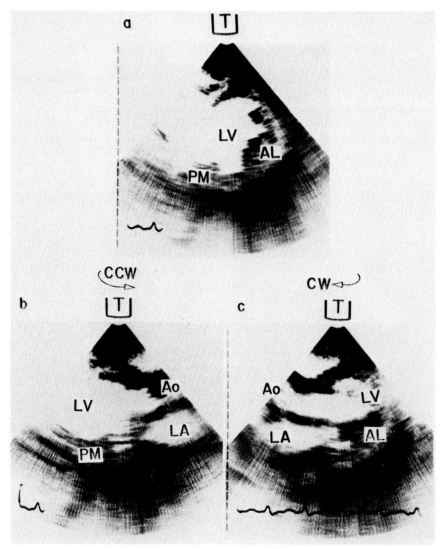

Figure 6.3 Echo cross-sections of anterolateral (AL), and posteromedial (PM) papillary muscles as viewed in short axis (*a*) and partial long axis (*b* and *c*) views. (*b*) and (*c*) are obtained by counter-clockwise (CCW) or clockwise (CW) rotations of the transducer (T) as shown. LV = Left ventricle; LA = left atrium; AO = aorta.

plane of the long axis of each papillary muscle and permit examination of changes in its length and spatial orientation.

Left ventricular and left atrial sizes and motions

M-mode as well as two-dimensional echocardiography are useful in quantitative assessment of the left heart chamber sizes. Chamber enlargement results from intrinsic mitral valve regurgitation, which in turn influences mitral valve function; hence the clinical dictum 'mitral regurgitation begets more mitral regurgitation'.

Functional anatomy of abnormally functioning but structurally normal mitral valve

Atrioventricular dissociation

Earlier experimental as well as more recent clinical observations utilizing echocardiography have demonstrated the important role played by atrial contraction followed by its subsequent relaxation on closure of the mitral valve. A clinical study in patients with complete A-V dissociation showed an exponential relationship between P-R interval and mitral valve closure to the next R wave interval for range of P-R from 0.2 to 0.6 s. This suggests that a P-R interval in excess of 0.2 s results in diastolic closure of the mitral valve, indicating no contribution of ventricular systole to this closure (*see Figure 6.4*). Effectiveness of this atriogenic valve closure has not been tested, although it may permit some brief reflux or regurgitation, presumably since the mitral annulus has not undergone its early systolic reduction. The diastolic closure of the mitral valve has been related to a reversal of the small normal atrioventricular pressure due to atrial contraction and a fall in atrial pressure due to its relaxation and partially emptied state.

The echocardiographic observations in man also showed that for P-R intervals of less than 0.1 s, timing of mitral valve closure was independent and consistently a systolic event (*see Figure 6.5*). This suggested that the valve closure for P-R intervals less than 0.1 s is a function of ventricular systole and the presence of the P wave is probably immaterial. For the P-R intervals between 0.1 and 0.2 s (as is normally seen), both atrial and ventricular mechanisms contribute to the valve closure. This is perhaps more effective, since the leaflet closure occurs in a setting of decreasing mitral annular size.

In patients with heart failure, a changing P-R interval does not influence timing of mitral valve closure despite A-V dissociation, either due to high left atrial pressure or weaker atrial contraction. This observation may be used potentially to define patients with elevated left atrial pressures.

Aortic regurgitation

Acute severe and occasionally chronic severe aortic regurgitation may be associated with a marked rise in left ventricular diastolic pressure, which when it exceeds left atrial pressure results in closure of the mitral valve. Thus, premature closure of the mitral valve may occur in mid or late diastole (*See Figure 6.6*). Such an occurrence indicates severe valvular regurgitation and a probable need for early surgical intervention. The timing of the P wave (atrial systole) must also be taken

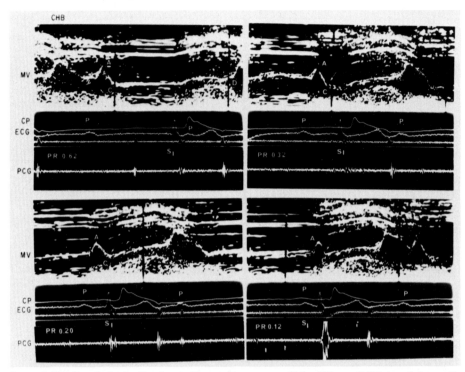

Figure 6.4 Timing of mitral valve closure (denoted by arrow at C) for different P-R intervals in a patient with complete A-V block. CP = Carotid pulse; ECG = electrocardiogram; PCG = phonocardiogram; S$_1$ = first heart sound. (Reproduced from Shah, P.M., *et al.* (1970), *Am. J. Cardiol.* by kind permission of authors and publishers.)

into consideration. Patients with aortic regurgitation may commonly have first-degree heart block, which may provide for atriogenic preclosure of the mitral valve. Thus, premature mitral closure can only be interpreted to indicate abnormally high left ventricular diastolic pressure when it occurs prior to the peak of the P wave on the EKG.

Additonal effects of chronic severe aortic regurgitation on the mitral valve complex would include: (1) mitral annular dilatation; (2) apical and lateral displacement of the papillary muscles; and (3) incomplete opening or early diastolic closure of the anterior mitral leaflet. The first two effects may result in 'functional' mitral regurgitation and the third may yield a 'functional' gradient across the mitral valve and the Austin–Flint diastolic murmur.

Aortic regurgitation results in a characteristic diastolic fluttering of the anterior mitral leaflet, which was thought to result from the impact of the regurgitant jet. A recent experimental observation suggests vortex formation as the basis of leaflet flutter in aortic regurgitation. This fluttering is not related to the genesis of the Austin–Flint murmur.

Dilated cardiomyopathy

Dilated cardiomyopathy produces a typical alteration in pattern of mitral valve motion that is best appreciated in the M-mode echocardiogram. Amplitude of

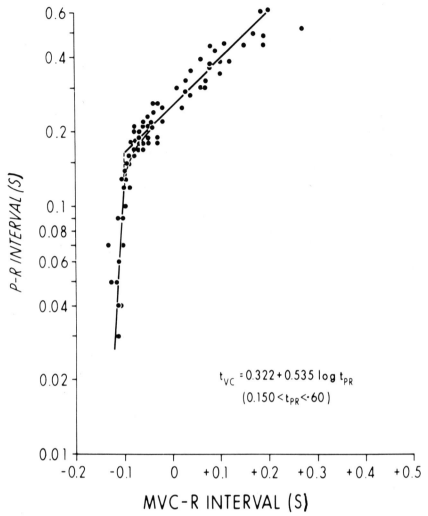

Figure 6.5 Correlation of P-R interval to mitral valve closure to onset of QRS (MVC-R) interval is demonstrated. *See* text for explanation. (Reproduced from Shah, P.M., *et al.* (1970), *Am. J. Cardiol.*, by kind permission of authors and publishers.)

leaflets opening is restricted, the degree of reduction being a function of stroke volume. The mitral valve area of maximum valve opening measured by two-dimensional echocardiography is smaller than normal but not as restricted as in mitral stenosis. In addition, early closing movement of the mitral valve at end-diastole is often interrupted by a prominent notch (termed the 'B' notch), the presence of which has been correlated with elevated left ventricular end-diastolic pressures. Neither M-mode nor two-dimensional echocardiography provides a ready explanation for development of mitral regurgitation in dilated cardiomyopathy.

Hence, a detailed quantitative analysis of mitral valve apparatus was undertaken

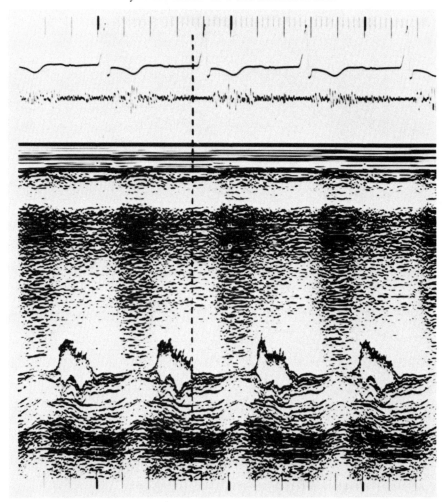

Figure 6.6 Diastolic fluttering and premature closure of the mitral valve are noted in a patient with chronic severe aortic regurgitation. The mitral valve closure (denoted by a dashed line), although occurring before QRS, actually follows the P wave. This is not necessarily indicative of high left ventricular diastolic pressure (*see* text).

in our laboratory in patients with dilated cardiomyopathy with and without mitral regurgitation (MR) using two-dimensional echocardiography. The two groups (i.e. the MR group and the no MR group) were matched for age, functional class and left ventricular function as assessed by ejection fraction. Briefly, the results demonstrated that mitral annular size at end-diastole was enlarged in dilated cardiomyopathies: 8.1 ± 1.0 for the MR group and 4.9 ± 1.0 for the non-MR group. The differences between the two group were highly significant ($p < 0.001$).

Left ventricular end-diastolic dimension was increased in all patients but the differences between the MR and the no MR group were less significant (7.4 ± 0.4 cm *vs.* 7.1 ± 0.5 cm; $p < 0.0.1$) and less pronounced. Other parameters studied, but not found significantly different between the two groups, were papillary muscle displacement and eccentricity and the 'central chordal' length. However, distance from mitral leaflet coaption point to mitral annular plane was significantly greater in the MR group (p < 0.001).

It was therefore concluded that the single best correlate of MR in dilated cardiomyopathy is the annular size. It would seem that larger combined surface area of the mitral leaflets would be needed for effective closure of the valve in the presence of a dilated orifice. This is further compounded by additional displacement of the coaptation point inferoapically into the left ventricle. These recent studies provide a clearer understanding of the mechanism of MR in dilated cardiomyopathy.

Hypertrophic cardiomyopathy

Hypertrophic cardiomyopathy, although primarily a myocardial disorder with massive and often asymmetric hypertrophy associated with a small hyperdynamic left ventricle, is often associated with anatomic as well as functional changes in the mitral valve. A subset of patients had narrowing of the left ventricular outflow space and functional or dynamic outflow 'obstruction' with accompanying involvement of the mitral valve. The anatomic changes include thickening of anterior leaflet, especially along its ventricular surface and elongation of the leaflets. The functional changes, studied best by two-dimensional echocardiography, contribute directly to the left ventricular outflow obstruction and associated mitral regurgitation. A previously reported observation from this laboratory showed abnormal coaption of the two mitral leaflets at onset of systole. As shown on the left panel in *Figure 6.11*, the normal coaptation of the leaflets as viewed by apical views on two-dimensional echocardiograms largely involves the tips or free margins of the leaflets. The abnormality noted in hypertrophic cardiomyopathy consists of a mid portion of the anterior leaflet coapting with the tip or mid portion of the posterior leaflet (*see Figure 6.7*). This leaves a distal portion of one or both leaflets within the left ventricular cavity in early systole. Subsequently in midsystole, 'residual' portion of the leaflet(s) angulate sharply toward the interventricular septum. This represents systolic anterior motion (SAM) of the mitral valve seen on M-mode echocardiography and denotes site and localization of left ventricular outflow obstruction. The SAM returns toward the closed leaflets in late systole prior to diastolic opening of the mitral valve. Amplitude of diastolic opening of the anterior leaflet is reduced as a result of narrow outflow space and the leaflet abuts the bulging interventricular septum. In addition, evaluation of mitral annular size in our laboratory shows that its maximal diastole size is similar to that of normal subjects; however, its early systolic reduction is increased.

The precise mechanism of abnormal valve coaptation remains to be elucidated. Two of the observed changes that may contribute are: (1) elongation of one or both leaflets; and (2) greater than normal reduction in the annular size in early systole (*see Figure 6.8*). This abnormal coaptation appears to be a necessary precondition for the development of leaflet SAM. Thus, the abnormal coaptation results in protrusion into the left ventricle, of a distal 'residual' portion of the mitral leaflet(s). Subsequently the hydrodynamic forces created by an early rapid ejection through narrowed outflow space results in sharp angulation of the distal leaflet along with the chordal attachments into the outflow space. This leaflet SAM is thought to be the most frequent cause of outflow obstruction. Although chordal

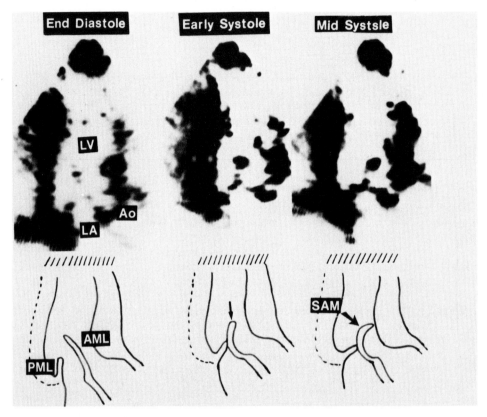

Figure 6.7 Three stop frames of apical cross-section by two-dimensional echo at end diastole, early systole and mid systole in a patient with hypertrophic obstructive cardiomyopathy illustrate the mechanism of systolic anterior motion (SAM).

buckling within the hyperdynamic left ventricle may result in 'chordal SAM', this does not result in outflow gradients.

Myocardial ischemia/infarction

Mitral regurgitation is known to accompany acute myocardial ischemia, acute infarction and old or healed infarction with possible chronic ischemia. The mechanisms of mitral regurgitation in coronary artery disease have been controversial. Mechanisms of MR are probably determined by the setting of myocardial ischemia. Functional anatomy of the mitral valve in coronary artery disease will be considered on the basis of clinical syndromes.

ACUTE MYOCARDIAL ISCHEMIA

Acute myocardial ischemia results in impairment of regional contractile function. Thus, ischemia of a papillary muscle would be expected to result in systolic malfunction of the mitral valve. However, failure of development of MR following

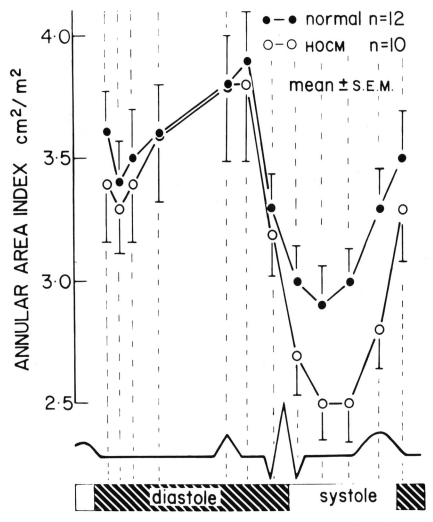

Figure 6.8 Mitral annular area index in normal and in hypertrophic obstructive cardiomyopathy (HOCM). Systolic reduction of the annular area in HOCM is significantly larger than normals.

infarction or necrosis of papillary muscle in the experimental animal has led to a suggestion that papillary muscle as well as adjacent ventricular wall dyskinesis is necessry for the occurrence of MR. A recent study in our laboratory utilizing brief coronary artery occlusions in closed-chest dogs resulted in MR in about 75% of the experiments and was associated with mitral valve prolapse in every instance (*see Figure 6.9*). This suggests to us that transient ischemia, as would be observed during an episode of angina, may result in mitral valve prolapse. Its mechanism may be a failure of papillary muscle contraction and possibly its elongation resulting in leaflet prolapse. The latter will involve a portion of one or both leaflets based on chordal anatomy. This mechanism of acute transient MR accompanying angina may be more common than is recognized.

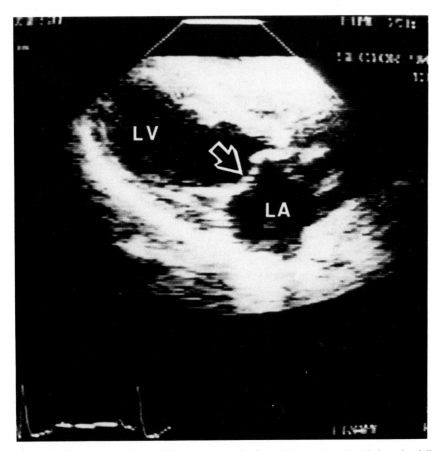

Figure 6.9 Mitral valve prolapse of the anterior leaflet (arrow) is seen in a closed-chest dog following occlusion of left anterior descending coronary artery.

ACUTE MYOCARDIAL INFARCTION

Three distinct pathogenetic mechanisms for MR accompanying acute myocardial infarction may be involved: (1) ischemic, resulting in mitral valve prolapse; (2) disruption or rupture of a papillary muscle at its tip, resulting in a flail mitral valve; (3) rupture of base of papillary muscle resulting in massive MR from flail mitral valve.

CHRONIC OR HEALED MYOCARDIAL INFARCTION

Healing of myocardial infarction results in an atrophic, fibrotic papillary muscle. When this is associated with akinesia or dyskinesia of adjacent ventricular wall, there may result an incomplete coaption of mitral valve leaflets from the latter being pulled into the left ventricular cavity during systole. This effect will be compounded when chronic ventricular dilatation supervenes and results in mitral annular dilatation. Mitral regurgitation in these patients with chronic ischemic disease may thus be associated with tethering of a leaflet into the ventricular cavity and annular dilatation.

Abnormally functioning, structurally abnormal mitral valve

Chronic rheumatic disease with pure or predominant mitral stenosis

Chronic rheumatic pathology with thickening and fusion of the two leaflets determines the characteristic pattern of valve opening and closure, whilst timings of cross-overs between left ventricular and left atrial pressures determine timings of these valvular events. A typical two-dimensional echocardiographic appearance in parasternal long axis view consists of reduced separation of the two leaflets along their free margins with a sudden ballooning of body of the anterior mitral leaflet toward the interventricular septum (*see Figure 6.10*). This results in a so-called 'hockey-stick' appearance of the anterior mitral leaflet in diastole. The leaflets lose their normal diastolic closing motion and are held in a relatively fixed, open position throughout diastole. The valve closure is as sudden as opening and the body of the anterior leaflet bulges somewhat toward the left atrium. This latter appearance is reminiscent of mitral leaflet prolapse. A parasternal short axis view shows the size of the anatomic mitral valve orifice at its tip. Thickening of the chordae tendineae, the papillary muscles or both may be best visualized in the apical views.

The anterior leaflet mobility is markedly restricted in the presence of heavy calcification. Mitral opening snap and closure sound (S1) is probably closely related to rapidity with which the anterior leaflet balloons out as it opens or returns to a closed position.

Chronic rheumatic disease with predominant mitral regurgitation

Rheumatic pathology involves thickening, calcification and fusion of the leaflets to a varying degree with frequent shortening of the chordal structures. It is difficult to assess degree of mitral regurgitation from the motion pattern or the echocardiographic appearance of the valve.

Mitral valve prolapse syndromes

DEFINITIONS

The term mitral valve prolapse should be reserved for functional abnormality characterized by projection or protrusion of a variable portion of the mitral valve into the left atrium, i.e. cephalad to the plane of the mitral annulus. Thus, mitral valve prolapse is a functional defect, not a clinical entity. A spectrum of clinical disorders associated with mitral valve prolapse may be described under a generic term of mitral valve prolapse syndromes. Three types of functional abnormalities that are readily distinguished by two-dimensional echocardiography include (1) mid-late systolic prolapse; (2) holosystolic prolapse; and (3) flail mitral valve syndrome. Besides the echocardiographic distinctions, these three types generally have some recognizable auscultatory features. The mid-late systolic prolapse is associated with one or more clicks, late systolic murmur and a normal first heart sound (S1). The holosystolic prolapse is distinguished by a loud S1 and generally a

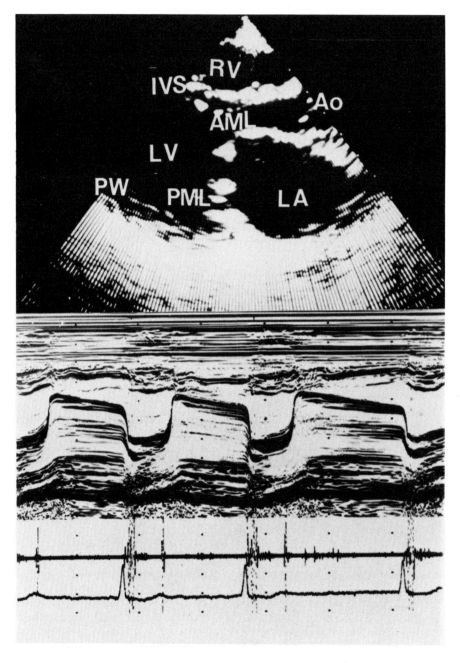

Figure 6.10 Two-dimensional (upper panel) and M-mode echo in mitral stenosis. Note the typical hockey-stick appearance due to anterior mitral leaflet (AML) body ballooning into the left ventricle (LV) in diastole.

holosystolic murmur, with or without additional systolic clicks. The flail mitral valve is characterized by a soft or absent S1 and holosystolic murmurs.

ETIOLOGICAL FACTORS

Etiologies of the first two types include: (1) idiopathic myxomatous degeneration; (2) Marfan's syndrome; (3) acute myocardial (papillary muscle) ischemia; (4) distorted left ventricular geometry as in ostium secundum atrial septal defect. The causes of flail mitral valve syndrome include: (1) idiopathic degeneration with elongation and/or rupture of chordae tendineae; (2) Marfan's syndrome with chordae elongation and/or rupture; (3) vegetative endocarditis; (4) trauma; (5) papillary muscle rupture.

FUNCTIONAL ANATOMY OF THE MITRAL VALVE

Functional anatomy of the first two types, i.e. late systolic and holosystolic mitral valve prolapse, is similar except for the timing of prolapse. Preliminary data indicate that approximately half of the patients with idiopathic degenerative etiology and nearly all with Marfan's syndrome have a dilated mitral valve annulus unrelated to size of the left atrium or the left ventricle. Thus, these show a structural defect in the form of primary ectasia of the mitral annulus. The valve leaflets are often thickened and redundant. The extent of this change varies from being focal to one scallop or segment of a valve leaflet to a generalized thickening of both the leaflets. The coaptation of the mitral valve leaflets at their tips, as visualized best from the multiple cross-sectional apical views by two-dimensional echocardiography, is normal. A variable portion of either or both leaflet(s) projects cephalad to a plane of the mitral annulus during ventricular systole (*see Figure 6.11*). This prolapse is seen coincident with initial valve closure and S wave of the EKG in the holosystolic variety, whilst it is observed in mid or late systole in the

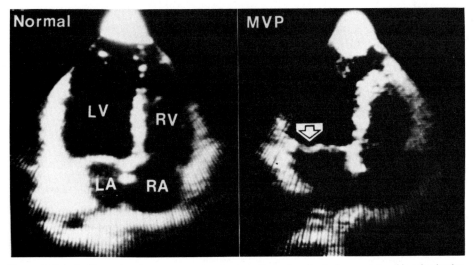

Figure 6.11 Apical four-chamber cross-sections by two-dimensional echo in normal and in mitral valve prolapse (MVP). The posterior leaflet is noted to billow into the left ventricle (arrow) in systole.

late systolic mitral valve prolapse. The timing of prolapse is often related to size and geometry of the left ventricle. Posterior leaflet prolapse comprises 60–70% of all cases of mitral prolapse. Thus, isolated anterior leaflet prolapse is by no means uncommon.

A flail mitral valve is generally associated with a detailed mitral annulus. This is out of proportion with the degrees of left ventricular and left atrial dilatation. It is not uncommon for the mitral annulus to be over three times the normal size. The valve leaflets and chordae tendineae are often thickened, redundant and elongated. A characteristic functional abnormality consists of failure of normal leaflet coaptation at their tips (*see Figure 6.12*). A portion or a whole valve leaflet as seen from one or more apical cross-sections by two-dimensional echocardiography is observed to prolapse into the left atrium in late diastole and early ventricular systole. The presystolic prolapse of a flail leaflet represents an unrestrained closing

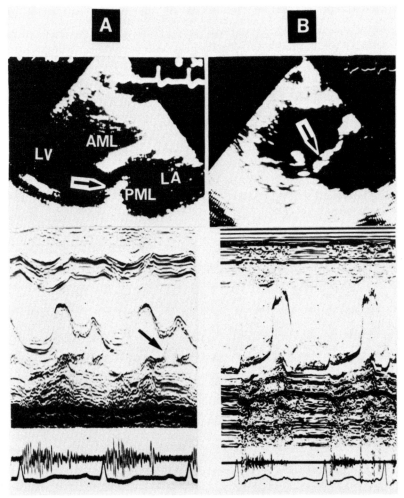

Figure 6.12 Flail valve involving the posterior leaflet (PML) in panel A and the anterior mitral leaflet (AML) in panel B are shown. The M-mode echo (lower panels) show chaotic motion.

motion which follows atrial contraction and relaxation. In our experience presystolic occurrence of prolapse is a common finding in the flail leaflet syndrome. The flail leaflet continues its progress farther into the left atrium during ventricular systole. In diastole the flail leaflet makes a whip-like motion as it opens into the left ventricular cavity. During ventricular filling it may exhibit coarse and chaotic flutter. A flail leaflet, especially following endocarditis, shows a diagnostic systolic fluttering (*see Figure 6.13*).

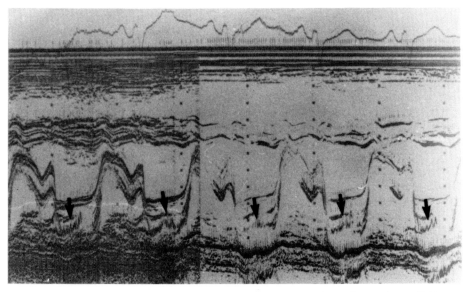

Figure 6.13 M-mode echo in a patient with flail mitral valve syndrome shows diagnostic systolic fluttering, leaflet thickening and abnormal diastolic movement.

Our finding of mitral annular dilatation in some patients with mitral valve prolapse without an associated enlargement of the left heart chambers confirms earlier pathological observations of annular dilatation in mitral valve prolapse. These patients with idiopathic mitral valve prolapse may exhibit genetic or acquired predisposition to myxomatous degeneration of the mitral valve, to leaflet redundancy, to dilatation of the annulus and elongation of chordae tendineae. This subset may be under risk of progression with increased mitral regurgitation, chordal rupture and flail mitral leaflet syndrome. It may be speculated that this subset is also likely to be a risk of endocarditis. Additional longitudinal follow-up studies will be needed to confirm these speculations as to the risk of progression and of infection.

Infective endocarditis

The destructive lesions of endocarditis may involve predominantly the leaflets of the chordae. Disruption of leaflet tissue results in mitral regurgitation without obvious motion abnormalities. On the other hand disruption of chordae tendineae results in flail mitral valve syndrome with accompanying mitral regurgitation.

Degenerative calcification of ageing

Annular and subannular calcification is common in the elderly. When extensive, it may interfere with normal annular 'contraction'. Thus, a larger effective systolic orifice may result in failure of complete coaptation and subsequent mitral regurgitation. Calcification may extend into the leaflets, rendering them rigid and less mobile. Although extensive valvular calcification of underlying rheumatic damage may be difficult to discern from advanced degenerative calcification, functional anatomy of the valve is generally characteristic. Calcification of degenerative etiology involves most often basal or annular attachment of the leaflets and extends to a variable degree into the leaflets. As a rule the free margins and the chordae tendineae are spared. Hence the leaflet movement is preserved at the tips even when the body of the leaflet may be restricted. In contrast, the rheumatic process most often results in commissural fusion involving tips of the leaflets and often affects chordae tendineae. Hence, a heavily calcified rheumatic valve is immobile both at the tip as well as the body of the leaflet. This differentiation in motion pattern may be readily made by two-dimensional echocardiography.

Congenital anomalies

Mitral atresia or mitral stenosis are rare congential anomalies. Leaflet fenestration accompanying atrioventricular cushion defects (e.g. ostium primum ASD) may be readily recognized in short axis views of the left ventricle by two-dimensional echocardiography.

Normally functioning, structurally abnormal valve

Libman–Sacks endocarditis

Vegetations in patients with systemic lupus erythematosis are small, granular and located near the basal margins of the leaflets. These do not produce significant functional derangement, although mild mitral regurgitation may be observed.

Marantic endocarditis

These have no known influence on functional anatomy of the mitral valve.

Acknowledgements

Dr Chuwa Tei is a Senior Investigator of the American Heart Association-Greater Los Angeles Affiliate supported in part by Group Investigatorship Award, The Arthur Dodd Fuller Foundation for Cardio-Vascular Research and Veterans Adminstration Medical Research Funds.

Bibliography

1. GRAMIAK, R. and SHAH, P.M. (1971). Cardiac ultrasonography. *Radiol. Clin. N. Am.*, **IX,** 469
2. SHAH, P.M., KRAMER, D.H. and GRAMIAK, R. (1970). Influence of the timing of atrial systole on mitral valve closure and on first heart sound in man. *Am. J. Cardiol.*, **26,** 231

3. SHAH, P.M. and GRAMIAK, R. (1975). Clinical usefulness of echocardiography. In *Non-Invasive Methods in Cardiology* (ed S. Zoneraich), Springfield, Il.: Charles Thomas

4. SHAH, P.M., GRAMIAK, P. and KRAMER, D.H. (1969). Ultrasound localization of left ventricular outflow obstruction in hypertrophic obstructive cardiomyopathy. *Circulation*, **40**, 3

5. SHAH, P.M. (1977). Echocardiography in the diagnosis of hypertrophic obstructive cardiomyopathy. *Am. J. Med.*, **62**, 830

6. SZE, K.C. and SHAH, P.M. (1976). Pseudoejection sound in hypertrophic subaortic stenosis: An echocardiographic correlative study. *Circulation*, **54**, 504–509

7. SHAH, P.M., TAYLOR, R.D. and WONG, M. (1981). Abnormal mitral valve coaptation in hypertrophic obstructive cardiomyopathy: Proposed role in systolic anterior motion of mitral valve. *Am. J. Cardiol.*, **48**, 258

8. CHILD, J.S., SKORTON, D.J., TAYLOR, R.D., KRIVOKAPICH, J., ABBASI, A.S., WONG, M. and SHAH, P.M. (1979). Cross-sectional and M-mode echocardiographic features of flail posterior mitral leaflets. *Am. J. Cardiol.*, **44**, 1383

9. ORMISTON, J.A., SHAH, P.M., TEI, C. and WONG, M. (1981). Size and motion of the mitral valve annulus in man. I: A two-dimensional echocardiographic method and findings in normal subjects. *Circulation*, **64**, 113

10. ORMISTON, J.A., SHAH, P.M., TEI, C. and WONG, M. (1982). Size and motion of the mitral valve annulus in man. II: Abnormalities in mitral valve prolapse. *Circulation*, **65**, 713

11. BURCH, G.E., DEPASQUALE, N.P. and PHILLIPS, J.H. (1963). Clinical manifestations of papillary muscle dysfunction. *Arch. Int. Med.*, **112**, 158

12. BURCH, G.E., DEPASQUALE, N.P. and PHILLIPS, J.H. (1968). The syndrome of papillary muscle dysfunction. *Am. Heart J.*, **75**, 399

13. BASHOUR, F.A. (1965). Mitral regurgitation following myocardial infarction: The syndrome of papillary mitral regurgitation. *Dis. Chest*, **48**, 113

14. MILLER, G.E., COHN, K.E., KERTH, W.J., SELZER, A. and GERBODE, F. (1968). Experimental papillary muscle infarction. *J. Thor. Card. Surg.*, **56**, 611

15. MITTAL, A.K., LANGSTON, M. JR., COHN, K.E., SELZER, A. and KERTH, W.J. (1971). Combined papillary muscle and left ventricular wall dysfunction as a cause of mitral regurgitation. *Circulation*, **44**, 174

16. SASAYAMA, S., TAKAHASI, M., OSAKADA, G., HIROSE, K., HAMASHIMA, H., NISHIMUSA, E. and KAWAI, C. (1979). Dynamic geometry of the left atrium and left ventricle in acute mitral regurgitation. *Circulation*, **60**, 177

17. PERLOFF, J.K. and ROBERTS, W. (1972). The mitral apparatus, functional anatomy of mitral regurgitation. *Circulation*, **46**, 227

18. ROBERTS, W.C. and COHEN, L.S. (1972). Left ventricular papillary muscles; description of the normal and a survey of conditions causing them to be abnormal. *Circulation*, **46**, 138

19. OGAWA, S., HUBBARD, F.E., MARDELLI, T.J., DREIFUS, L.S. and MEIXELL, L.M. (1979). Cross-sectional echocardiographic spectrum of papillary muscle dysfunction. *Am. Heart J.*, **97**, 312

20. SHELBOURNE, J.C., RUBINSTEIN, D. and GORLIN, R. (1969). A reappraisal of papillary muscle dysfunction. *Am. J. Med.*, **46**, 862

21. GODLEY, R.W., WANN, S., ROGERS, E.W., FEIGENBAUM, H. and WEYMAN, A.E. (1981). Incomplete mitral leaflet closure in patients with papillary muscle dysfunction. *Circulation*, **63**, 565

22. BOLTWOOD, C.M., TEI, C., TRIM, P., WONG, M. and SHAH, P.M. (1982). The mechanism of mitral regurgitation in nonischemic dilated cardiomyopathy (Abstr). *Circulation*, **66**, Suppl. II, 213

23. TEI, C., SAKAMAKI, T., SHAH, P.M., MEERBAUM, S., SHIMOURA, K., KONDO, S. and CORDAY, E. (1982). Induction of mitral valve prolapse with regurgitation in experimental acute ischemia. *Circulation*, **66**, Suppl. II: 87

24. HENRY, W.L., GRIFFITH, I.M., MICHAELIS, L.L., MCINTOSH, C.L., MORROW, A.G. and EPSTEIN, S.E. (1975). Measurement of mitral orifice area in patient with mitral valve disease by real-time, two-dimensional echocardiography. *Circulation*, **51**, 827

25. WANN, L.S., WEYMAN, A.E., FEIGENBAUM, H., DILLON, J.C., JOHNSTON, K.W. and EGGELTON, R.C. (1978). Determination of mitral valve area by cross-sectional echocardiography. *Ann. Int. Med.*, **88**, 337

26. GILBERT, B.W., SCHATZ, R.A., VONRAMM, O.T., BEHAR, V.S. and KISSLO, J.A. (1976). Mitral valve prolapse; two-dimensional echocardiographic and angiographic correlation. *Circulation*, **54**, 716

27. DEMARIA, A.N., NEUMANN, A., LEE, G. and MASON, D.T. (1977). Echocardiographic identification of the mitral valve prolapse syndromes. *Am. J. Med.*, **62**, 819

7

Left atrial function in mitral valve disease

Shigetake Sasayama and Chuichi Kawai

The left atrium is a muscular contractile chamber located in the inflow path to the ventricle which provides transportation of blood from pulmonary veins to the ventricle in various ways. The left atrium serves as a conduit for left ventricular filling. It also serves as a volume reservoir receiving blood from the pulmonary veins during left ventricular systole. When the elastic chamber dilates during filling, energy is absorbed in stretching the wall with elevation of atrial pressure; acting in this way the chamber serves as a passive energy reservoir. The potential energy stored during ventricular systole becomes kinetic energy which is released by atrial emptying. With the onset of atrial systole, the atrium performs the function of active energy transport[1]. The booster pump action of atrial systole allows more volume and pressure delivered than would be discharged by the passive energy reservoir alone. However, it may be difficult to separate clearly the contribution of the individual function, because all of these functions operate with varying degrees of influence upon ventricular filling, depending upon the loading condition of the atrium.

Importance of atrial transport has been demonstrated repeatedly by the intensified depression of ventricular performance with the sudden loss or reversal of the normal sequence of atrioventricular contraction[2, 3]. Some pathologic cardiac states in which diminished compliance of the left ventricle with increased resistance to ventricular filling increases dependence on the atrial contribution to ventricular filling[4, 5].

Significant increase in cardiac output has been demonstrated after successful cardioversion from atrial fibrillation[6]. On the other hand, patients with atrial fibrillation do not always reveal cardiac symptoms, and restoration of normal sinus rhythm by cardioversion was shown to have little effect on cardiac output[7]. Killip et al.[8] postulated that the mechanism of the failure to increase cardiac output was underlying atrial myocardial disease—'left atrial failure'.

Despite such existing evidence on the hemodynamic function of the left atrium, studies concerning the changes in atrial geometry throughout the cardiac cycle under different hemodynamic conditions are limited. It will be the purpose of this review to describe atrial function directly measured in the intact animal and to discuss the relative atrial contribution to ventricular filling in the presence either of

96

mitral valve dysfunction induced by inflow obstruction with balloon inflation, or valves rendered incompetent by sectioning chordae tendineae.

Atrial function in normal cardiac cycle

To measure phasic changes of left atrial diameter throughout the cardiac cycle directly in the canine heart and relate them to ventricular filling and ejection, we employed the ultrasonic approach which has proved to be highly suitable for the continuous measurement of dynamic changes in the several cardiac dimensions subtended by a pair of crystals simultaneously[9, 10]. We placed one pair of ultrasonic crystals externally on the anterior and posterior epicardial surfaces of the left atrium for the measurement of transverse chamber diameter, and another pair in the left ventricular wall subendocardially in a circumferential plane for the measurement of segment length. Left atrial and left ventricular pressure was also recorded simultaneously. Subsequent to the P wave of the electrocardiogram, (see Figure 7.1) left atrial pressure increases to form a small a wave. Twenty 50ms after the onset of the atrial pressure rise, the left atrial wall begins to shorten and the left atrial diameter decreases by an average of 4.6% from the end-diastolic value of 19.7 mm. With atrial contraction, the left ventricle is expanded to a certain extent. The nadir of the atrial chamber shortening is during the isovolumic contraction phase of the left ventricle. With the onset of ventricular contraction, the left atrium begins to expand, rapidly in the beginning and slowly at the end, until the opening of the mitral valve. The atrial diameter averaged 20.5 mm at the point of peak v wave in the atrial pressure.

After mitral valve opening, the left atrial diameter remains constant until the beginning of the next atrial contraction or decreases rapidly coincidentally with y descent of the v wave of the atrial pressure (see Figure 7.1). Payne et al.[11] studied the phasic changes in atrial dimension in the conscious dog with this same ultrasonic method and documented an increase in atrial diameter during isovolumic ventricular systole and a decrease during ventricular ejection. They explained the former change by the reversed mitral flow due to bulging of the mitral leaflets into the atrium. The latter change was attributed to the downward displacement of the mitral annulus. We observed that the onset of atrial expansion after active shortening is not always coincident with the beginning of the isovolumic systole, depending on the heart rate and atrioventricular conduction time. The initial left atrial expansion is more likely to be related to the rapid storage of blood due to damming up of the blood stream by the closure of mitral valve.

Our data are in accord with angiographic observations which showed that the atrium has a spherical shape and decreases uniformly in size with active atrial contraction and expands during ventricular ejection. The changes in atrial circumference are generally symmetrical but the variations in the anteroposterior dimension are always eccentric, almost entirely due to valve ring displacement. Thus, the left atrium is regarded as a cylinder which achieves piston-like displacement of the mitral annulus with only little movement of the dorsal part of the wall which is firmly anchored to the veins. The ventricular contraction directly stretches and lengthens the atrial wall. Nevertheless, the same contraction pattern was observed in multiple diameters with changes of practically equal magnitude in the length of anteroposterior diameter as in the two different circumferential diameters[12, 13].

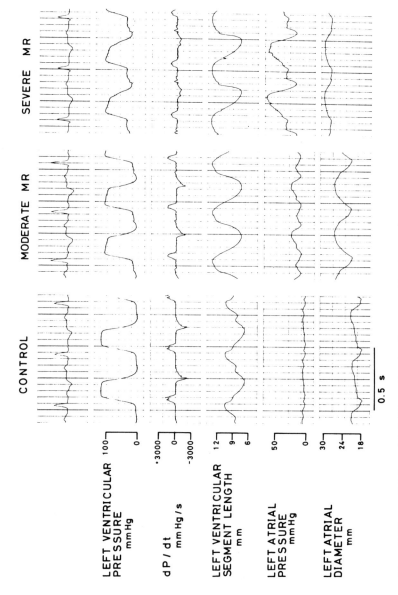

LEFT VENTRICULAR PRESSURE mmHg

dP/dt mmHg/s

LEFT VENTRICULAR SEGMENT LENGTH mm

LEFT ATRIAL PRESSURE mmHg

LEFT ATRIAL DIAMETER mm

CONTROL MODERATE MR SEVERE MR

0.5 s

Figure 7.1 Sequential changes in left heart function from control levels to graded mitral regurgitation (MR) induced by sectioning the chordae tendineae. Normal waveforms at control state are shown at the left, recordings at initial moderate MR in the middle, and at the later severe stages at the right. The top line of traces are standard ECGs.

Atrial function in acute mitral regurgitation

Following control recordings, the mitral valve was rendered incompetent by sectioning the chordae tendineae via the transventricular route. With the onset of moderate regurgitation, the left ventricular cavity was significantly enlarged with a marked augmentation of stroke excursion. There was comparable increase in end-diastolic pressure. The peak left ventricular pressure decreased significantly with more rapid decline during ejection. This pronounced alteration in the pressure pulse contour together with more rapid reduction in ventricular size due to regurgitation of the blood into the atrium accelerates the reduction in the ventricular systolic wall stress via the Laplace relation, with further increase in the velocity and extent of shortening. However, despite an enhanced total stroke excursion, the changes in effective forward flow were variable, depending on the amount of the regurgitation.

End-diastolic diameter of the atrial cavity was also increased, associated with an augmented atrial shortening and expansion. The most prominent change in left atrial pressure was not only its elevation but also typical modification of the pressure pulse contour with a distinct *a* wave followed by a more prominent *v* wave (*see Figure 7.1*).

When mitral regurgitation was rendered more severe by additional chordal rupture, the left ventricular end-diastolic pressure was elevated even higher, and the end-diastolic dimension and stroke excursion of the left ventricular chamber continued to increase. The left atrial pressure was makedly elevated, with an abbreviation of the *x* descent and striking increase in *v* wave with early onset of its ascent. The latter change was somewhat more prominent than the mean pressure changes. More severe regurgitation produced a further increase in the atrial diameter but was associated with a decreased atrial wall motion which did not appear to be effectively compensated for by the geometrical advantage of the enlarged chamber to eject a larger volume with less diameter change (*see Figure 7.2*).

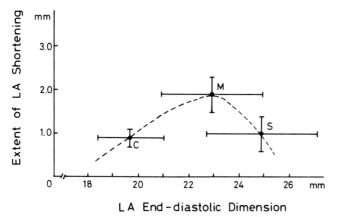

Figure 7.2 The relationship between the extent of left atrial (LA) shortening and the end-diastolic left atrial diameter, obtained during progression of mitral regurgitation. There is a striking enhancement of atrial shortening with the initial increase in atrial diameter; however, less marked wall motion is associated with further enlargement of left atrial chamber in later stages. The data indicate that the behaviour of the left atrium is in accordance with the Frank–Starling principle, with a prominent descending limb at extreme atrial dilation. C = control; M = moderate; S = severe stages of mitral regurgitation.

These results are quite consistent with the Starling curves obtained in rabbit atria by relating stroke work of isobaric contraction to diastolic volume which always exhibited a descending limb at very high volumes[14]. Williams *et al.* [15] also determined the active length–tension curves of the atrial muscle in anesthetized open-chest dogs and demonstrated that active tension developed by atrial muscle increased as a function of initial muscle length with maximum tensions at muscle lengths that exceeded the initial length by 50–60%; extension of length beyond this point resulted in a decline in active tension (*see Figure 7.3*). The response is analogous to the Frank–Starling mechanism of the ventricular myocardium. Though the absolute pressures generated by the atria are far less than those produced by the ventricle, the maximum active tension of the atrium is similar to the maximum force generated by the ventricular myocardium, when appropriate corrections were made for differences in the cross-sectional areas of these tissues.

In order to analyze the behaviour of the left atrium in response to gradually increased volume load by pressure–diameter relation, the left atrial pressure was

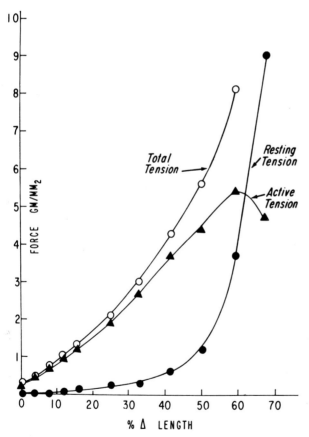

Figure 7.3 Resting, active and total tension recorded directly in the right atrium of an anesthetized open-chest dog at increased muscle lengths using an adjustable strain-gauge arch. At any given contractile state, the active tension developed by atrial myocardium was found to increase as a function of initial length, while contraction of the atria above the peak of the length–active tension curve resulted in the decrease in force. The response is analogous to the Frank–Starling mechanism of ventricular myocardium. (Reproduced from reference 15, by kind permission of authors and publishers.)

fed into a storage oscilloscope on the *y*-axis and left atrial diameter signal on the *x*-axis in each cardiac cycle. The loops obtained during the control period and after production of mitral regurgitation of graded severity were superimposed on one photograph (*see Figure 7.4*). In the control period, atrial pressure before the onset of atrial systole was low and diameter change was associated with minimal alteration in pressure, resulting in a relatively flat P-D loop (lower left, *Figure 7.4*). When left atrial diameter and pressure were moderately increased with the production of acute mitral regurgitation, enhanced booster function of the atrium was evident from the augmented initial counterclockwise loop. As the mitral regurgitation increased, the left atrium became to operate on a higher and steeper

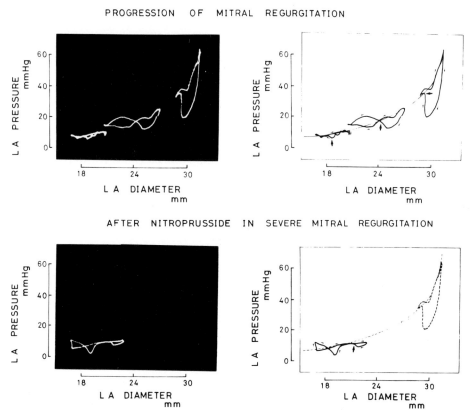

Figure 7.4 The upper panel illustrates the superimposed atrial pressure–diameter loops in the control state and at two stages of graded mitral regurgitation. The original display is schematized in the right panel to indicate the end-diastolic point (thick arrow) and the direction of rotation (thin arrow). The single resting length–tension curve of the left atrium is delineated by the ascending limb of the *v* wave and the corresponding diameter change of the three loops. The left atrium with moderate mitral reg-urgitation operates on the lower flat portion of this curve and the enhanced booster function is evident by the augmented initial counterclockwise loops. With progression of mitral regurgitation, the left atrium moves up to the higher steep portion of the same curve, where the diameter changes little with a considerable change in pressure, indicating the predominant conduit function. The lower panel shows the pressure–diameter loop of the same dog after administration of nitroprusside, which moves down the same curve delineated during the progression of mitral regurgitation (superimposed by the dotted curve) to a more compliant lower flat portion.

po...ion of its passive pressure–length relationship, which was delineated by the ascending limb of each v wave and the concomitant diameter change. Here, there was little change in the diameter and a considerable alteration in pressure throughout the cardiac cycle. Under these circumstances, effective further elongation of sarcomere lengths cannot occur with further increases in regurgitation.

Thus, the decrease in atrial shortening in severe mitral regurgitation can be related to an increased afterload to atrial contraction due to an elevated left ventricular filling pressure when the limit of preload reserve of the atrial myocardium has been reached[16].

Factors modifying regurgitant volume

Nitroprusside infusion in experimental acute mitral regurgitation produced a remarkable fall in left atrial pressure accompanied by a significant decrease in left ventricular systolic and end-diastolic pressures. The left atrial diameter was markedly diminished with a considerable augmentation of active atrial contraction. Left ventricular chamber size was also remarkably decreased. There was no detectable change in the total stroke volume, while forward stroke volume was substantially augmented (*see Figure 7.5*). All of these findings indicated a reduction in the regurgitant volume.

On the contrary, the increase in systolic blood pressure with methoxamine caused a significant rise in left atrial pressure with enhancement of the v wave. Left ventricular end-diastolic pressure was also markedly elevated. There was a significant enlargement of the left atrial as well as left ventricular chambers. Accompanying the latter changes there was a considerable reduction in left ventricular wall motion (*see Figure 7.6*).

Chatterjee *et al.* [17] first demonstrated potential benefit of administrating nitroprusside in patients with clinically significant mitral regurgitation due to dysfunction of the subvalvular apparatus. Subsequently, similar results have been reported in several groups[18–20]. However, the precise mechanism of reduction in regurgitation still remains controversial. Earlier investigators postulated that the decrease in systemic vascular resistance is the primary factor responsible for the improvement of mitral regurgitation. The importance of lowering arterial impedance has been supported by the subsequent observation of the same salutary effect of hydralazine which selectively acts on the arteriolar resistance bed in patients with severe mitral regurgitation[21].

It has generally been accepted that ventricular emptying could be enhanced by reducing impedance to ejection by vasodilator therapy, particularly when the ventricle is over-distended and the preload reserve is fully utilized. However, in the presence of mitral regurgitation, overall pump function is unchanged by vasodilating agents because afterload reduction has already been afforded by the low impedance pathway via the regurgitant leak[22] and an accelerated decline of the ventricular wall stress during ejection[23].

Accordingly, augmentation of forward stroke volume appeared to be a result of redistribution of the left ventricular output so that a greater portion was directed forward by virtue of its selective lowering of aortic impedence. Reduced regurgitation decreased the left atrial chamber size. Being released from overstretch, the left atrium moved down the single passive-pressure–diameter

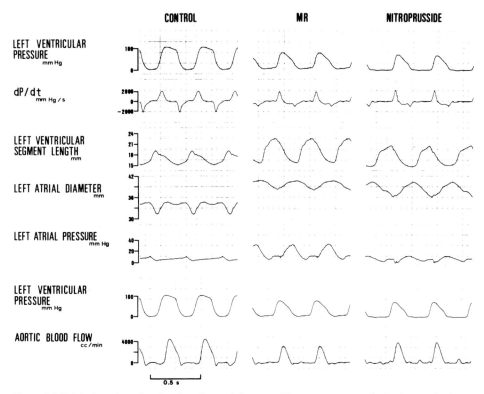

Figure 7.5 Original tracings showing the effects of nitroprusside at severe stage of mitral regurgitation (MR). In addition to the recordings of pressure and dimension of the left atrium and the left ventricle in the upper panel, the aortic blood flow is illustrated in the lower panel. Following the control recording (left panel), severe mitral regurgitation was produced, which was characterized by the marked distension of atrial cavity and decreased wall motion (middle panel). Nitroprusside caused an augmentation of forward stroke volume associated with no significant change in stroke excursion of the left ventricle from a decreased end-diastolic dimension. There was a significant fall in atrial pressure with striking reduction in the *v* wave. Left atrial diameter decreased with a significant restoration of atrial shortening (right panel).

curve to a more complaint, lower, flat portion, thereby substantially restoring the atrial shortening (*see Figure 7.4*).

Chatterjee *et al.*[17] also called attention to the reduction of left ventricular volume as an additional factor to improve valvular competence. More recently, Yoran *et al.* clearly demonstrated that the regurgitant flow was more dependent on the size of the mitral orifice [24], and nitroprusside was assumed to reduce regurgitation primarily by decreasing the regurgitant orifice size as a result of the reduction in ventricular volume[25]. Alternatively, augmentation of left ventricular afterload was associated with an increase in regurgitation primarily by increasing the regurgitant orifice size.

Likewise, increased contractility reduced the regurgitant volume on account of decrease in mitral valve area as a result of diminished left heart chamber size, improvement of the atrial pump function and enhanced contraction of the muscular portion of the annular margin[9].

Thus, the factors that tend to diminish left heart cavity size will reduce mitral

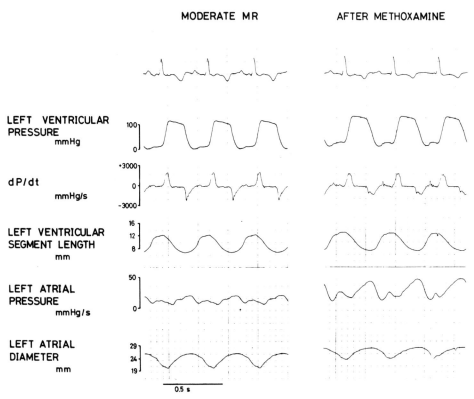

Figure 7.6 Original tracings obtained in one dog showing the effect of methoxamine administered at a moderate stage of mitral regurgitation (MR). When methoxamine was slowly infused intravenously, the heart rate changed little. There was significant elevation of left ventricular systolic and end-diastolic pressures. Left atrial and left ventricular chambers were markedly enlarged and the wall motions of both chambers were severely depressed. Mean left atrial pressure was progressively elevated and accompanied by a more marked *v* wave, indicating an augmented regurgitant volume.

regurgitation independent of the transvalvular pressure gradient which has previously been regarded as the dominant determinant of regurgitant flow.

Atrial function in mitral stenosis

The effect of active atrial contraction on left ventricular filling in patients with mitral stenosis has been the subject of considerable investigation and continued to evoke interest and controversy.

Experimental studies on mitral stenosis have been limited because of the difficulties in establishing a realistic model without introducing secondary changes in the circulation. In another series of experiments, we attempted to augment outflow resistance of the left atrium by introducing a balloon catheter at the mitral orifice through the appendage in open-chest dogs instrumented with ultrasonic dimension gauges to measure the transverse diameter of the left atrium and the left ventricular segment length, together with intracavitary pressures of both chambers. With inflation of the balloon, the left atrial pressure was gradually elevated with a more prominent *a* wave in the pressure pulse (*see Figure 7.7*). The left atrial chamber was progressively expanded with greater increase in magnitude of left atrial contraction. This observation also indicated the behaviour of the left atrium in accordance with the Frank–Starling principle. The relevance of these findings in experimental animals to naturally occurring mitral stenosis in man is not certain and hemodynamic studies in man have demonstrated much more variable results than encountered here in the dog.

Cohn and Mason[26] analyzed the height of the left atrial contraction wave in patients with pure mitral stenosis and sinus rhythm and showed that the relative height of the *a* wave varied inversely with the hemodynamic severity of the mitral obstruction and the left atrial size. According to these data, it was assumed that in any given patient, as the mitral stenosis becomes more severe or longstanding, left atrial contraction may become weaker and make a smaller contribution to left ventricular filling.

The *v* wave of the left atrial pressure pulse in mitral stenosis is generally considered to be small[27]. However, this is not always the case in the clinical settings in which dominant *v* waves are often associated with decreased distensibility of the atrium. Obviously, left atrial distention contributes substantially to the augmentation of atrial contraction in patients with mitral stenosis; however, additional factors such as hypertrophy of atrial myocardium or pathological changes may also modify this process.

Carleton and Graettinger[28] studied the hemodynamic role of the atria in a group of patients with and without mitral stenosis, by comparing cardiac output obtained during sequential A-V packing with well-placed atrial contraction to that obtained after elimination of effective atrial contraction by synchronous A-V pacing. They stated that effective atrial systole augmented left ventricular output by approximately 20% in patients without valvular disease; however, atrial systole made no significant contribution in the presence of mitral stenosis. The major factor for the reduced effect of atrial systole in augmenting stroke volume in patients with severe mitral stenosis might be the stenotic valve itself; in the absence of a fixed resistence to left ventricular inflow, the energy produced by atrial contraction is transmitted to the ventricle, shifting the ventricular position upward on the pressure–volume curve. In the presence of mitral valve obstruction, raising atrial pressure by atrial contraction fails to augment the diastolic valve flow, for the kinetic energy is dissipated in overcoming the resistance across the valve[28–30].

A number of investigators have suggested that an abnormality of the left atrial myocardium, i.e. atrial failure, could be a significant contributory factor to impairment of ventricular filling[4, 7, 31]. Patients with mitral valve disease and atrial fibrillation often exhibit a surprisingly small atrial contraction wave in the atrial pressure tracings, upon restoration of atrial repolarization wave by condioversion. Such weak atrial contraction is not likely to influence ventricular filling significantly, and an increase in cardiac output after cardioversion would not be anticipated[4, 7]. The depression of atrial contracion fails to maintain lower levels of mean left atrial pressure for any given left ventricular end-diastolic pressure and may play a role in the genesis of the elevated venous pressure in congestive heart failure[31].

On the other hand, when little time had been afforded for compensatory homeostatic mechanisms to come into play to maintain cardiac output during acute interventions, atrial contraction augmented the end-diastolic transmitral valvular gradient by approximately 40% in patients with mitral stenosis with a resultant

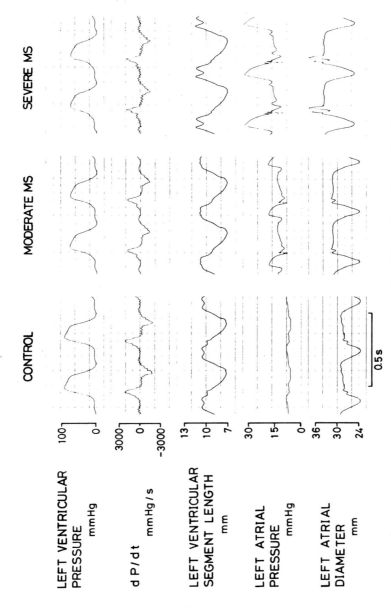

Figure 7.7 Original tracings showing normal waveforms (left panel) and changes due to increased outflow resistance of the left atrium by inflating balloon at the mitral orifice (middle and right panels). The left atrial pressure was gradually elevated with more prominent *a* wave. The left atrial chamber was progressively enlarged with greater increase in magnitude of atrial contraction. The left ventricular function remained unchanged throughout the course. MS = mitral stenosis.

increase in diastolic flow across the stenotic mitral valve and corresponding enhancement of ventricular filling[8, 32–34]. In the presence of even severe mitral stenosis, diastolic flow and cardiac output could be augmented by atrial contraction at both fast and slow rates[32]. Likewise, withdrawal of effective atrial transport decreases the diastolic flow per beat and cardiac output by 20%[32]. However, according to the Gorlin formula, flow across the stenotic valve depends on the square root of the mean diastolic pressure gradient and directly on the mitral valve area. Thus, the atrial contribution to the mean mitral valve gradient does not augment flow across the severely stenotic mitral valve as much as it would in a less stenotic valve.

Our acute experiment showed that despite the outflow obstruction of the left atrium, augmented atrial contraction provided adequate filling of the ventricle as evidenced by unchanged left ventricular end-diastolic pressure and fiber length, thus allowing equal amounts of left ventricular systolic shortening. Thus, activated atrial performance in mitral stenosis may well be an early adaptive response to maintain cardiac output.

Summary

The left atrium is a muscular contractile chamber located in the inflow path to the ventricle and performs transport functions in various ways. The relative importance of such atrial functions appears to vary depending upon the loading condition of the atrium at any given moment. Accordingly, we studied dynamic geometry of the left atrium in open-chest dogs subjected to acute mitral regurgitation and mitral stenosis using ultrasonic dimension gauge and high-fidelity micromanometers.

In the control state, three definite phasic changes of the left atrial diameter were observed during one cardiac cycle: shortening with atrial contraction, expansion during ventricular ejection and restoration of its end-diastolic dimension by the onset of the next atrial contraction.

Acute onset of mitral regurgitation initially induced a remarkable augmentation of atrial shortening with chamber dilation; however, with the further progression of mitral regurgitation, the atrial wall motion was significantly reduced. These findings indicated that the left atrium also behaved in accordance with the Frank–Starling principle and an extreme atrial dilation produced a prominent descending limb, conduit function thereby predominating over active atrial transport.

The amount of regurgitation was highly dependent on the geometry of the mitral orifice, and factors that decreased the size of the left heart cavity diminished the regurgitation by increasing competence of the components of mitral apparatus.

When the atrial outflow tract was obstructed to simulate mitral stenosis, there occurred significant elevation of left atrial pressure with a more prominent *a* wave and enlargement of the left atrial chamber with greater increase in magnitude of atrial contraction. The left ventricular dimension and function were thereby not significantly altered. Thus, activated atrial performance in mitral stenosis may well be an early adaptive response to maintain ventricular filling.

Acknowledgements

This project was supported by Scientific Research Grant Nos. 244044, 457240, 412001 and 5670332 from the Ministry of Education, Science and Culture, Japan, and a Japan Heart Foundation Research Grant.

References

1. LEONARD, J.J., SHAVER, J. and THOMPSON, M. (1980). Left atrial transport function. *Trans. Am. Clin, Climatol. Assoc.*, **92**, 133–141
2. COHEN, S.I. and FRANK, H.A. (1982). Preservation of active atrial transport. An important clinical consideration in cardiac pacing. *Chest*, **81**, 51–54
3. HAAS, J.M. and STRAIT, G.B. (1974). Pacemaker-induced cardiovascular failure. Hemodynamic and angiographic observations. *Am. J. Cardiol.*, **33**, 295–299
4. BRAUNWALD, E. (1964). Symposium on cardiac arrhythmias. With comments on the hemodynamic significance of atrial systole. *Am. J. Med.*, **37**, 665–669
5. GROSSMAN, W. and MCLAURIN, L.P. (1976). Diastolic properties of the left ventricle. *Ann. Int. Med.*, **84**, 316–326
6. MORRIS, J.J., ENTMAN, M., NORTH, W.C., KONG, Y. and MCINTOSH, H. (1965). The changes in cardiac output with reversion of atrial fibrillation to sinus rhythm. *Circulation*, **31**, 670–678
7. GRAETTINGER, J.S., CARLETON, R.A. and MUENSTER, J.J. (1964). Circulatory consequences of change in cardiac rhythm produced in patients by transthoracic direct-current shock. *J. Clin. Invest.*, **43**, 2290–2302
8. KILLIP, T. and BAER, R.A. (1966). Hemodynamic effects after reversion from atrial fibrillation to sinus rhythm by precordial shock. *J. Clin. Invest.*, **45**, 658–671
9. SASAYAMA, S., TAKAHASHI, M., OSAKADA, G., HIROSE, K., HAMASHIMA, H., NISHIMURA, E. and KAWAI, C. (1979). Dynamic geometry of the left atrium and left ventricle in acute mitral regurgitation. *Circulation*, **60**, 177–186
10. SASAYAMA, S., TAKAHASHI, M. and KAWAI, C. (1981). Left atrial function in acute mitral regurgitation. Factors which modify the regurgitant volume. *Herz*, **6**, 156–165
11. PAYNE, R.M., STONE, H.S. and ENGELKEN, E.J. (1971). Atrial function during volume loading. *J. Appl. Physiol.*, **31**, 326–331
12. GRIBBE, P., LIND, J., LINKO, E. and WEGELIUM, C. (1958). The events of the left side of the normal heart as studied by cineradiography. *Cardiologia.*, **33**, 293–304
13. TSAKIRIS, A.G., PADIYAR, R., GORDON, D.A. and LIPTON, I. (1977). Left atrial size and geometry in the intact dog. *Am. J. Physiol.*, **232**, H167–H172
14. BLINKS, J.R. (1961). Method for study of contraction of isolated heart muscle under various physical conditions. *Circ. Res.*, **9**, 342–348
15. WILLIAMS, J.F. JR., SONNENBLICK, E.H. and BRAUNWALD, E. (1965). Determinants of atrial contractile force in the intact heart. *Am. J. Physiol.*, **209**, 1061–1069
16. ROSS, J. JR., FRANKLIN, D. and SASAYAMA, S. (1976). Preload, afterload and the role of afterload mismatch in the descending limb of cardiac function. *Europ. J. Cardiol.*, **4**, 77–86
17. CHATTERJEE, K., PARMLEY, W.S., SWAN, H.J.C., BERMAN, G., FORRESTER, J. and MARCUS, H.S. (1973). Beneficial effects of vasodilator agents in severe mitral regurgitation due to dysfunction of subvalvar apparatus. *Circulation*, **48**, 684–690
18. GOODMAN, D.J., ROSSEN, R.M., HOLLOWAY, E.L., ALDERMAN, E.L. and HARRISON, D.C. (1974). Effect of nitroprusside on left ventricular dynamics in mitral regurgitation. *Circulation*, **50**, 1025–1032
19. HARSHAW, C.W., GROSSMAN, W., MUNRO, A.B. and MCLAURIN, L.P. (1975). Reduced systemic vascular resistence as therapy for severe mitral regurgitation of valvular origin. *Ann. Int. Med.*, **83**, 312–316
20. SASAYAMA, S., OHYAGI, A., LEE, J.D., NONOGI, H., SAKURAI, T., WAKABAYASHI, A., FUJITA, M. and KAWAI, C. (1982). Symposium on current problems in valvular heart disease. Effect of the vasodilator therapy in regurgitant valvular disease. *Jpn. Circ. J.*, **46**, 433–441
21. GREENBERG, B.H., MASSIE, B.M., BRUNDAGE, B.H., BOTVINICK, E.H., PARMLEY, W.W. and CHATTERJEE, K. (1978). Beneficial effects of hydralazine in severe mitral regurgitation. *Circulation*, **58**, 273–279
22. ECKBERG, D.L., GAULT, J.H., BOUCHARD, R.L., KARLINER, J.S. and ROSS, J. JR. (1973). Mechanics of left ventricular contraction in chronic severe mitral regurgitation. *Circulation*, **47**, 1252–1259
23. URSCHEL, C.W., COVELL, J.W., SONNENBLICK, E.H., ROSS, J. JR. and BRAUNWALD, E. (1968). Myocardial mechanics in aortic and mitral valvular regurgitation: The concept of instantaneous impedance as a determinant of the performance of the intact heart. *J. Clin. Invest.*, **47**, 867–883
24. YORAN, C., YELLIN, E.L., BECKER, R.M., GABBAY, S., FRATER, R.W.M. and SONNENBLICK, E.H. (1979). Dynamic aspects of acute mitral regurgitation: Effects of ventricular volume, pressure and contractility on the effective regurgitant orifice area. *Circulation*, **60**, 170–177
25. YORAN, C., YELLIN, E.L., BECKER, R.M., GABBAY, S., FRATER, R.W.M. and SONNENBLICK, E.H. (1979). Mechanism of reduction of mitral regurgitation with vasodilator therapy. *Am. J. Cardiol*, **43**, 774–777
26. COHN, L.H. and MASON, D.T. (1966). Determinants of the height of the left atrial contraction wave in mitral stenosis. *Am. J. Cardiol.*, **18**, 724–729

27. MORROW, A.G., BRAUNWALD, E., HALLER, J.A. and SHARP, E.H. (1957). Left atrial pressure pulse in mitral valve disease. A correlation of pressure obtained by transbronchial puncture with the valvular lesion. *Circulation*, **16**, 399–405

28. CARLETON, R.A. and GRAETTINGER, J.S. (1967). The hemodynamic role of the atria with and without mitral stenosis. *Am. J. Med.*, **42**, 532–538

29. STOTT, D.K., MARPOLE, D.G.F., BRISTOW, J.D., KLOSTER, F.E. and GRISWOLD, H.E. (1970). The role of left atrial transport in aortic and mitral stenosis. *Circulation*, **41**, 1031–1041

30. KENDALL, M.E., WALSTON, A. II, COBB, E.R. and GREENFIELD, J.C. JR, (1971). Pressure-flow studies in man: Effect of atrial systole on ventricular function in mitral stenosis. *J. Clin. Invest.*, **50**, 2653–2659

31. MITCHELL, J.H. and SHAPIRO, W. (1969). Atrial function and the hemodynamic consequences of atrial fibrillation in man. *Am. J. Cardiol.*, **23**, 556–567

32. THOMPSON, M.E., SHAVER, J.A. and LEON, D.F. (1977). Effect of tachycardia on atrial transport in mitral stenosis. *Am. Heart. J.*, **94**, 297–306

33. HEIDENREICH, F.P., THOMPSON, M.E., SHAVER, J.M. and LEONARD, J.J. (1969). Left atrial transport in mitral stenosis. *Circulation*, **40**, 545–554

34. HEIDENREICH, F.P., SHAVER, J.A., THOMPSON, M.E. and LEONARD, J.J. (1970). Left atrial booster function in valvular heart disease. *J. Clin. Invest.*, **49**, 1605–1618

8

The dynamics of acute experimental mitral regurgitation

Chaim Yoran, Robert W.M. Frater, Edmund H. Sonnenblick and Edward L. Yellin

Introduction

The function of the mitral valve depends on the integrity of the valve leaflets, chordae tendineae, papillary muscles, mitral annulus and the contraction of the subvalvular left ventricular wall. The regurgitant flow across the incompetent mitral valve is determined by the systolic pressure gradient between the left ventricle and left atrium, the regurgitant orifice size and the duration of regurgitation or the length of ventricular systole[1, 2]. It has been accepted that the regurgitant orifice size is fixed under different hemodynamic states[1] except in the clinical syndrome of papillary muscle dysfunction in which the properties of the supporting structures may change with time[3–5]. However, studies from this laboratory[6–8] and elsewhere[9] have demonstrated that the regurgitatant orifice size varies directly with the size and shape of the left ventricle.

Methods

Animal preparation

Six mongrel dogs weighing 20–30 kg were anesthetized with sodium pentobarbitol and artificially ventilated. The animal preparation was described previously[10]. Briefly, after a midline sternotomy and left thoracotomy, the pericardium was opened and the heart was supported in a pericardial cradle. Left ventricular and left atrial pressures were measured with microtip catheters (Millar). Aortic pressure was measured with a Stratham gauge (P23De). All three transducers were adjusted to equal sensitivity and a common baseline. An electromagnetic flow probe (Carolina Medical Electronics) was placed around the ascending aorta.

The left atrium was opened during a cardiopulmonary bypass and under direct vision acute mitral regurgitation was produced by excising a triangular portion of the free edge of the anterior mitral leaflet. A toroidal electromagnetic flow probe with a soft mobile Dacron sleeve was sutured around the mitral annulus with special care taken to avoid interference with cusp and ring movement. Annular mobility was verified at autopsy. In a control study designed to provide an analog of a fixed regurgitant orifice, a Bjork–Shiley tilting-disc prosthesis (17 mm annulus diameter) with a 25 mm^2 hold in the occluder was inserted in series with the flow probe in one dog. The left atrium was then closed, normal sinus rhythm was restored (DC defibrillation when necessary) and the animal was weaned from bypass. Phasic mitral and aortic flows were measured with a two-channel square-wave flowmeter (Carolina Medical Electronics). The two flows, LV, LA and aortic pressures, LV *dp/dt* and ECG were recorded at high gain and a paper speed of 100 mm/s on an oscillographic recorder (Electronics for Medicine DR-12).

Calculations

The mean systolic pressure gradient (SPG) between the left ventricle and left atrium was calculated from simultaneous LV and LA pressure curve using a sonic digitizer (Science Accessories GP-3) coupled to a digital computer (PDP 11/34). Filling volume (FV) regurgitant volume (RV) and forward stroke volume (SV) were calculated by digitizing the flow curves. The average of 3–5 determinations was used for each calculation. Zero mitral flow was determined initially while the animal was still in ventricular fibrillation; during the experiment by producing long postextrasystolic diastolic periods; and again at the end of each experiment by arresting the heart with potassium chloride. The mean area of the regurgitant orifice (MRA) during ventricular stystole was calculted from a modified Gorlin equation[6–8].

Interventions

Nitroprusside:—IV infusion (average dose 100 μg/min) to lower systolic pressure by 10–20 mm Hg.
  Norepinephrine:—IV infusion (4–10 μg/min).
  Volume infusion—200–400 ml blood rapidly infused to increase LVEDP to approxmately 18 mm Hg.
  Angiotension—IV infusion (5–10 μg/min).

Results

Vasodilation

The hemodynamic effects of nitroprusside are summarized in *Table 8.1*. During the administration of nitroprusside the systemic vascular resistance decreased from 2767 ± 72 to 2331 ± 85 dynes/s/cm^{-5} ($p < 0.005$). There were substantial reductions in regurgitant volume, filling volume, LVEDP and left atrial 'V' wave (*see Figure 8.1*). The reduction in both peak LV and LA pressure resulted in an unchanged SPG (*see Figures 8.1* and *8.2* panel C). The regurgitant fraction (RF; RF = RV/SV total) and MRA decreased. If the MRA had remained unchanged the calculated regurgitant volume associated with the decreased SPG would have been more than the measured RV (11 ml and 9 ml, respectively). Thus, of the total reduction in regurgitation volume, 37.5% is due to decrease of the SPG while 62.5% is due to the reduction of MRA (*see Figure 8.2*, panel D).

Increased myocardial contractility

Table 8.1 and *Figures 8.3* and *8.4* show the hemodynamic effects of norepinephrine infusion. LV *dp/dt* increased from 2050 ± 160 to 3760 ± 290 mm Hg/s. Despite the

TABLE 8.1. Hemodynamic effects of nitroprusside: contractility, volume loading and increased arterial pressure

	LVSP (mm Hg)	LVEDP (mm Hg)	LAV (mm Hg)	CO (l/min)	SV (ml)	SV/RV
Nitroprusside:						
C	120.3 ± 6.9	14.7 ± 1.0	41.4 ± 2.0	2.46 ± 0.22	14.6 ± 1.5	1.45 ± 0.32
NP	109.0 ± 7.1	10.3 ± 1.2	26.3 ±2.1	2.42 ± 0.20	13.7 ± 1.4	1.83 ± 0.36
p	<0.02	<0.001	<0.001	NS	NS	<0.001
Volume loading:						
C	108.2 ± 5.6	8.9 ± 0.8	20.2 ± 1.7	1.79 ± 0.16	10.8 ± 0.9	1.65 ± 0.24
V	120.7 ± 5.7	16.7 ± 1.3	43.1 ± 3.3	2.53 ± 0.20	15.7 ± 1.2	1.55 ± 0.19
p	<0.001	<0.001	<0.001	<0.001	<0.001	NS
Angiotensin:						
C	101.8 ± 7.7	11.0 ± 1.0	26.2 ± 1.7	2.08 ± 0.25	13.1 ± 1.4	1.44 ± 0.37
A	135.7 ± 9.1	16.3 ± 1.9	31.5 ± 3.6	1.57 ± 0.19	10.4 ± 1.0	0.85 ± 0.21
p	<0.01	<0.01	NS	<0.05	NS	<0.05
Norepinephrine:						
C	94.1 ± 3.4	12.0 ± 2.3	24.9 ± 3.9	1.66 ± 0.14	10.2 ± 1.0	1.21 ± 0.29
NE	126.6 ± 5.2	8.6 ± 1.9	20.0 ± 2.7	2.17 ± 0.12	12.7 ± 0.8	1.70 ± 0.34
p	<0.01	<0.01	<0.02	<0.001	<0.05	<0.001

Values are means ± SEM. C = Control; CO = cardiac output; LAV = left atrial V wave; LVEDP = left ventricular end-diastolic pressure; LVSP = left ventricular systolic pressure; NP = nitroprusside; V = volume loading; A = angiotensin; N = norepinephrine; NS = not significant; RV = regurgitant volume; SV = forward left ventricular stroke volume.

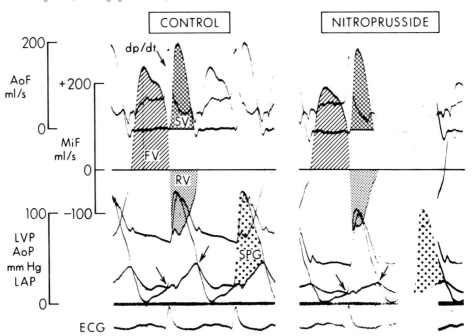

Figure 8.1 Effects of nitroprusside infusion: oscillographic records during control period and nitroprusside infusion. AoF = Aortic blood flow; LVP = left ventricular pressure; Aop = aortic pressure; LAP = left atrial pressure; MiF = mitral blood flow; *dp/dt* = first derivative of LVP; FV = filling volume; RV = regurgitant volume; SV = forward stroke volume; RT = regurgitant time. Note a decrease in regurgitant volume. The decrease in both peak systolic pressure and left atrial pressure resulted in an unchanged systolic pressure gradient.

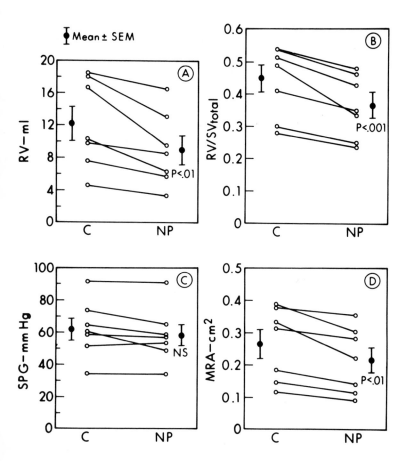

Figure 8.2 Effects of nitroprusside infusion. C = Control; NP = nitroprusside; RV = regurgitant volume; RV/SV total = calculated ratio of RV to the total left ventricular stroke volume; SPG = mean systolic pressure gradient between the left ventricle and left atrium; MRA = calculated area of the effective regurgitant orifice. Vertical bars are means ± SEM. NS = Not significant. (Reproduced from reference 6, by kind permission of authors and publishers.)

51% increase in SPG after norepinephrine infusion the RV remained unchanged. If the MRA had remained unchanged the increase of SPG would have increased the RV. These results are due to a 17% decrease in MRA (*see Figure 8.4*, panel D).

Volume loading

The hemodynamic effects of volume loading are shown in *Table 8.1* and *Figures 8.5* and *8.6*. The increase in peak LV pressure was associated with a rise in left atrial pressure and therefore the SPG increased by only 5% (*see Figure 8.6*, panel C). MRA increased by 31% (*see Figure 8.6*, panel D). If the regurgitant area had remained unchanged by volume loading the small increase in SPG would have accounted for only a 10% increase in RV. The increase of the MRA alone accounted for an increase of 34% in RV.

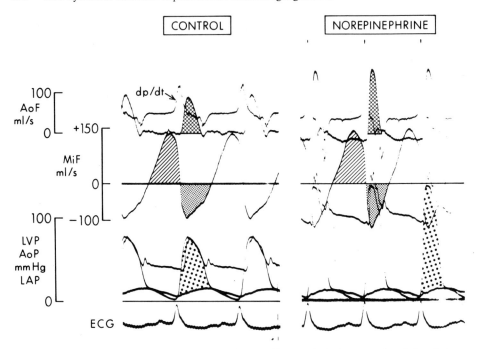

Figure 8.3 Effects of norepinephrine infusion: oscillographic records during control period and norepinephrine infusion. Note the unchanged regurgitant volume (RV) despite a large increase in systolic pressure gradient (SPG). Abbreviations as in *Figure 8.1*.

Increment of systolic pressure

The hemodynamic effects of angiotensin infusion are shown in *Table 8.1, Figures 8.7* and *8.8*. RV increased by 41% and regurgitant fraction increased by 35% (*see Figure 8.8*, panels A and B). SPG rose by 39% and MRA increased by 14% (*see Figure 8.8*, panels C and D). If the MRA remained unchanged it would have accounted for a 23% increase in RV. The further increase in RV to 41% was due to the increase in MRA.

Spontaneous changes of regurgitant orifice during ejection

During ventricular systole the mitral regurgitant area was calculated at four instants of time: one preceding peak regurgitant flow, one at peak flow MRA (p) and two following the peak flow. The instantaneous MRA (t) normalized by MRA (p) is plotted against time (t) normalized by regurgitant time (RT) (*see Figure 8.9 (left)*). The regression line showing the trend is based on 187 individual observations. The slope differs significantly from zero ($p < 0.001$) which represents no change in time. During ventricular systole there was a 41% reduction in MRA between 10% and 80% of the normalized regurgitant time. Typical aortic flow and regurgitant mitral flow curves were integrated and the volume changed (normalized by FV) was plotted as a function of time (*see Figure 8.9 (right)*). The resulting curve is sigmoidal with substantial linearity during mid systole. Thus MRA decreases with time in proportion to the decrease in ventricular volume.

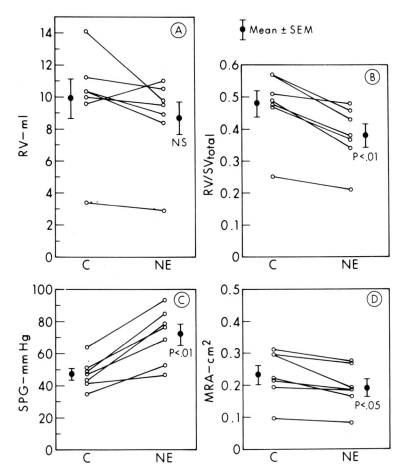

Figure 8.4 Effects of norepinephrine infusion: NE = Norepinephrine; other abbreviations as in *Figure 8.2*. (Reproduced from reference 7, by kind permission of authors and publishers.)

In the dog with the fixed regurgitant orifice size (Bjork–Shiley tilting prosthesis; *see Figure 8.10*) the measured MRA was $30\,mm^2$ ($25\,mm^2$ for the hole and $5\,mm^2$ for the perioccluder space). The calculated MRA derived from the hydraulic formula was $26 \pm 1\,mm^2$ and did not change during ejection. The normalized results are plotted in *Figure 8.9* (left, filled circles).

Discusssion

In previous studies of acute mitral regurgitation the role of the mitral apparatus was eliminated either because an extracardiac cannula between the left atrium and the left ventricle was used[11], or because a perforated tube was advanced from the left atrial appendage through the mitral valve into the left ventricle[12]. In other studies the regurgitant volume was calculated from two different and non-simultaneous methods: applying angiographic methods for the determination of the total cardiac

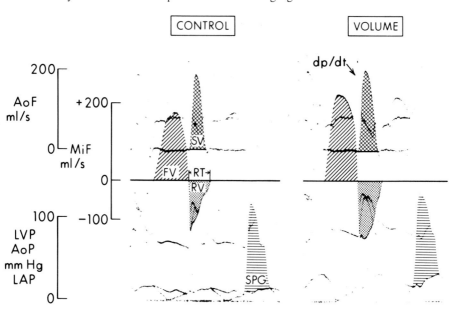

Figure 8.5 Effects of volume loading. Oscillographic records during control and volume loading. Abbreviations as in *Figure 8.1*. Note the large increase in regurgitant volume despite unchanged SPG.

output and dye dilution for the forward cardiac output[9]. In our studies the direct measurement of phasic transmitral flow was obtained by an electromagnetic flow probe placed around the mitral annulus. When combined with measurements of ventricular and atrial pressures and aortic flow we were able to determine filling volume, stroke volume, regurgitant volume, and the effective regurgitant orifice size on a beat-to-beat basis[6-8]. We demonstrated that in acute mitral regurgitation during ventricular systole the effective MRA decreases in a linear fashion to an estimated 59% of its initial value (*See Figure 8.9 (left)*). The decrease in MRA parallels the decrease in left ventricular volume during ejection (*see Figure 8.9 (right)*). The fixed orifice-size study yielded a constant value for the MRA during ventricular ejection. Since the natural valve study did not, we are confident that the probe did not interfere with mitral apparatus function. Moreover, any impairment of annulus mobility would have tended to minimize the changes in MRA.

The decrease in systemic vascular resistance or the decreased impedence to left ventricular ejection is considered by many to be the primary mechanism of the reduction of mitral regurgitation by nitropusside[13, 16]. Our studies indicate that nitroprusside caused a reduction of both peak systolic pressure and left atrial pressure. Thus the systolic pressure gradient was only slightly reduced. The decrease in regurgitation volume cannot be attributed to the small reduction of the SPG. Thirty eight per cent of the decrease in regurgitant volume is due to a decrease in SPG, whereas 62% can be explained by a reduction in the effective MRA. The decrease in left atrial pressure and left ventricular end-diastolic pressure by nitroprusside suggests a reduction in ventricular volume. Thus the venodilation action on the capacitance bed and reduction of ventricular volume by

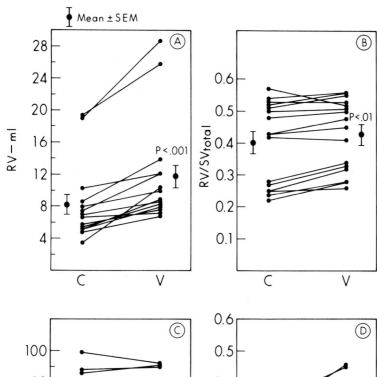

Figure 8.6 Effects of volume loading. V = Volume; other abbreviations as in *Figure 8.2*. (Reproduced from reference 7, by kind permission of authors and publishers.)

nitroprusside and the secondary decrease of the effective regurgitant orifice size is the major mechanism of reduction of mitral regurgitation by nitroprusside[6].

Norepinephrine infusion resulted in a significant increase in the systemic blood pressure and reduction of LVEDP. Despite a substantial increase in the SPG, regurgitant volume remained unchanged. This can be explained only by the significant decrease in MRA (*see Figure 8.4*). The magnitude of mitral regurgitation is related directly to the product of the effective MRA and the square root of the ventricular–atrial pressure gradient. Thus, factors altering the MRA will affect the regurgitation relatively more than similar changes in the SPG. The reduction of ventricular volume (as evidenced by a decrease of LVEDP) is probably the major mechanism which explains the unchanged regurgitant volume despite a significant

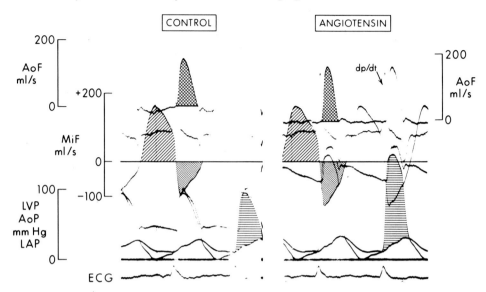

Figure 8.7 Effects of angiotensin infusion. Oscillographic records during control period and angiotensin infusion. Other abbreviations as in *Figure 8.1*. Note the large increases in the systolic pressure gradient (SPG) and regurgitant volume (RV).

increase of SPG by norepinephrine. It has been shown that the mitral leaflets contain muscle fibers which contract synchronously with atrial systole[17, 18] and that at least two-thirds of the mitral valve ring is attached to the base of the left ventricle[19, 20]. It is therefore reasonable to assume that norepinephrine may have a direct effect on the size of the mitral annulus.

Volume loading resulted in a significant increase of the regurgitant volume despite an unchanged SPG (*see Figures 8.5* and *8.6*). The increase in RV which was measured directly from the mitral flow probe could not be derived from the hydraulic formula if the regurgitant orifice remained unchanged. The significant increase of the effective MRA is the only way to explain the substantial increase in RV during volume loading. Thus, the increased mitral regurgitation during volume expansion is due primarily to an increase in the effective MRA secondary to an increase in ventricular volume as inferred from an increase in LVEDP. These findings are in agreement with those of Borgenhagen *et al.*[9].

The administration of angiotensin resulted in significant increases of both peak left ventricular systolic and end diastolic pressures. It has been shown that increased left ventricular afterload changed ventricular geometry. At end diastole the left ventricle became more globular[21] and ejection fraction decreased[22, 23]. With increased LVEDP and reduced ejection fraction the end systolic volume increased, perhaps preventing complete systolic coaptation of the mitral valve leaflets. The increase of ventricular volume and changes in ventricular configuration by angiotensin is the probable mechanism of the increase of the effective MRA which explains the increase of the regurgitant volume not accounted for by the increase of the SPG.

Our findings indicate that in experimental acute mitral insufficiency the regurgitant orifice is not a fixed structure; it can be altered by different hemodynamic factors. The MRA decreases monotonically with time during

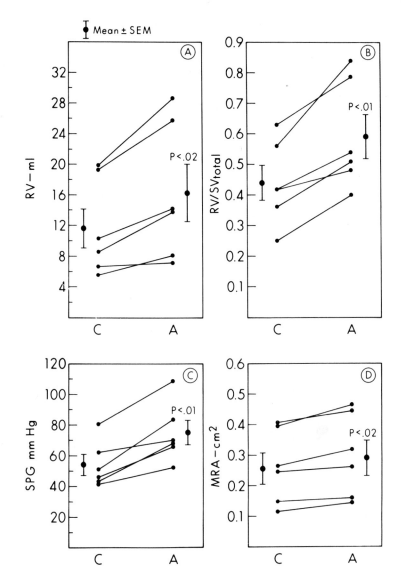

Figure 8.8 Effects of angiotensin infusion. C = Control; A = angiotensin. Other abbreviations as in *Figure 8.2*. (Reproduced from reference 7, by kind permission of authors and publishers.)

ventricular ejection. Increases of ventricular afterload and/or preload enlarges the ventricle, widens the annulus and the regurgitant orifice and increases mitral regurgitant flow. Conversely, reduction in ventricular volume and increased contractility narrows the mitral annulus and the MRA and decreases the regurgitant flow. The relation of this experimental model of acute mitral regurgitation to clinical conditions is only speculative. Nevertheless, it resembles the clinical syndrome of acute mitral regurgitation due to ruptured chordae tendineae of various origins. Our findings support the clinical view that maintaining

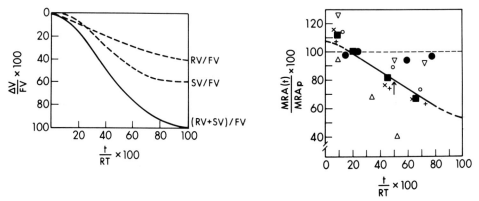

Figure 8.9 (Left) The instantaneous MRA (t) normalized by MRA (p) at peak mitral flow is plotted against time (t) normalized by regurgitant time (RT). The filled squares are the mean values of all points. The SE is too small to show. The data for the fixed orifice (filled circles) are not significant from 100, indicating no change during ejection. *Right:* Changes in ventricular volume during ejection. The change in volume is obtained by adding the regurgitant volume (RV) and forward stroke volume (SV) expressed as a fraction of filling volume (FV). (Reproduced from reference 8, by kind permission of authors and publishers.)

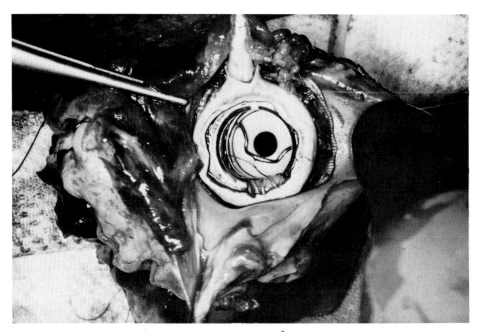

Figure 8.10 A Bjork–Shiley tilting disc prosthesis with 25 mm^2 hole.

a small left ventricle with sustained myocardial contractility will reduce mitral regurgitant flow particularly when the leaflets are mobile.

Acknowledgements

This work could not have been done without the skilled technical help of Messrs A.

Leon, P. Bon and F. Rivera. We thank Ms M. Olivera for typing the manuscript. This work was supported in part by USPHS Grants HL-19391 and HL-24638.

References

1. GORLIN, R. and DEXTER, L. (1952). Hydraulic formula for the calculation of the cross sectional area of the mitral valve during regurgitation. *Am. Heart J.*, **43**, 188
2. SILVERMAN, M.R. and HURST, J.W. (1968). The mitral complex. *Am. Heart J.*, **76**, 399
3. BURCH, G.E., DEPASQUALE, N.P. and PHILLIPS, J.H. (1963). Clinical manifestation of papillary muscle dysfunction. *Arch. Intern. Med.*, **112**, 112
4. BURCH, G.E., DEPASQUALE, N.P. and PHILLIPS, J.H. (1968). The syndrome of papillary muscle dysfunction. *Am. Heart J.*, **75**, 399
5. SHELBURNE, J.C., RUBENSTEIN, D. and GORLIN, R. (1968). The significance of papillary muscle dysfunction in coronary artery disease. *Clin. Res.*, **16**, 249
6. YORAN, C., YELLIN, E.L., BECKER, R.M., GABBAY, S., FRATER, R.W.M. and SONNENBLICK, E.H. (1979). Mechanism for reduction of mitral regurgitation with vasodilator therapy. *Am. J. Cardiol.*, **43**, 773
7. YORAN, C., YELLIN, E.L., BECKER, R.M., GABBAY, S., FRATER, R.W.M. and SONNENBLICK, E.H. (1979). Dynamic aspects of mitral regurgitation: Effects of ventricular volume, pressure and contractility on the effective regurgitant orifice area. *Circulation*, **60**, 170
8. YELLIN, E.L., YORAN, C., SONNENBLICK, E.H., GABBAY, S. and FRATER, R.W.M. (1979). Dynamic changes in the canine mitral regurgitant orifice area during ventricular ejection. *Circulation Research*, **45**, 677
9. BORGENHAGEN, D.M., SERUR, J.R., GORLIN, R., ADAMS, D. and SONNENBLICK, E.H. (1977). The effects of the left ventricular load and contractility on mitral regurgitation orifice size and flow in the dog. *Circulation*, **56**, 106
10. LANIADO, S., YELLIN, E.L., MILLER, H. and FRATER, R.W.M. (1973). Temporal relation of the first heart sound to closure of the mitral valve. *Circulation*, **47**, 1006
11. BRAUNWALD, E., WELCH, G.H., JR and SARNOFF, S.J. (1957). Hemodynamic effects of quantitatively varied experimental mitral regurgitation. *Circ. Res.*, **5**, 539
12. BRAUNWALD, E., WELCH, G.H. and MORROW A.G. (1958). The effects of acutely increased systemic resistance on the left atrial pressure pulse: A method for the clinical detection of mitral insufficiency. *J. Clin. Invest.*, **37**, 35
13. CHATTERJEE, K., PARMLEY, W.W., SWAN, H.J.C., BERMAN, G., FORRESTER, J. and MARCUS, H.S. (1973). Beneficial effects of vasodilator agents in severe mitral regurgitation due to dysfunction of subvalvular apparatus. *Circulation*, **48**, 684
14. GOODMAN, D.J., ROSSEN, R.M., HOLLOWAY, E.L., ALDERMAN, E.L. and HARRISON, D.C. (1974). Effect of nitroprusside on left ventricular dynamics in mitral regurgitation. *Circulation*, **50**, 1025
15. HARSHAW, C.W., GROSSMAN, W., MUNRO, A.B. and MCLAURIN, L.P. (1975). Reduced systemic vascular resistance as therapy for severe mitral regurgitation of valvular origin. *Ann. Intern. Med.*, **83**, 313–316
16. CHATTERJEE, K. and PARMLEY, W.W. (1977). The role of vasodilator therapy in heart failure. *Prog. Cardiovasc. Dis.*, **19**, 301
17. SONNENBLICK, E.H., NAPOLITANO, L.M., DAGGETT, W.M. and COOPER, T. (1967). An intrinsic neuro-muscular basis for mitral valve motion in the dog. *Circ. Res.*, **21**, 9
18. FENOGLIO, J.J., JR, PHAM, T.D., WIT, A.L., BASSETT, A.L. and WAGNER, B.M. (1972). Canine mitral complex: ultrastructure and electromechanical properties. *Circ. Res.*, **31**, 417
19. FRATER, R.W.M. and ELLIS, F.H. JR (1961). The anatomy of the canine mitral valve: with notes on function and comparisons with other mammalian mitral valves. *J. Surg. Res.*, **1**, 171
20. FRATER, R.W.M. (1961). Mitral valve anatomy and prosthetic valve design. *Mayo Clin. Proc.*, **36**, 582
21. LIEDTKE, A.J., PASTERNAC, A., SONNENBLICK, E.H. and GORLIN, R. (1972). Changes in canine ventricular dimensions with acute changes in preload and after load. *Am. J. Physiol.*, **223**, 820
22. TSAKIRIS, A.G., VANDENBERG, R.A., BANCHERO, H., STRUM, R.E. and WOOD, E.H. (1968). Variations of left ventricular end diastolic pressure, volume, and ejection fraction with changes in outflow resistance in anesthetized intact dogs. *Circ. Res.*, **23**, 213
23. CARLETON, R.A. and CLARK, J.G. (1968). Measurement of left ventricular diameter in the dog by cardiac catheterization. Validation and physiologic meaningfulness of an ultrasonic technique. *Circ. Res.*, **22**, 545

9

Uses and limitations of echocardiography in the examination of the mitral valve

Nelson B. Schiller

In institutions where echocardiography is competently performed, it is often the first method employed when mitral valve disease is clinically suspected. The purpose of this chapter will be to examine the capabilities and limitations of echocardiography as a method of examining and characterizing the normal and morbid appearance and behavior of the mitral valve and its supporting apparatus.

Echocardiography and the mitral valve: Historical aspects

In 1953, Edler and Hertz[1] reported the first clinical experience with the use of pulsed ultrasound to image cardiac structures. Using so-called M-mode methods, reflections resulting from the interaction of a single beam of ultrasound with a cardiac target could be photographically traced. These tracings clearly recorded the rapid motion of the mitral valve and led to the observation that mitral stenosis predictably and reliably altered this pattern. Although the observations of Edler and Hertz were later validated by many workers, it was 15 years before initial acceptance of their methods. As late as 1971, prominent investigators were still expressing doubt concerning the validity of echocardiography as a tool for evaluating the mitral valve[2]. In 1964, just 10 years after their classic paper, Hertz published the first pictures of a system designed to produce two-dimensional real-time images of the heart[3]. It was 10 years after this demonstration that rapid proliferation of the two-dimensional technique began. Today, M-mode and two-dimensional methods are used in tandom for the routine clinical evaluation of the mitral valve.

Echocardiograpy of the normal mitral valve

An adequate echocardiographic examination should consist of both an M-mode tracing and a real-time two-dimensional interrogation of cardiac structures[4].

In our laboratory, we examine patients through a variety of anatomic 'windows'. These windows are loci in the suprasternal notch, thorax and abdomen through which ultrasonic energy can travel to the target, reflect and return to the sending/receiving transducer. The most important requirement for such windows is that there be a minimum of bone, air or air-containing tissue (lung, bowel, etc.) between the transducer and the target. We routinely use the precordial parasternal, precordial apical and subcostal windows to image the mitral valve. M-mode echo which consists of a single beam of ultrasound with a high repetition rate (1000/s) is used to demonstrate motion of individual leaflets or scallops and two-dimensional echocardiography is used to look at the integrated motion of larger portions of the valve and its relation to surrounding structures. The two-dimensional imaging format has the advantage of presenting anatomy as real-time, moderately well-resolved tomographic slices and the disadvantage of a relatively slow frame rate (30 frames/s or less).

The normal mitral valve is very difficult to image by other methods. Angiography sometimes shows the valve as a linear filling defect while scintigraphy or conventional radiographic techniques cannot image it at all. Conversely, because of its position normal to the ultrasound beam and acoustic properties the mitral valve is one of the easiest targets in the heart from which to detect reflected sound waves. On M-mode examination, the normal valve exhibits a rather complex motion pattern which accurately reflects the phasic nature of ventricular filling. The familiar M-shaped motion pattern of the mitral valve is shown in *Figure 9.1*. The early large opening movement of the valve (movement toward the top of the picture is anterior) is the result of early passive rapid filling and the second reopening the result of atrial contraction. Note that the valve has assumed a nearly

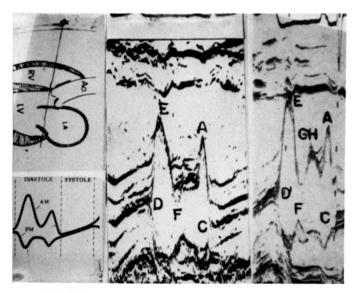

Figure 9.1 Left: Diagrammatic representation of the long axis of the heart showing a single M-mode beam of ultrasound traversing both inferior and posterior mitral leaflets. Schematically shown below is a diagram of the M-mode echographic pattern resulting from the interaction of the ultrasound beam with the anterior (am) and posterior (pm) leaflets. The valve moves in diastole in an M-shaped pattern but in systole both leaflets are applied to one another and migrate slightly from posterior to anterior. In the right two panels are shown actual echographic tracings of two mitral valves. The letters identify various events in the complex diastolic motion pattern. In particular, the E point is the peak anterior valve motion during the early passive phase of diastole. The A wave is the result of active atrial contraction just prior to the onset of systole. The F, G and H waves are diastasis waves best seen at slow heart rates.

closed position in the middle of diastole, reflecting near parity between atrial and ventricular pressures.

The two-dimensional appearance of the mitral valve depends somewhat upon the projection from which it is viewed. For example, in the short axis plane, the valve presents itself as an ovoid orifice while on long axis it assumes the appearance of clapping hands, with the upper hand longer and more mobile than the lower. *Figure 9.2* is a long axis view of the mitral valve taken during systole. *Figure 9.3 (left)* shows the longer anterior leaflet (aortic leaflet) in coaptation with the shorter posterior (mural). This image of the valve was taken in the apical four chamber long axis view.

In general, the normal mitral valve should appear as a mobile two-leaflet structure which moves freely enough to respond to the normal flux of diastolic

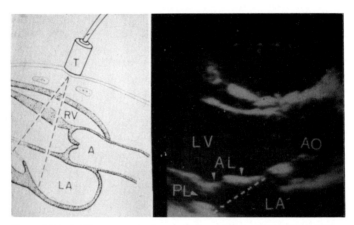

Figure 9.2 Left: Diagrammatic, long axis view of the ventricle obtained from the precordium. *Right:* Echogram obtained during systole. Note that the aortic leaflets are open while the mitral leaflets (AL and PL) are closed. The line was drawn along the plane of the mitral annulus. Note that the mitral leaflets normally close on the ventricular side of this line. In fact, there is usually a small volume of atrial blood on the ventricular side of this line. In mitral prolapse, the posterior and anterior leaflets may cross this line and enter the left atrium during systole.

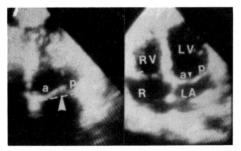

Figure 9.3 The anterior (a) and posterior (p) leaflets are shown in a normal individual on the left and in an individual with mitral prolapse on the right. Both images were obtained from the apical four-chamber view. In the normal individual the coaptation of the leaflets occurs on the ventricular side of the line drawn along the plane of the mitral annulus. Also, the posterior leaflet is much shorter than the anterior. In the mitral prolapse patient the valve is inverted and traverses the mitral annulus so that all or part of the valve is situated on the atrial side of the annulus during systole. Note that the posterior leaflet is prominent when compared with the normal.

filling (i.e. rapid filling, conduit phase and atrial contraction) but which forms a stable coaptation plane in systole without entering the left atrium. In fact, in normal cardiac function, the mitral valve remains on the ventricular side of the annular plane and descends towards the apex against the pressure gradient as the longitudinal ventricular muscle fibers shorten in the long axis of the chamber. This descent of the base, of which the mitral valve is an essential element, is probably the most important contributor to atrial filling.

Other anatomic features of the mitral apparatus appreciated on two-dimensional echographic examiation are the papillary muscles and glimpses of the chordae tendineae. Skill in visualizing the papillary muscles can contribute to the assessment of subvalvular rheumatic changes.

Pathologic alterations of the mitral valve recognizable by echocardiography

Lesions with inflow obstruction

MITRAL STENOSIS, ACQUIRED

One of the first lesions to be recognized by echocardiography was rheumatic mitral stenosis. The changes in the appearance and pattern of motion induced by chronic rheumatic scarring are easily recognized in that they produce primary alterations in the valve's echocardiographic appearance and secondary changes in other structures. *Figure 9.4* contrasts the appearance of a normal mitral valve in the upper panel with that of a rheumatic valve. Among the earliest observations by

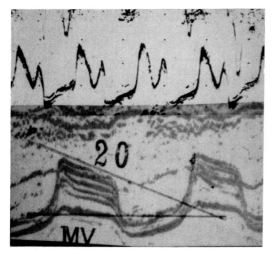

Figure 9.4 Upper panel depicts the anterior leaflet of a normal mitral valve. The lower panel depicts the anterior and posterior leaflets of a stenotic mitral valve. Note that the single thin line representing the anterior leaflets has been replaced by five parallel lines of increased density. Note also that the posterior leaflet moves in parallel with these five lines rather than independently. The method for computing the slope of the valve is shown. By extending the diastolic posterior closing motion of the stenotic valve for a full second the number of millimetres in the anterior to posterior direction which the valve traverses per second can be calculated. In this valve, the early diastolic filling slope was computed at 20 mm/s.

Edler[5] was that mitral stenosis was associated with a decreased early diastolic anterior mitral leaflet passive closing velocity. He also noted that the degree of closing slope slowing was a rough guide to the severity of stenosis. Our own research[4] suggests that the only way to improve the reliability of the mitral diastolic slope as a predictor of mitral stenosis severity is to take into account respiratory cycle influence on mitral slope (additive or subtractive effect of gross cardiac motion simultaneous with valve opening) by measuring slope at the same part of the respiratory cycle. *Figure 9.4 (lower)* demonstrates the method of measuring mitral slope by extrapolating diastolic motion over 1 s and calculating the anterior to posterior motion in mm per second. In this example, the slope is 20 mm/s. Note also that the abnormal valve in the lower panel also differs from the normal because it gives rise to multiple echoes rather than a single linear reflection and that it has lost the second reopening deflection (*a*-wave) of atrial contraction. The loss of presystolic reopening can occur in the presence of sinus rhythm, although in this situation the rheumatic valve will usually have slight pre-systolic anterior motion.

Secondary changes appearing on echographic studies of patients with mitral stenosis are left atrial enlargement, decreased left ventricular cavity dimension and tricuspid thickening. These changes and the primary alterations in valve appearance form a constellation of redundant information introducing considerable certainty into the diagnosis of mitral stenosis and assessment of its severity.

When Henry[6] demonstrated that two-dimensional echocardiography could accurately measure the stenotic mitral valve orifice, this technique received an important stimulus toward its acceptance. *Figure 9.5* demonstrates Henry's method of valve planimetry performed by digitizing the stop-frame video image of an early diastolic short axis frame of the valve. The minicomputer controlled analysis system displays the arc length of the valve orifice perimeter and the area it subtends. This latter value is the valve area and is a measurement that has been repeatedly validated as probably being the single most reliable method of assessing the severity of mitral stenosis. In fact, its only shortcoming appears to be that in 10–15% of patients adequate studies for measurement cannot be obtained. In these individuals either the valve is not imaged well or the valve is too heavily calcified to allow clear delineation of the valve's limiting orifice. In *Figure 9.5*, the valves depicted range in orifice area from $1.5\,cm^2$ to $4\,cm^2$. In the largest valve the degree of narrowing is trivial and the major hemodynamic abnormality is mitral regurgitation. In rheumatic mitral regurgitation the echocardiogram shows failure of valve leaflet coaptation, the degree of which is proportional to the severity of regurgitation[7].

Does the ability of two-dimensional echocardiography to measure accurately the mitral valve orifice overturn the use of M-mode echocardiography in recognizing the pattern of mitral stenosis? Our own experience suggests that the answer is no. In most cases of moderate to severe mitral stenosis, the two-dimensional appearance of a small left ventricle sitting atop a spherical, enlarged left atrium provides an important qualitative clue to the diagnosis.

Figure 9.6 shows a long axis image from a patient with mitral stenosis. The large left atrium, small left ventricle and thickened valve leaflets can be appreciated. However, the appearance of the valve in a stop-frame two-dimensional image suggests rather subtle abnormalities. A simultaneous M-mode study shown in the lower panel demonstrates the typical appearance of the mitral valve which confirms the diagnosis of rheumatic mitral stenosis. Stenosis severity can be assessed by planimetry of the short axis early diastolic orifice. Thus, the combination of two-dimensional and M-mode methods are additive and not competitive.

OTHER LESIONS CAUSING INFLOW OBSTRUCTION

Calcified mitral annulus is a very common echocardiographic entity which is usually not associated with hemodynamically important mitral insufficiency or stenosis. This degenerative condition is most strongly associated with age, although IHSS and secondary hyperparathyroidism of renal disease have also been associated with annular calcification. In a few patients the degree of calcification and the extent of infiltration into the valve leaflets and other portions of the valve apparatus becomes so severe that hemodynamically significant inflow obstruction (sometimes severe) can result. Except for demonstrating severe distortion of the valve apparatus by dense persistent echoes, two-dimensional echocardiography is not highly effective in differentiating extensive annulus disease without inflow obstruction from the same condition with obstruction.

Congenital conditions that result in mitral stenosis are relatively rare. However, in adults conditions are encountered such as cor triatriatum. Parachute mitral valve (single papillary muscle) and supravalvar mitral stenosis are almost exclusively problems of pediatric populations. Echocardiography is highly effective in diagnosing these conditions as well as other obstructive lesions such as left atrial myxoma, large obstructive vegetation or mitral stenosis resulting from bronchial carcinoid syndrome. Although the carcinoid syndrome is 'rare' we have encountered 18 of these individuals in the past 9 years, two of whom had bronchial carcinoid.

Echocardiography of mitral valve abnormalities associated with mitral regurgitation

Stenotic lesions alter the diastolic motion pattern of the mitral valve and are readily identifiable by M-mode echocardiography. Conversely, lesions associated with mitral insufficiency are often associated with subtle abnormalities of the mitral valve elements and are commonly not recognizable. Furthermore, since mitral motion during systole is normally minimal and since dysfunction of small, localized portions of the valve can result in significant regurgitation, M-mode echocardiography may miss the abnormality and two-dimensional imaging may fail to resolve it. Doppler ultrasound flow analysis and detection techniques can locate small, high-velocity, regurgitant jets and with further validation may emerge as the method of choice for the positive identification of mitral insufficiency.

RHEUMATIC MITRAL REGURGITATION

Usually, the scarring associated with the rheumatic process results in characteristic alterations in the valve's M-mode motion pattern. Even when stenosis is minimal or undetectable, the valve area is usually sufficiently reduced to alter its closure rate, sufficiently thickened to alter its echographic appearance and sufficiently narrowed to separate it readily from normal. Finally, failure of coaptation can be seen during systole on a short axis image and its extent is proportional to the severity of regurgitation. Unfortunately, rheumatic mitral regurgitation is the only regurgitant lesion identifiable by inspection of the two-dimensional systolic appearance of the valve. *Figure 9.5* is a case of rheumatic mitral regurgitation and shows a valve area of $4\,cm^2$. Since normal mitral valves in individuals with normal cardiac output have valve areas of $6–8\,cm^2$, this valve is anatomically but not hemodynamically stenotic. In the lower panel of *Figure 9.5(c)*, note that coaptation of most of the valve

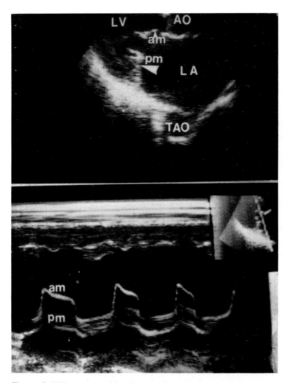

Figure 9.6 Upper panel is a long axis two-dimensional stop-frame image taken during diastole. In comparison with *Figure 9.2*, note the left atrium is considerably enlarged relative to the size of the left ventricle and aorta. The thoracic aorta (TAO) is also clearly seen. An M-mode beam has been passed through the anterior and posterior mitral leaflets, and lower panel clearly shows the rheumatic pattern of motion. Once again, the anterior and posterior mitral leaflets (am and pm) are moving in parallel during diastole rather than independently.

inapparent, in a significant number it was associated with discomfort, disability, or even sudden death.

The accumulation of experience with the echocardiographic diagnosis of mitral prolapse has also seen the emergence of a number of problems that attended its use. Some of these problems can be eliminated by the addition of two-dimensional echocardiographic techniques.

Research by Markiewicz et al.[12] provided information relating to the sensitivity of M-mode echo in mitral prolapse. They showed that if one considers the presence of a late systolic murmur, click, or both as evidence of mitral prolapse, then M-mode echocardiography was falsely negative about 40% of the time. This group, among others, also drew attention to the potential of apocryphally producing an echocardiographic prolapse pattern by having the ultrasound beam intercept the mitral valve from a superior angle.

Work by Bon Tempo et al.[13] and Salomon et al.[14] pointed out that chest wall deformities in mitral prolapse are very common. In fact, up to 75% of individuals with prolapse have radiographic evidence of a thoracic skeletal abnormality. In our experience, such deformities frequently frustrate our attempts to gain proper transducer placement and are a major cause of technically inadequate single-beam M-mode studies.

Among other deficiences of M-mode echocardiography are its inability to evaluate comprehensively leaflet thickening and deformity, its insensitivity to tricuspid prolapse, its inability to detect aortic valve prolapse and its limited ability to evaluate the aortic root. The failings are significant because they limit appreciation of the spectrum of related and, at times, clinically important abnormalities in persons with mitral prolapse.

In our own laboratory, we have been impressed with the number of patients who, in addition to mitral prolapse, have prolapse of both their aortic and tricuspid valves. This combination of abnormalities has been termed the multiple myxomatous valve syndrome. It is estimated by Rippe et al.[15], perhaps conservatively, that 3% of individuals with mitral prolapse have this syndrome.

Finally, it has been our experience that although an obvious mitral prolapse pattern on M-mode studies, in the absence of pericardial effusion, is diagnostic of the condition, many persons present mitral systolic motion patterns that are ambiguous. In some of these persons a well-recorded mid systolic click or late murmur can influence interpretation of these patterns. In persons with normal auscultatory findings, however, no diagnosis can or should be made.

Given both the incomplete information provided by an M-mode echocardiographic study and its lack of sensitivity, the accelerating availability of two-dimensional echocardiographic techniques has been a welcome occurrence that directly affects our approach to the non-invasive evaluation of patients suspected of having mitral valve prolapse.

This modality allows the production of two-dimensional tomographic images of the mitral valve from at least five standard views. Thus, it is possible to view virtually every portion of the valve in relationship to other internal landmarks, such as the atrioventriuclar ring. The initial descriptions of the two-dimensional echocardiographic findings were made independently by both Gilbert et al.[16] and Sahn et al.[17], who in 1976 described the behaviour of prolapsing valves that were imaged in the long axis, tomographic views from a precordial window. From this view, which images the mitral leaflets and atrioventricular ring attachments in the plane of the aortic root, these groups observed displacement of the point of systolic leaflet coaptation, from its normal location in the ventricle, toward the atrioventricular ring or across it into the left atrium. They also observed that in the process of abnormal posterior valve displacement, the leaflets buckle, or arch, the anterior leaflet forming an abnormal angle with the aortic posterior wall. They also commented on the hyperdynamic appearance of the posterior mitral annulus. Additionally, we have observed that in systole the valve appears to develop an elastic appearance as it protrudes into the mitral annulus. Normally, the mitral valve descends, with the base and the atrioventricular ring, toward the left ventricular apex. Since a prolapsing mitral valve moves in the opposite direction, that is, toward the atrium, an illusion of hypermobility is created. This illusion is analogous to the sensation of increased speed that occurs in rail passengers when a train passes in the opposite direction.

We have found the apical two-chamber and four-chamber views (see Figure 9.3) particularly helpful in the diagnosis of prolapse but not necessarily superior to the precordial long axis view.

Leaflet thickening and deformity, particularly of the posterior leaflet scallops and the chordal insertions, can be very marked in mitral prolapse. Although the implications of marked deformity of the valve have not been studied, it is our impression that such patients form a subset with higher morbidity. Two-dimensional imaging clearly identifies patients with deformed valves.

In patients with involvement of other valves, two-dimensional echocardiography also allows detection of tricuspid and aortic valve prolapse. In patients suspected of having Marfan's syndrome, detection of dilatation limited to the root of the aorta can be almost diagnostic of the condition. Mitral prolapse is common in atrial defects[18] and in Ebstein's anomaly. Two-dimensional echocardiography is effective in excluding the possibility of such defects. Segmental wall motion abnormalities associated with ischemic heart disease can occasionally be accompanied by late systolic murmurs. Segmental wall abnormalities associated with previous myocardial infarction can be effectively detected by two-dimensional echocardiography, and these patients differentiated from those with prolapse. Confirming earlier experience, Barnett et al.[19] have recently reported that, of patients under 45 years of age who have had a cerebrovascular ischemic event, 40% have M-mode evidence of mitral prolapse. Other workers using two-dimensional echocardiography have recently reported detecting small mobile masses, presumed to be embologenic thrombi at the posterior mitral valve leaflet base[20].

The capabilities of the two-dimensional technique in mitral prolapse must be weighed against its limitations. Although the superior time resolution of M-mode echocardiography can often provide a firm diagnosis of mitral prolapse, the two-dimensional echocardiogram imposes the difficult requirement that rapidly moving structures be evaluated qualitatively. Although it is reasonable to assume that a quantitative approach to the behaviour of the mitral valve would facilitate the diagnosis of prolapse, the lack of an acceptable reference standard for the diagnosis of prolapse makes the development of a quantitative method very difficult. As stated earlier, M-mode echocardiography not infrequently presents findings that are ambiguous. Although two-dimensional echocardiography often provides clarification in these situations, the two-dimensional study can also be ambiguous. Since it is not known whether mitral prolapse is in a continuum with normal or an all-or-none entity, the dividing line between normal and abnormal findings is simply not known. Two-dimensional studies falling between those that are obviously normal and those that are not are of necessity ambiguous.

M-mode echocardiography does not have a monopoly on technical problems. Although two-dimensional echocardiography greatly reduces the number of patients in whom technical problems, such as chest deformities, prevent adequate evaluation, it has many pitfalls for the inexperienced. For example, only one scallop of the posterior leaflet may be abnormal. As this scallop may be seen only in one view, failure to perform a complete examination may introduce error. Another common error is confusing the mitral annulus with the coapted leaflets and falsely concluding that the coapted leaflets are posteriorly displaced.

Provocative maneuvers for mitral valve prolapse, performed with M-mode echocardiography, have been proposed but are generally unsuccessful. The major problem with these maneuvers is that it is difficult to maintain transducer position during the peak effect of the maneuver. For example, if the patient is instructed to squat, there is usually a change in the orientation of the heart and in the pattern of respiration. If, while the patient is squatting, it is possible to obtain an echocardiogram of the mitral valve, one cannot be assured that the orientation of the ultrasonic beam employed in the resting tracing was maintained during provocation. Administration of amyl nitrite may cause the patient to cough or become somewhat restless, introducing difficulties in obtaining adequate images.

Our experience suggests that the most productive time for imaging the valve occurs after the initial tachycardia induced by amyl nitrite has subsided.

In conclusion, after an experience of almost 5 years, we believe that two-dimensional echocardiography will have a growing role in the evaluation of mitral valve prolapse because it is the single most effective tool available for this purpose. Its effectiveness is enhanced when it is used in conjunction with M-mode echocardiography, particularly when the latter is combined with simultaneous phonocardiography. It must be emphasized that technical expertise in this application of two-dimensional echocardiography is mandatory, and it is further emphasized that even under ideal circumstances a number of studies will be ambiguous. Finally and most importantly, the application of ultrasound imaging to the evaluation of patients suspected of mitral valve prolapse and the interpretation of the results must be completely governed by thorough evaluation of the patient and by sound clinical judgement.

CALCIFICATION OF THE MITRAL ANNULUS

Calcification in and around the mitral annulus is extremely common in patients over 60 years of age. Echocardiography effectively identifies this condition but often fails in assessing the severity of associated mitral regurgitation. Secondary evidence of mitral insufficiency such as atrial enlargement can occasionally be helpful in assessing the severity of regurgitation, but associated conditions such as hypertrophy or atrial fibrillation often weaken this evidence. Also, calcification of the mitral ring appears to be more common in conditions such as hypertrophic obstructive cardiomyopathy and secondary hyperparathyroidism of renal disease. In our experience, older individuals with marked annulus calcification and mitral regurgitation are often found on echocardiography to have associated mitral valve prolapse. Thus, the identification of annular calcification is in no way tantamount to identifying the cause of mitral regurgitation or its severity.

MITRAL INSUFFICIENCY ASSOCIATED WITH ISCHEMIA OR INFARCTION OF THE LEFT VENTRICLE

It is well known that coronary artery disease can alter the integrity of the mitral apparatus by interfering with the contractility of muscle groups associated with chordal support[2]. When the ventricular wall to which the papillary muscle is attached becomes ischemic or is infarcted, systolic chordal tension levels necessary for maintaining mitral coaptation do not develop and various degrees of mitral insufficiency ensue. Perversion of the muscular component of mitral support can occur when the base of support of the muscle is temporarily ischemic during angina and can be associated with transient mitral insuffiency. It can also occur when myocardial infarction permanently damages the wall supporting the papillary muscle in which case the mitral regurgitation is permanent and can range from mild to severe in degree.

Finally, necrotic disruption of the mitral valve (ruptured papillary muscle) can lead to severe, often fatal, mitral insufficiency. In our experience, the appearance of the papillary muscle itself seldom gives any clue to the presence or severity of papillary muscle disorders. Calcification of the muscle tips, while common, is seldom associated with mitral regurgitation. On the other hand, the presence of a large inferior basal dyskinetic wall segment, particularly if it surrounds or reaches the base of the papillary muscle, is strong evidence for an ischemic origin of clinically detected mitral regurgitation. In addition to malalignment of the papillary muscles, we have found an apically displaced mitral coaptation point to be of little help in differentiating patients with ischemic mitral regurgitation from those with 'cardiogenic' regurgitation arising from diffuse cardiomyopathy. Our views are consistent with the work of Cohen *et al.*[24-24], who observed that ligation of the papillary muscle was not sufficient to cause mitral insufficiency. Since ischemic mitral insufficiency almost always suggests involvement of a fairly large segment of myocardium, the term papillary muscle dysfunction[25] is probably a misnomer.

DISRUPTION OF THE MITRAL VALVE DUE TO INFECTION OF CHORDAL RUPTURE

Vegetations arising in association with endocarditis of the mitral valve can cause mitral insufficiency by interfering with closure of the valve or by causing disruption of leaflet and/or chordal continuity. Usually, patients with endocarditis and valve disruption can be identified by a constellation of findings. Prominent among these findings is the detection of a mass on the valve. Such masses are often assumed to represent vegetations but, on occasion, a healed vegetation, an area of myxomatous change or a torn leaflet can mimic a true vegetation. The clinical setting can often be of considerable importance in determining the importance of an echographically detected mass lesion. On the other hand, many patients with endocarditis who are early in the course of their illness may have an entirely normal echographic examination.

In the examination of mitral mass lesions or suspected endocarditis, M-mode echocardiography is extremely helpful in that disrupted portions of the mitral valve usually exhibit systolic vibrations of the limited portion of the leaflet that has become untethered or flail.

Figure 9.7 demonstrates a leaflet tip vegetation attached to the posterior leaflet. During diastole (D) a mobile, dense echo moves into the left ventricular cavity. During systole, the mass crosses the AV ring and enters the left atrium. This latter finding is typical of mitral disruption. In this case a diagnosis of endocarditis was correctly made because of clinical considerations and because of the fluffy appearance of the valve. However, a chronic vegetation (i.e. healed and fibrous or calcified) or a chorda attached to a detached myxomatously thickened valve fragment can mimic the appearance of an active bulky vegetation. When vegetation with local valve destruction is suspected, it is important to obtain an M-mode tracing through the diseased portion of the valve. Systolic vibrations of a thickened and freely mobile portion of a valve are diagnostic of vegetation and/or disruption. Visual inspection of a 30 frames/s two-dimensional image cannot usually detect these diagnostically important systolic vibrations. M-mode, with a sampling frequency of 1000/s, is ideally suited to this application.

CARDIOGENIC MITRAL INSUFFICIENCY

When the left ventricle dilates and becomes hypokinetic, poor systolic emptying leaves the papillary muscles in a position where they exert lateral tension on the mitral valve rather than tension along the ventrical axis of the ventricle[21]. This malalignment leads to mitral insufficiency, often well-appreciated on physical examination but almost impossible to detect with conventional M-mode and two-dimensional techniques. Regardless of whether mitral insufficiency is present,

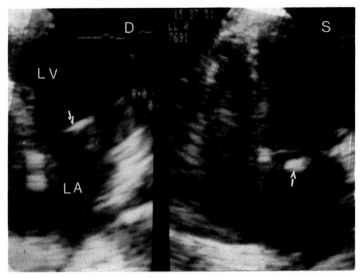

Figure 9.7 In the left panel the arrow points to a thickened portion of the tip posterior mitral leaflet which probably is an attached vegetation. In the systolic panel at the right this mobile, fluffy structure has moved from the ventricle across the mitral annulus and is now seen prolapsed into the left atrium. Notice that the anterior leaflet still appears to be in the correct position just above the mitral annulus. When one leaflet moves well beyond the systolic position of the other, a ruptured chordae tendineae is almost always present.

the ventricles of patients with cardiomyopathy are spherical rather than elliptical and have poor mitral excursion. The combination of poor mitral opening into a large residual end-systolic volume leads to significant mitral septal separation. In 'pure' mitral insufficiency and a normal ventricle, the mitral valve opens onto the septal endocardium. Thus, a dilated, poorly contracting left ventricle with mitral septal separation in a patient with a mitral regurgitation murmur is highly suggestive, if not diagnostic, of cardiomyopathy with secondary mitral insufficiency. On the other hand, a dilated, hyperdynamic ventricle with a large anterior mitral excursion is highly suggestive of valvular mitral insufficiency.

In ischemic heart disease, mitral insufficiency often arises when there is extensive inferobasal myocardial infarction. In these patients the base of attachment for the posteromedial papillary muscle is damaged or destroyed and no longer offers an appropriately timed and sufficiently strong contraction necessary for valve competence.

Quantitative echocardiography in the evaluation of mitral insufficiency

An extensive discussion about the quantitative aspects of echocardiography and about their application to patients with mitral valve disease is beyond the scope of this chapter. A number of studies have established that echocardiography can measure the size of the left ventricle and atrium[26, 27]. In order to use the measurement capabilities of ultrasound, one must be aware of normal population echocardiographic data and with correlation of echocardiographic and angiographic studies. Very recently, normal data became available[28, 29] and can now be used to assess degree of departure from normality in a given patient.

In conclusion, echocardiography is an extremely powerful tool for the study of the mitral valve. It has both clinical and research applications and, when mitral valve disease is suspected, should function as one of the first diagnostic modalities employed.

References

1. EDLER, I. and HERTZ, C.H. (1954). The use of the ultrasonic reflectoscope for the continuous recording of movements of heart walls. *Kungl Fysiogr Sallsk Lund Forhandl*, **24**, 5
2. DOCK, W. (1971). Ultrasonic echoes (Letter). *Circulation*, **44**, 487
3. HERTZ, C.H. (1964). Ultrasonic heart investigation. *Med. Electron. Biol. Eng.*, **2**, 39
4. SCHILLER, N.B. (1981). Interactions of M-mode and two-dimensional echocardiography. In *Diagnostic Echocardiography* (eds. J.W. Linhart and C.R. Joyner). St. Louis, Mo: Mosby Co.
5. EDLER, I. and GUSTAFSON, A. (1957). Ultrasonic cardiogram in mitral stenosis: Preliminary communication. *Acta. Med. Scandinav.*, **159**, 85
6. HENRY W.L., GRIFFITH, J.M., MICHAELIS, L.L., *et al.* (1975). Measurement of mitral orifice area in patients with mitral valve disease by real-time, two-dimensional echocardiography. *Circulation*, **51**, 827
7. WANN, L.S., FEIGENBAUM, H., WEYMAN, A.E. and DILLON, J.C. (1978). Detection of rheumatic mitral regurgitation using cross-sectional echocardiography. *Am. J. Cardiol.*, **41**, 1258
8. BARLOW, J.B. and BOSMAN, C.K. (1966). Aneurysmal protusion of the posterior leaflet of the mitral valve. *Am. Heart J.*, **71**, 166
9. DILLON, J.C., HAINE, C.L., CHANG, S. and FEIGENBAUM, H. (1971). Use of echocardiography in patients with prolapsed mitral valve. *Am. J. Cardiol.*, **43**, 503
10. KERBER, R.E., ISAEFF, D.M. and HANCOCK, E.W. (1971). Echocardiographic patterns in patients with the syndrome of systolic click and late systolic murmur. *N. Engl. J. Med.*, **284**, 691
11. SHAH, P.M. and GRAMIAK, R. (1970). Echocardiographic recognition of mitral valve prolapse (abstract). *Circulation*, **42** (Suppl. 3), 45
12. MARKIEWICZ, W., STONER, J., LONDON, E., *et al.* (1976). Mitral valve prolapse in one hundred presumably healthy young females. *Circulation*, **53**, 464
13. BON TEMPO, C.P., RONAN, J.A., JR., DE LEON, A.C., JR. and TWIGG, H.L. (1975). Radiographic appearance of the thorax in systolic click-late systolic murmur syndrome. *Am. J. Cardiol.*, **36**, 27
14. SALOMON, J, SHAH, P.M. and HEINLE, R.A. (1975). Thoracic skeletal abnormalities in idiopathic mitral valve prolapse. *Am. J. Cardiol.*. **36**, 32
15. RIPPE, J.M., ANGOFF, G., SLOSS, L.J., *et al.* (1979). Multiple floppy valves: an echo-cardiographic syndrome. *Am. J. Med.*, **66**, 817
16. GILBERT, B.W., SCHATZ, R.A., VON RAMM, O.T., *et al.* (1976). Mitral valve prolapse: two-dimensional echocardiographic and angiographic correlation. *Circulation*, **54**, 716
17. SAHN, D.J., ALLEN, H.D., GOLDBERG, S.J. and FRIEDMAN, W.F. (1976). Mitral valve prolapse in children: a problem defined by real-time cross-sectional echocardiography. *Circulation*, **53**, 651
18. LEACHMAN, R.D., COKKINOS, D.V. and COOLEY, D.A. (1976). Associate of ostium secundum atrial septal defects with mitral valve prolapse. *Am. J. Cardiol.*, **38**, 167
19. BARNETT, H., BOUGHNER, D., TAYLOR, D., *et al.* (1980). Further evidence relating mitral valve prolapse to cerebral ischemic events. *N. Engl. J. Med.*, **302**, 139
20. ROTHBARD, R.L., NANDA, N.C., FLECK, G. and HEINLE, R.A. (1980). Mitral valve prolapse and stroke: detection of potential emboli by real-time two-dimensional echo-cardiography (abstract). *Circulation*, **60** (Suppl. 2), 382
21. ROBERTS, W.C. and PERLOFF, J.K. (1972). Mitral valvular disease: A clinicopathologic survey of the conditions causing the mitral valve to function abnormally. *Ann. Intern. Med.*, **77**, 939–975
22. MILLER, G.E., JR., COHN, K.E., KERTH, W.J., *et al.* (1968). Experimental papillary muscle infarction. *J. Thorac. Cardiovasc. Surg.*, **56**, 611–616
23. TSAKIRIS, A.G., RASTELLI, G.C., AMORIM, D., *et al.* (1970). Effect of experimental papillary muscle damage on mitral valve closure in intact anestetized dogs. *Mayo Clin. Proc.*, **45**, 275–285
24. MITTAL, A.K., LANGSTON, M. JR., COHN, K.E., *et al.* (1971). Combined papillary muscle and left ventricular wall dysfunction as a cause of mitral regurgitation. An experimental study. *Circulation*, **44**, 174–180

25. NOREN, G.R., RAGHIB, G., MOLLER, J.H. *et al.* (1964). Anomalous origin of the left coronary artery from the pulmonary trunk with special reference to the occurrence of mitral insufficiency. *Circulation*, **30**, 171–179

26. SCHILLER, N.M., ACQUATELLA, H., PORTS, T.A., DREW, D., GOERKE, J., RINGERTZ, H., SILVERMAN, N.H., BRUNDAGE, B., BOTVINICK, E.H., BOSWELL, R., CARLSSON, E. and PARMLEY, W.W. (1979). Left ventricular volume from paired biplane two-dimensional echocardiographs. *Circulation*, **60**, September

27. SILVERMAN, N.H., PORTS, T.A., SNIDER, A.R., SCHILLER, N.B., CARLSSON, E. and HEILBRON, D.C. (1980). Determination of left ventricular volume in children: echocardiographic and angiographic comparisons. *Circulation*, **62**, 548–557

28. WANG, Y., HEILBRON, D., GUTMAN, J., WAHR, D. and SCHILLER, N.B. (1982). Clinical quantitative echocardiography I: End systolic atrial volume in a normal adult population. *Am. J. Cardiol.*, **49**, 905

29. WAHR, D., WANG, Y. and SCHILLER, N.B. (1982). Clinical quantitative echocardiography II: Left ventricular volume in a normal adult population. *Am. J. Cardiol.*, **49**, 906

10

Vasodilator therapy for mitral regurgitation

Kanu Chatterjee

Introduction

The fact that resistance to left ventricular ejection influences the severity of mitral regurgitation has been known for more than half a century. In 1922, Wiggers and Fell[1] demonstrated that increased arterial pressure is associated with marked augmentation of the regurgitant V wave in the left atrial pressure tracing, in experimental mitral regurgitation. Although the severity of mitral regurgitation is primarily determined by the degree of the anatomic and functional derangement of the structural components of the mitral valve apparatus, resistance to left ventricular ejection also contributes to the severity of mitral regurgitation and its hemodynamic consequences[2-4]. Increased aortic impedance enhances the regurgitant fraction and causes a further decrease in forward stroke volume. Conversely, reduction in impedence to left ventricular ejection is associated with decreased regurgitant volume and increased forward stroke volume. Mechanical systolic unloading with the use of intra-aortic balloon counterpulsation decreases the magnitude of the regurgitant V wave and increases cardiac output. Reduction of left ventricular ejection impedance, however, can also be accomplished with the use of vasodilator agents capable of reducing systemic vascular resistance. It is not surprising, therefore, that the vasodilator agents have been used to alter the dynamics of mitral regurgitation favorably and to minimize the adverse hemodynamic consequences[5-9].

Vasodilator agents in mitral regurgitation

Several vasodilator agents produce beneficial hemodynamic effects in patients with mitral regurgitation. The hemodynamic effects of nitroprusside infusion in patients with mitral regurgitation are summarized in *Table 10.1*[5]. Two of the eight patients in this study developed severe mitral regurgitation following acute myocardial infarction; the remaining six patients had severe chronic mitral regurgitation. In the group, as a whole, cardiac index and forward stroke volume index increased by 50% and 56%, respectively, with a decrease in systemic vascular resistance by an average of 39%. There was also a significant decrease in pulmonary vascular resistance. Despite a modest decrease in arterial pressure, heart rate decreased.

TABLE 10.1 Hemodynamic effects of nitroprusside in mitral regurgitation[9]*

Variable	Control			Nitroprusside			p
Heart rate (beats/min)	101	±	5.9	95	±	4.9	0.01
Arterial pressure (mean) (mm Hg)	83	±	3.8	70	±	3.3	0.005
Pulmonary arterial pressure (mean) (mm Hg)	45	±	2.4	29	±	2.4	0.0005
Pulmonary capillary wedge pressure (mean) (mm Hg)	33	±	1.8	16	±	1.4	0.0005
V wave (mm Hg)	50	±	4.5	19	±	2.9	0.0005
Cardiac index (l/min/m^2)	2.2	±	0.35	3.3	±	0.47	0.005
Forward stroke volume index (ml/m^2)	23	±	4.4	36	±	6.6	0.005
Stroke work index (g-m/m^2)	16	±	3	29	±	6	0.01
Systemic vascular resistance (dynes/s/cm^5)	1802	±	331	1102	±	241	0.005
Pulmonary vascular resistance (dynes/s/cm^5)	263	±	45	163	±	26	0.025

*Results are given as means ±SE (eight observations).

During nitroprusside infusion, there was a dramatic decrease in the magnitude of the peak V wave and mean capillary wedge pressure (*see Figure 10.1*). Reduction of the regurgitant V wave suggests a decrease in the regurgitant volume. Left ventricular volumes were calculated by cine angiography in some of these patients. Regurgitant volume was calculated by subtracting the forward stroke volume, determined by the thermodilution technique, from the angiographically determined left ventricular total stroke volume. In all patients, regurgitant volume decreased and the forward stroke volume increased. End-diastolic and end-systolic

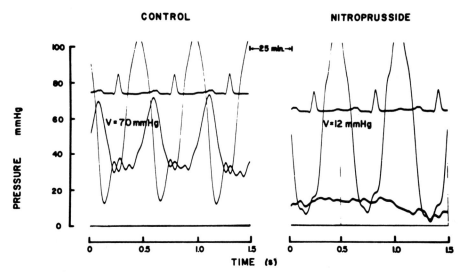

Figure 10.1 Effects of nitroprusside in acute severe mitral regurgitation. In a representative patient, the effects of nitroprusside on pulmonary capillary wedge and left ventricular pressures are illustrated. Before nitroprusside infusion, left ventricular end-diastolic pressure was 32 mm Hg and the magnitude of the peak V wave in the wedge pressure tracing was 70 mm Hg. After infusion of nitroprusside, left ventricular end-diastolic pressure and pulmonary capillary wedge pressure markedly decreased and the V waves were only 12 mm Hg. During nitroprusside infusion, the systolic pressure gradient between left ventricle and left atrium also increased. (Reproduced from Chatterjee, K., Parmley, W.W., Swan, H.J.C., *et al.* (1973). Beneficial effects of vasodilator agents in severe mitral regurgitation due to dysfunction of subvalvular apparatus, *Circulation*, **48**, 684, by kind permission of authors and publishers.)

volume decreased, but the total stroke volume remained unchanged (*see Table 10.2*)[5]. The calculated left ventricular ejection fraction tends to increase because the ventricle has a smaller end-diastolic volume. Thus, it appears that during nitroprusside infusion there is a redistribution of the total stroke volume of the left ventricle, with more blood ejected forward into the aorta and less blood ejected backward into the left atrium.

TABLE 10.2. Left ventricular volumes both before and during nitroprusside infusion in four patients with mitral regurgitation[9]*

	EDV (ml/m²)	ESV (ml/m²)	TSV (ml/m²)	FSV (ml/m²)	RV(%)	EF	EDP (mm Hg)
Control	238 ± 51	140 ± 33	96 ± 24	31 ± 7	64 ± 8	0.41 ± 0.07	30 ± 2.5
Nitroprusside	206 ± 46	113 ± 32	93 ± 20	49 ± 9	44 ± 11	0.47 ± 0.08	14 ± 2.3
p value	<0.01	<0.005	NS	<0.25	<0.05	<0.05	<0.005

EDV = End-diastolic volume; ESV = end-systolic volume; TSV = total stroke volume; FSV = forward stroke volume; RV = regurgitant volume; EF = ejection fraction; EDP = end-diastolic pressure; NS = not significant.
*Reproduced with permission from Grossman, W., Broadie, B., Mann, T., *et al.* (1975). Effects of sodium nitroprusside on left ventricular diastolic pressure–volume relations. *Circulation*, **52**, II. 35

As systemic vascular resistance and arterial pressure decrease, the decrease in regurgitant volume is likely to be due to decreased aortic impedance. Furthermore, lower intraventricular pressure and smaller end-diastolic volume is associated with decreased left ventricular wall stress. Reduced wall stress (afterload) should be associated with augmented myocardial fiber shortening, which might contribute to increased forward stroke volume.

However, reduction in regurgitant volume during nitroprusside infusion might not be entirely due to decreased aortic impedance and left ventricular afterload. Improved competence of the mitral valve apparatus may also be a contributing factor. This is suggested by the observed increase in the systolic pressure gradient between the left ventricle and pulmonary capillary wedge pressure (*see Figure 10.1*). Reduction of ventricular size might also improve the functional integrity of the subvalvular structures, thereby improving functional competence of the mitral valve apparatus. Furthermore, a decrease in heart rate and left ventricular wall stress may relieve papillary muscle ischemia and improve mitral valve competence. Although the relative contributions of these mechanisms in individual patients cannot be determined, it is apparent that nitroprusside produces beneficial hemodynamic effects and can be useful for the management of patients with mitral regurgitation.

Hydralazine, another direct-acting vasodilator, also produces beneficial hemodynamic effects in patients with mitral regurgitation. The acute hemodynamic effects of intravenous hydralazine (0.3 mg/kg), in a group of patients with severe chronic mitral regurgitation, are summarized in *Table 10.3*[8]. The average heart rate did not change; however, there was a small but statistically significant fall in mean arterial pressure. Systemic vascular resistance decreased by an average of 44% and this was accompanied by a substantial increase in cardiac index (50%) and forward stroke volume index (50%). Left ventricular total stroke volume, however, remained unchanged. Although there was no change in left ventricular end-diastolic pressure, mean pulmonary capillary wedge pressure decreased significantly, mostly due to a reduction in the amplitude of the regurgitant V wave (*see Figure 10.2*). Decreased amplitude of the V wave suggests decreased

TABLE 10.3 Hemodynamic effects of intravenous hydralazine in mitral regurgitation[9]

Variable	Control			Hydralazine			p
Heart rate	90	±	7 (SEM)	90	±	5	NS
MAP (mm Hg)	99	±	5	87	±	5	<0.001
PAP (mm Hg)	47	±	6	41	±	5	<0.01
PCW (mm Hg)	33	±	4	25	±	3	<0.005
PCW V wave (mm Hg)	48	±	6	33	±	6	<0.005
LVEDP (mm Hg)	21	±	3	18	±	3	NS
Forward CI (l/min/m^2)	2.0	±	0.1	3.0	±	0.2	<0.001
Forward SVI (ml/m^2)	22	±	2	33	±	3	<0.001
SVR (dyne/s/cm^5)	2100	±	170	1290	±	90	<0.001
EDVI (ml/m^2)	130	±	14	120	±	12	NS
ESVI (ml/m^2)	67	±	12	63	±	11	NS
Total SVI (ml/m^2)	62	±	6	60	±	5	NS
Regurgitant SVI (ml/m^2)	40	±	6	27	±	6	<0.001
Regurgitant fraction (%)	61	±	5	42	±	5	<0.001
Ejection fraction (%)	51	±	5	52	±	5	NS

MAP = mean arterial pressure; PAP = mean pulmonary artery pressure; PCW = mean pulmonary capillary wedge pressure;
LVEDP = left ventricular end-diastolic pressure; CI = cardiac index; SVI = stroke volume index; SVR = systemic vascular resistance;
EDVI = end-diastolic volume index; ESVI = end-systolic volume index; NS = not significant.

regurgitant volume, following intravenous hydralazine. Indeed, the calculated regurgitant fraction decreased in almost all patients, although left ventricular ejection fraction remained unchanged in the majority of patients (*see Figure 10.3*).

Oral hydralazine also produces similar hemodynamic effects in patients with chronic mitral regurgitation during short-term therapy (*see Table 10.4*). Systemic vascular resistance, mean pulmonary capillary wedge pressure and V wave amplitude all tend to decrease, while forward stroke volume and forward cardiac output increase substantially. In these patients, there was no significant change in heart rate, mean arterial pressure, pulmonary artery pressure and pulmonary

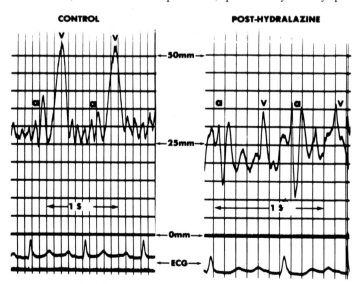

Figure 10.2 Marked decrease of pulmonary capillary wedge V wave amplitude following intravenous hydralazine. C = control; H = hydralazine.

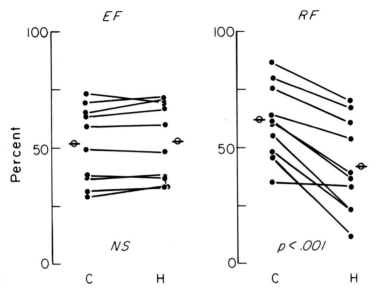

Figure 10.3 Overall ejection fraction (EF) did not change after intravenous hydralazine, but regurgitant fraction (RF) decreased from 61% to 39%. C = control; H = hydralazine; NS = not significant.

vascular resistance. In contrast to sodium nitroprusside, hydralazine did not cause any change in left ventricular end-systolic or end-diastolic volumes and ejection fraction, although the regurgitant fraction decreased consistently (*see Figure 10.4*). It needs to be emphasized, however, that changes in left ventricular volumes and dynamics, after long-term hydralazine therapy, might be different than those observed after short-term therapy. As hydralazine consistently decreases regurgitant volume, it is conceivable that following long-term hydralazine therapy,

TABLE 10.4 Hemodynamic changes after 48 hours of oral hydralazine in five patients with severe mitral regurgitation[9]

Variable	Control			Oral hydralazine			p
Heart rate (beats/min)	88	±	8	88	±	6	NS
Mean arterial pressure (mm Hg)	96	±	6	87	±	4	NS
Mean pulmonary artery pressure (mm Hg)	53	±	9	44	±	9	NS
Mean pulmonary capillary wedge pressure (mm Hg)	35	±	6	22	±	5	< 0.05
V wave (mm Hg)	61	±	7	36	±	4	< 0.05
Forward cardiac index (l/min/m^2)	2.1	±	0.3	3.7	±	0.4	< 0.005
Forward stroke index (ml/m^2)	23	±	4	42	±	5	< 0.002
Systemic vascular resistance (dynes/s/cm^5)	1780	±	270	940	±	78	< 0.05
Pulmonary vascular resistance (dynes/s/cm^5)	360	±	98	280	±	53	NS
End-diastolic volume index (ml/m^2)	152	±	22	149	±	17	NS
End-systolic volume index (ml/m^2)	83	±	17	79	±	14	NS
Total stroke volume index (ml/m^2)	69	±	10	70	±	6	NS
Regurgitant stroke volume index (ml/m^2)	46	±	9	28	±	6	< 0.05
Regurgitant fraction (%)	65	±	5	39	±	5	< 0.002
Ejection fraction (%)	46	±	5	49	±	5	NS

NS = Not significant.

left ventricular end-diastic volume may eventually decrease, which might cause further improvement in mitral valve competence.

It is apparent that although the hemodynamic effects of sodium nitroprusside and hydralazine are qualitatively similar, important differences exist between the acute hemodynamic effects of these two agents. Forward stroke volume index increases

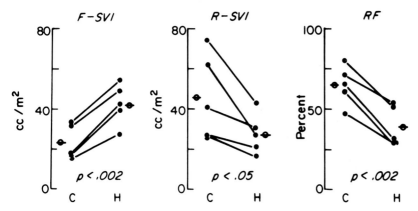

Figure 10.4 Effect of oral hydralazine on forward stroke volume index (FSVI), regurgitant stroke volume index (R-SVI), and regurgitant fraction (RF) in five patients with chronic mitral regurgitation. With hydralazine, FSVI increased as R-SVI and RF decreased. C = Control; H = hydralazine. (Reproduced from Greenberg, B.H., *et al.* (1978). Beneficial effects of hydralazine in severe mitral regurgitation, *Circulation*, **58**, 273.)

with both drugs. However, reduction in end-diastolic volume occurs with nitroprusside and not with hydralazine. Thus, although the pulmonary capillary wedge pressure decreases with both agents, the change observed with sodium nitroprusside is usually greater, and probably reflects both a decrease in left ventricular end-diastolic pressure and in the regurgitant V wave; with hydralazine, it primarily reflects the change in the amplitude of the regurgitant V wave. Since both agents appear to have similar effects on the degree of mitral regurgitation, it is likely that the changes in left ventricular end-diastolic pressure, produced by nitroprusside, result from its additional vasodilating action on the venous bed and the consequent increase in venous compacitance.

Reduction of left ventricular diastolic volume might be of considerable importance in mitral regurgitation, particularly when it is due to dysfunction of the subvalvular apparatus. Increased left ventricular diastolic volume causes a worsening of mitral regurgitation. Decreased left ventricular chamber size might improve valvular competence either directly, by improving coaptation of the valve leaflets during systole, or indirectly, by reducing myocardial ischemia. However, as hydralazine usually does not cause any significant decrease in left ventricular diastolic volume, the improvement in mitral regurgitation is likely to be related to reduction of aortic impedance.

The addition of nitrates or nitroglycerin to hydralazine decreases left ventricular diastolic volume, and, therefore, combined nitrate and hydralazine therapy can produce changes in the dynamics of mitral regurgitation similar to those of sodium nitroprusside.

The hemodynamic effects of prazosin, an α-1 receptor blocking agent, were evaluated in a limited number of patients with chronic mitral regurgitation. A substantial reduction in pulmonary capillary wedge pressure and an increase in forward cardiac output have been observed. However, the changes in left ventricular volumes and dynamics of mitral regurgitation with prazosin have not been evaluated.

Clinical application

It is apparent that vasodilator therapy has the potential to decrease the severity of mitral regurgitation and to improve hemodynamics, suggesting that such therapy might be useful in the clinical management of patients with mitral regurgitation. However, specific clinical indications still need to be defined. In patients with acute severe mitral regurgitation, such as following recent myocardial infarction or due to ruptured chordae, sodium nitroprusside can cause marked hemodynamic and clinical improvements. Thus, intravenous vasodilator therapy with sodium nitroprusside appears to be a rational therapeutic intervention for immediate symptomatic relief and to reverse the adverse hemodynamic conseqences. However, the clinical experience suggests that such therapy is effective only for a short period of time, and surgical correction of the mitral valve dysfunction is eventually required to achieve sustained improvement. Thus, in patients with acute mitral regurgitation, vasodilator therapy should be employed only as a measure to prepare the patient for surgical correction.

In patients with chronic mitral regurgitation, the role of vasodilator therapy also remains unclear. In symptomatic patients, mitral valve replacement or repair is the treatment of choice. However, there are some clinical situations where surgery could be delayed or possibly avoided. In patients with markedly depressed left ventricular function, mitral valve surgery is associated with considerable operative mortality, and the post-operative results are often not satisfactory. In such patients, a trial of vasodilator therapy is indicated. In patients with associated medical problems prohibiting surgery, vasodilator therapy may provide long-term benefits.

As progressive left ventricular dilation causes further worsening of mitral regurgitation, prevention of ventricular dilation with the use of some vasodilator agents is an alternative therapeutic rationale to prevent progression of mitral insufficiency. However, without controlled studies, this therapeutic approach remains speculative.

References

1. WIGGERS, J. and FEIL, H. The cardio-dynamics of mitral insufficiency. *Heart*, **9**, 149
2. ROBARD, S., KRAUSE, S., LOWENTHAL, M. and KATZ, L.N. (1956). Acute dynamic effects of a shunt between a systemic artery and the left atrium. *Am. J. Physiol.*, **187**, 458
3. BRAUNWALD, E., WELCH, G.H., JR. and SARNOFF, S.J. (1957). Hemodynamic effects of quantitatively varied experimental mitral regurgitation. *Circ. Res.*, **5**, 539
4. JOSE, A.D., TAYLOR, R.R. and BERNSTEIN, L. (1964). The influence of arterial pressure on mitral incompetence in man. *J. Clin. Invest.*, **43**, 2094
5. CHATTERJEE, K., PARMLEY, W.W., SWAN, H.J.C., BERMAN, G., FORRESTER, J. and MARCUS, H.S. (1973). Beneficial effects of vasodilator agents in severe mitral regurgitation due to dysfunction of subvalvular apparatus. *Circulation*, **48**, 684
6. GOODMAN, D.J., ROSEN, R.M., HOLLOWAY, E.L., ALDERMAN, E.L. andd HARRISON, D.C. (1974). Effect of nitroprusside on left ventricular dynamics in mitral regurgitation. *Circulation*, **50**, 1025
7. HARSHAW, C.W., GROSSMAN, W., MUNRO, A.B. and MCLAURIN, L.P. (1975). Reduced systemic vascular resistance as therapy for severe mitral regurgitation of valvular origin. *Ann. Intern. Med.*, **83**, 312

8. GREENBERG, B.H., MASSIE, B.M., BRUNDAGE, B.H., BOTVINICK, E.H., PARMLEY, W.W. and CHATTERJEE, K. (1978). Beneficial effects of hydralazine in severe mitral regurgitation. *Circulation*, **58**, 1978
9. CHATTERJEE, K., PORTS, T.A. and PARMLEY, W.W. (1979). Nitroprusside: Its clinical pharmacology an application in acute heart failure. In *Vasodilator Therapy for Cardiac Disorders* (ed. L. Gould and C.V.R. Reddy), p. 25. New York: Futura

The determinants and implications of pump and myocardial function in mitral valve disease

11

The use of quantitative angiocardiography in mitral valve disease

J. Ward Kennedy

In this chapter, I shall discuss the quantitative angiographic studies of the left atrium (LA) and left ventricle (LV) as they relate to different types of mitral valve disease and present data on the changes measured with these techniques before and after successful surgical treatment of mitral valvular disease and indicate which of these measurements have been useful in the understanding of the long-term prognosis in patients who have medical or surgical management of their disease.

It may be useful to spend a moment considering the historical development of the diagnostic methods we use today. Mitral stenosis was the first form of valvular disease to undergo routine diagnostic cardiac catheterization. In the early 1950s Gorlin and Gorlin developed a formula for the calculation of the size of the orifice of the stenotic mitral valve.[1]

This formula, or modification of it, is still in use today. The period of the 1950s was to a great extent devoted to use of measurements of pressure and flow to define the severity of disease. By 1960, considerable development had been made in cardiac angiography, and the era of quantitative measurements of the cardiac chambers was ushered in by the classic papers of Drs Sandler, Dodge and colleagues in this country, and that of Arvidsson in Sweden.[2, 3] These workers defined reliable methods for the measurements of the volume of the left ventricle and left atrium in man. A few years later these techniques were further developed to allow the estimation of LV mass.[4] Others became interested in this area of investigation and adapted these methods to cine-filming techniques, which are now in routine use in laboratories throughout the world.[5, 6]

This period, from around 1960 to the mid-1970s, was dominated by angiographic investigation. There is little doubt that since the mid-1970s echocardiography and nuclear cardiology have undergone tremendous development. It has been interesting to watch our echocardiographic and nuclear medicine colleagues attempt to make the same measurements and derive the same information with their non-invasive methods that we did earlier with angiographic techniques. To a great extent their efforts have been successful. Although echocardiographic results are difficult to quantify, they provide more information about mitral valvular anatomy than do angiographic methods. For patients with mitral valve disease, the methods currently available in nuclear cardiology are diagnostically less useful than echocardiographic techniques. The exception to this is the use of serial blood-pool scans to evaluate the course of LV function in patients with mitral insufficiency.

149

I shall limit my presentation to data derived from quantitative angiographic methods in patients with mitral valve disease.

Methods

The volumetric data presented in this chapter were derived from the methods developed by Sandler and Dodge working at the Seattle V.A. Hospital in the early 1960s. At this time, angiographic filming was initially done at six frames per second using biplane roll film changers. Later, faster changers were developed to allow 12 frames/second filming. The volume for each pair of films was calculated by the length–area method and the sequence of volumes was then arranged into a time-volume curve using the ECG as the time reference. Reasonable volume curves could be derived from three successive cardiac cycles with 6 frames/second filming techniques and from one to two cycles with 12 frames/second filming.

The LV pressure was often recorded simultaneously during the filming sequence, and a pressure–volume curve was derived by plotting the LV pressure on the vertical axis and the volume on the horizontal axis. From these pressure–volume curves one can derive LV work and compartmentalize work into systolic stroke work and work done on the LV during diastole. These methods, therefore, allowed rather complete characterization of the LV as a pump. With the help of Rackley, Dodge and Sandler extended these methods to determine the mass of the LV myocardium.[4] With knowledge of the diastolic volume of the LV and the thickness of the free wall of the ventricle, it was possible, assuming that the average thickness was represented by the free wall, to calculate LV mass. These measurements were verified with autopsy studies. We believe this is still the best indirect method for the quantification of LV hypertrophy mass in man.[4, 7]

One of the most important needs at that time was the development of a reliable method for determining the severity of valvular regurgitation. With knowledge of the LV stroke volume derived from the angiogram and forward stroke from the Fick or green dye dilution method for determining cardiac output, total regurgitant stroke volume was determined and shown. We routinely employ this technique in patients and believe it is of critical importance in the evaluation of many patients with mitral regurgitation, especially when there is an element of LV dysfunction. Unfortunately, the method is not widely used elsewhere because it requires careful calibration of the cine-angiographic system to derive actual LV volume and not simply the ejection fraction (EF).

Results

Beginning in 1964, quantitative antiographic methods were routinely applied to patients undergoing cardiac catheterization and left atrial or left ventricular angiography in the laboratories of the Seattle V.A. and the University of Washington Hospitals. We reported the results of the quantitative angiographic evaluations of 100 patients with mitral valve disease in 1970, and the comparison of the findings in patients with acute and chronic mitral regurgitation in 1973.[8, 9] *Figure 11.1* displays the end-diastolic volume/m^2 in patients with mitral stenosis (MS), combined mitral stensosis and regurgitation (MS and MR) and pure mitral regurgitation (MR). Pure MS was defined as a calculated mitral valve area of less

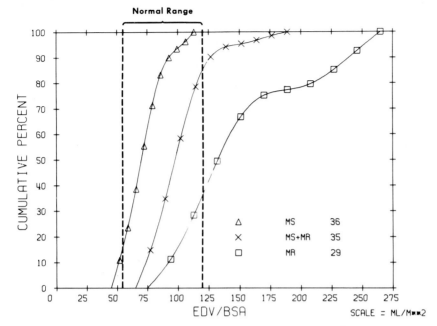

Figure 11.1 Cumulative distribution plot for end-diastolic volume, (ml/m²), in patients with mitral stenosis, mitral regurgitation and combined lesions. The normal range is indicated by vertical dashed lines.

than $2.5\,cm^2$ and less than $1.0\,l$/min of calculated regurgitation. Isolated MR was defined as more than $2.0\,l$/min of calculated regurgitation and a valve orifice of more than $4.0\,cm^2$ or no mitral gradient. Combined MS and MR was defined as a valve area of less than $4.0\,cm^2$ and regurgitant flow of more than $1.0\,l$/min. About 85% of patients with MS have a normal end-diastolic volume, while the other 15% have abnormally small ventricles. Since this experience was reported, we have seen an occasional patient with MS who has a dilated ventricle and a low ejection fraction. This situation is best explained by the combined presence of a cardiomyopathic process superimposed on chronic rheumatic heart disease.

Interestingly, the volume abnormalities in patients with MS and MR more closely resemble those with MS than those with isolated regurgitation About 65% of the patients with pure MR have increased end-diastolic volumes, and in most patients the degree of LV enlargement is closely related to the severity of regurgitation. *Figure 11.2* displays the cumulative plots of the EF for those patients. There is a group of patients with MS who have reduced EF, while this was relatively uncommon among these patients with MS and MR or MR. This pattern is no longer true. Today we often evaluate patients who have mitral regurgitation of non-rheumatic etiology who have significant LV dysfunction. *Figure 11.3* presents the cumulative distribution plots of LV mass in these patients. About 70% of the patients with MR have increased LV mass, compared to 40% of these with MS and MR and about 5% of those with MS. There are a few patients with MS who have very small values for LV mass and could be defined as having LV atrophy. This situation usually occurs in women who have long-standing disease with severe symptoms that have resulted in a prolonged period of reduced physical activity.

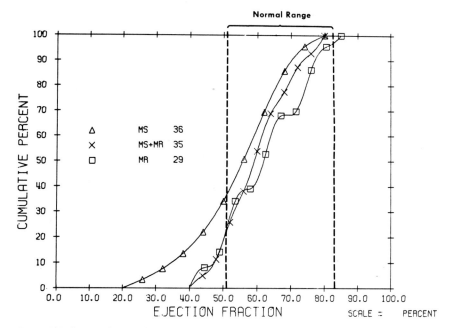

Figure 11.2 Cumulative distribution plot for ejection fraction in patients with mitral stenosis, mitral regurgitation and combined lesions. The normal range is indicated by vertical dashed lines.

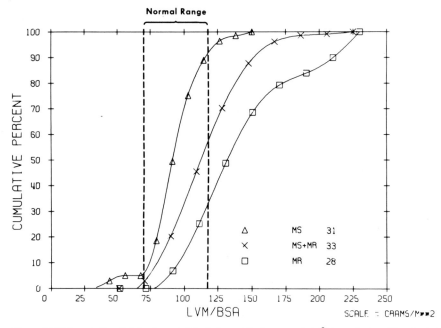

Figure 11.3 Cumulative distribution plot for left ventricular mass (g/m^2) in patients with mitral stenosis, mitral regurgitation and combined lesions. The normal range is indicated by vertical dashed lines.

The severity of MR for each patient group is shown in *Figure 11.4*. This demonstrates that few patients with MS and MR have severe regurgitation, with about 85% having less than 2.5 l/min/m², whereas about 80% of those with pure MR have more than 2.5 l/min/m² regurgitation. The largest volume of regurgitation in this series was about 12 l/min/m².

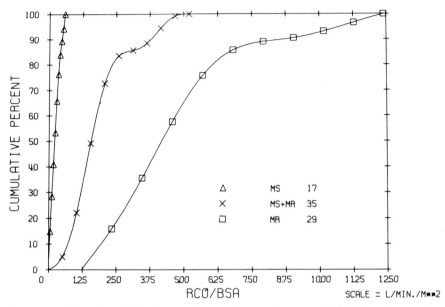

Figure 11.4 Cumulative distribution plot for regurgitant cardiac output in *l*/min in patients with mitral stenosis, mitral regurgitation and combined lesions.

Figure 11.5 presents the cumulative distribution for LA volume changes in these patients. These values are derived by subtracting the maximum from the minimum atrial volume measured during the cardiac cycle. From our experience in normals, we determined that the normal LA volume change during the cardiac cycle was up to 30 ml/m² of body surface area.[10] Most of the patients with mitral stenosis fall in this range, but about 70% of those with pure MR have atrial volume change greater than this value. This is due to systolic expansion of the atrium during LV ejection into the LA. The change in atrial volume is correlated with the volume of calculated LV regurgitant stroke volume (r = 0.785).[8]

Acute and chronic mitral regurgitation

The data here presented are no longer readily available to the clinician because LA volume is no longer easily measured with modern biplane cine systems if the atrium is significantly enlarged due to limitation of the field of view covered by nine inch image amplifiers. Baxley *et al.* reported their experience in acute and chronic MR. In that paper they presented the cumulative distribution plots for LA size in patients with acute MR and chronic MR, as shown in *Figure 11.6*. It is clear that those patients with recent-onset MR have smaller LA volumes than those with

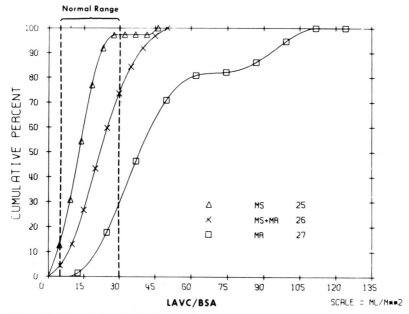

Figure 11.5 Cumulative distribution plot for left atrial volume in patients with mitral stenosis, mitral regurgitation and combined lesions.

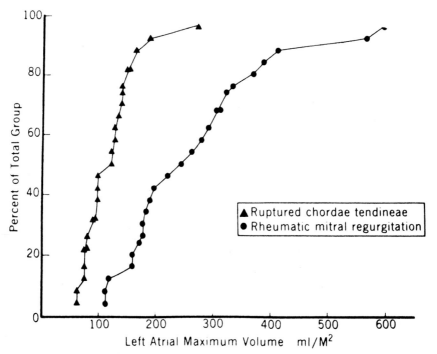

Figure 11.6 The cumulative distribution of left atrial volume for patients with acute and chronic mitral regurgitation.

chronic MR. This results in the transmission of higher pressures into the atrium during ventricular systole and often results in acute pulmonary edema. Baxley also showed that patients with acute MR have higher peak LA pressures, reduced LA compliance, and less LV hypertrophy than those with chronic MR.

I would now like to summarize the data accumulated on 19 patients who underwent successful mitral valve repair (eight patients) or replacement (11 patients) between 1969 and 1974.[11] These patients were selected from a larger group who had postoperative cardiac catheterization and angiography because they were shown to have hemodynamically well-functioning valves and had complete quantitative angiographic pressure and flow data for analysis. All patients had right heart, transeptal, and retrograde left heart catheterization. Postoperatively, eight patients improved one functional class, eight improved two functional classes, and one patient went from a Class IV to a Class I. There were two patients with MR who did not improve postoperatively.

There were no changes in LV volume, mass, ejection fraction or stroke work between the preoperative and postoperative evaluations for patients with MS or MS and MR. For the seven patients with MR, the EDV/m^2 fell from 124 ml $\pm$ 36 to 96 $\pm$ 35 (p < 0.01) and the stroke volume decreased significantly. The end-systolic volume/m^2 did not change significantly and the ejection fraction (EF) decreased from 55% $\pm$ 12 preoperatively to 43% $\pm$ 15 postoperatively (p $\pm$ 0.05). Stroke work also fell following surgery, but there was no decrease in LV mass. This lack of regression in LV hypertrophy is in contrast to the marked reduction of LV mass observed in patients following successful aortic valve replacement.[12] Of more importance is the fall in EF which occurred following surgery. We believe that this change is the result of the increased afterload placed on the LV following mitral valve repair or replacement for MR. This appears to unmask previously inapparent LV dysfunction.

The changes in EF for these seven patients and for two additional patients studied at the University of Alabama are shown in *Figure 11.7*. As can be seen, six of the patients had a decrease in the EF, whereas three of them had no decrease in the EF. Note that the two patients who had an EF below 50% preoperatively had a fall in the EF to below 30%. Patients with an EF in this range usually have symptoms of congestive heart failure.

From this experience and that of others, we believe that patients with predominant MR should be treated surgically prior to the onset of LV dysfunction. When they are still relatively asymptomatic but have significant volume overload and normal or high EF they can probably be followed safely with radionuclide measurements of EF or serial follow-up with two-dimensional echocardiography. We favor the former because it is more quantitative, and in our hands more reproducible. At the first evidence of a decrease in LV function, these patients should be carefully considered for valve replacement.

Prediction of late survival in patients with mitral valve disease

In the last section of this discussion, I would like to review the information that we have accumulated on the use of quantitative angiographic information to evaluate long-term prognosis in patients with mitral valve disease. We were in a unique position to do this study at the University of Washington because of the availability of quantitative angiographic information, starting in the early 1960s. From a

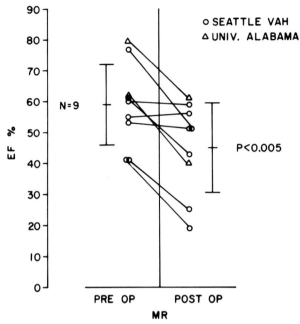

Figure 11.7 The change in ejection fraction (EF) before and after mitral valve surgery in patients with mitral regurgitation. The data for two of the patients were provided by Dr William Baxley from the University of Alabama.

complete review of the catherterization records at the Seattle V.A. Hospital and the University of Washington Hospital for the years 1960 through 1969, 249 patients were identified who had undergone complete hemodynamic and quantitative angiographic assessment of their mitral valve disease.

Seven angiographic, ten hemodynamic, three exercise, six clinical and five demographic variables were collected on each patient. Variables were categorized into levels of severity of abnormality. For example, patients were divided into three groups according to EF: > 50%, 31–50%, and < 30%. *Figure 11.8* displays the survival curves for the 177 surgically treated and the 72 medically treated patients.

There is a significant difference in survival between the two groups favouring those treated surgically. On examination of the two groups to determine whether they were different on entry, it was shown that they were similar in nine categories and significantly different in six. With the exception of sex, they were different in functional class, exercise limitation, pulmonary arterial pressure, pulmonary wedge pressure and an index of severity of mitral valve disease. In each of these categories, those treated surgically had more severe abnormalities. Of those treated surgically, 54% were women, and of those treated medically 38% were women. This sex difference probably relates to the fact that there were more women with severe mitral stenosis. Patients with MS were most likely to be treated surgically.

There were three subgroups of patients who had improved survival with surgical management: patients with combined MS and MR, those with MR, and those with mitral valve disease of all types with an EF between 31 and 50%. The survival curves are displayed for these subgroups in *Figures 11.9* and *11.10*. As seen in

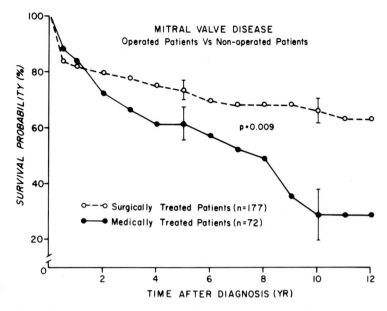

Figure 11.8 Actuarial survival curves of 177 surgically treated and 72 medically treated patients with mitral valve disease, demonstrating improved survival in the surgical cohort.

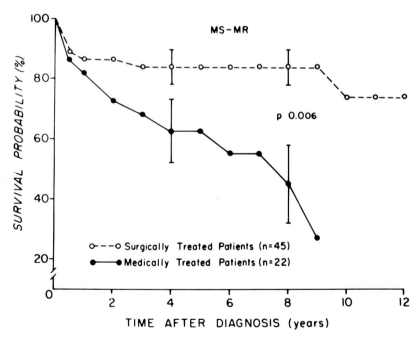

Figure 11.9 Actuarial survival curves of 45 surgically treated patients and 22 medically treated patients with mixed mitral stenosis and regurgitation (MS-MR), demonstrating improved survival in the surgical cohort.

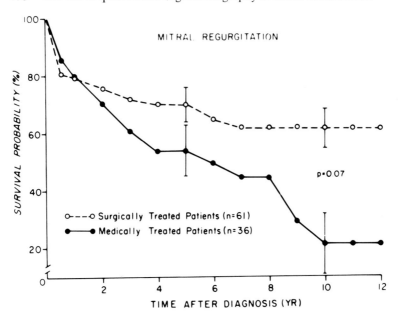

Figure 11.10 Actuarial survival curves of 61 surgically treated patients and 36 medically treated patients with mitral regurgitation, demonstrating improved survival of borderline significance in the surgical cohort.

Figure 11.9, the group of patients with MS and MR who were treated surgically had an excellent prognosis, with a 12-year survival of about 75%, whereas the patients who received medical therapy did very poorly, with about a 30% survival at 9 years. The other subgroups receiving surgical therapy have had similar results. Of note are those with MR, in whom the 5-year survival was only about 55%. Patients treated with mitral valve repair had an improved early survival as compared with those who underwent valve replacement, who had a much lower operative mortality. By 5 years, however, there was a trend favoring those with valve replacement.

In reviewing these data, we need to ask ourselves whether, in 1982, this early experience is relevant. Univariate analysis was utilized to evaluate these several variables relative to their ability to predict survival. Then were predictive. These were then examined multivariately, and only three were found to be predictive of outcome—arteriovenous oxygen difference and end-diastolic volume in the medically treated patients and age in the surgical cohort.

It should be remembered that these results were obtained in an era when the surgical management of these patients was much less satisfactory than it is today. This is especially true for those requiring mitral valve replacement. The overall surgical mortality was 12% and was 28% in the 43 patients who had mitral valve replacement. Reparative procedures carried an operative mortality of 7.0%. Today we anticipate an operative mortality in mitral valve surgery in the range of 2–4%, with the vast majority of these procedures being valve replacement. Despite these vast changes in operative mortality, we believe that this experience is relevant today. It indicates that the patient with relatively mild mitral valve disease has a poor prognosis if treated over the long term with medical therapy. This experience suggests that these patients should be carefully followed up and referred to surgery when their symptoms become significant or they develop evidence of LV dysfunction. Fortunately, we now have excellent methods to follow up these patients non-invasively with echocardiography and/or radionuclide techniques. With better methods of evaluation and improved surgical techniques, patients with mitral valve disease have a far better outlook than was true 10–20 years ago. We believe that quantitative angiographic techniques have played an important role in our gaining a better understanding of the hemodynamics of mitral valve disease and the results of medical and surgical management, and in the identification of patients who have a decreased long-term prognosis.

References

1. GORLIN, R. and GORLIN, S.G. (1951). Hydraulic formula for calculation of the area of the stenotic mitral valve, other cardiac valves and central circulatory shunts. *Am. Heart J.*, **1**, 41
2. DODGE, H.T., SANDLER, H., BALLEW, D.W., *et al.* (1960). The use of biplane angiocardiography for the measurement of left ventricular volume in man. *Am. Heart J.*, **60**, 762
3. ARVIDSSON, H. (1958). Angiocardiographic observations in mitral valve disease. *Acta Radiol. Suppl.*, **158**
4. RACKLEY, C.E., DODGE, H.T., COBLE, Y.D., JR. and HAY, R.E. (1964). A method for determining left ventricular mass in men. *Circulation*, **29**, 666–667
5. BUNNELL, I.L., GRANT, C. and GREENE, D.C. (1965). Left ventricular function derived from the pressure-volume diagram. *Am. J. Med.*, **39**, 881–894
6. KENNEDY, J.W., TRENHOLME, S.E. and KASSER, I.S. (1967). Left ventricular volume by one-plane cineangiography. *Circulation*, **35**, 61–69
7. KENNEDY, J.W., REICHENBACH, D.D., BAXLEY, W.A. and DODGE, H.T. (1967). Left ventricular mass. A comparison of angiocardiographic measurements with autopsy weight. *Am. J. Cardiol.*, **19**, 221
8. KENNEDY, J.W., YARNALL, S.R., MURRAY, J.A., *et al.* (1970). Quantitative angiocardiography: IV. Relationships of left atrial and ventricular pressure and volume in mitral valve disease. *Circulation*, **41**, 817
9. BAXLEY, W.A., KENNEDY, J.W., FIELD, B. and DODGE, H.T. (1973). Hemodynamics of ruptured chordae tendineae and chronic rheumatic mitral regurgitation. *Circulation*, **48**, 1288
10. MURRAY, J.A., KENNEDY, J.W. and FIGLEY, M.M. (1968). Quantitative angiocardiography: II. The normal left atrial volume in man. *Circulation*, **37**, 800
11. KENNEDY, J.W., DOCES, J.G. and STEWART, D.K. (1979). Left ventricular function before and following surgical treatment of mitral valve disease. *Am. Heart J.*, **97**, 592–598
12. KENNEDY, J.W., TWISS, R.D., BLACKMAN, J.R., *et al.* (1968). Hemodynamic studies one year following homograft aortice valve replacement. *Circulation*, **37** (Suppl. II), 110

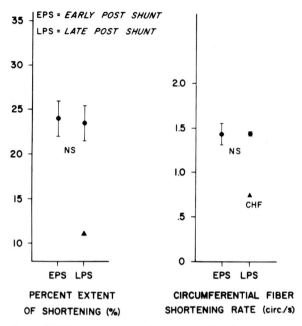

Figure 12.2 Responses to experimental chronic volume overloading early and late after the creation of chronic arteriovenous fistula. Normalized relations of left ventricular function remain normal, and unchanged early and late post-shunt. A single animal in which severe congestive heart failure developed is indicated by the triangles which show depressed relations late post-shunt. (Reproduced from reference 2, by kind permission of authors and publishers.)

pressures in excess of 20 mm Hg sarcomere lengths were similar to those during acute volume overloading, approximately 2.2 μm, although ventricular volume was increased (*see Figure 12.3*)[4]. Electron micrographs showed hypertrophy of the myocardial fibers and some loss of array of the Z-lines of adjacent sarcomeres (perhaps due to slippage, or to the pattern of myocardial hypertrophy) but there was no evidence of elongation of sarcomeres beyond approximately 2.2 μm[4]. This finding indicated that the Frank–Starling mechanism at the sarcomere level was not utilized in the adaptation that occurred from the acute to the chronic volume overload state; rather it was accomplished by eccentric hypertrophy with more sarcomeres being developed in series.

In *Figure 12.4(a)*, a hypothetical curve for the relation between left ventricular volume and left ventricular circumference is shown, and the measured changes from end-diastole to end-systole of the acutely volume-overloaded heart and the heart after its adaptation to chronic volume overload are superimposed. Notice that the chronically dilated heart is operating on a flatter portion of the volume-circumference relation, and this geometric change allows it to deliver a much larger stroke volume with the same percentage shortening of the circumference. If we consider the sarcomere as the smallest unit of circumference (*see Figure 12.4(b)*) it can be seen that, since end-diastolic sarcomere length remains constant, the ventricle should be able to deliver a larger stroke volume with normal shortening of each sarcomeric unit.

These adaptations to volume overloading in the experimental animal appear to resemble those observed after more long-standing chronic volume overload, with

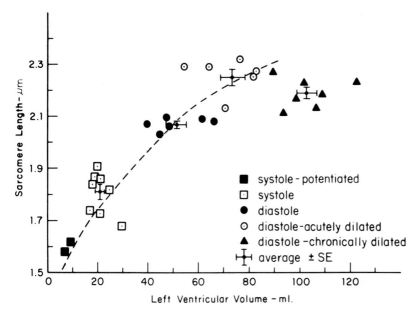

Figure 12.3 Relations between left ventricular volume and sarcomere length at the midwall in the dog. The hypothetical curve for an ellipse is shown by the dashed line and the volume–sarcomere length relations at various ventricular volumes are shown. The solid triangles indicate the diastolic sarcomere length–volume relations in the chronically dilated ventricle due to chronic volume overload. (Reproduced from reference 4, by kind permission of the authors and publishers.)

compensated eccentric hypertrophy, in the human subject. During severe experimental mitral regurgitation, we have shown that when the peak wall stress does not rise appreciably, there is a substantial alteration of the dynamics of ejection such that lowered wall stress early and late in systole results in more myocardial fiber shortening with increased stroke volume[7]. In chronic volume overloading due to mitral regurgitation in man, clinical studies suggest that eccentric hypertrophy results in some increased wall thickness, so that the ratio of left ventricular diameter to wall thickness remains normal[8]; therefore, allowing normal fractional shortening and velocity of shortening, and a normal or elevated ejection fraction[8]. Even when a fall in mean VCF suggests early left ventricular dysfunction, the left ventricular ejection fraction may remain normal in chronic mitral regurgitation due to the low impedance leak into the left atrium[9].

The responses to chronic volume overload may be summarized as follows: in the early stages of volume overloading there is an increase in fiber length and sarcomere length which help to increase the stroke volume. As progressive left ventricular dilatation and eccentric hypertrophy occur, the myocardial fibers continue to increase in length yielding an increased number of sarcomeres in series, but without further increase in diastolic sarcomere length. A modest increase in left ventricular wall thickness allows the ventricle to maintain a relatively normal afterload. In the compensated ventricle these adaptations lead to maintenance of normal or enhanced measures of left ventricular function (VCF, ejection fraction) and suggest that myocardial inotropic state is normal, as shown in studies on isolated muscle after chronic volume overload[10]. Thus, increases in stroke volume

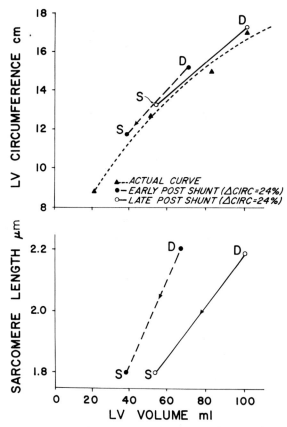

Figure 12.4 (a) Average values for left ventricular circumference at the minor equator and calculated left ventricular volumes at end-diastole (D) and end-systole (S) early (closed circles) and late (open cirlces) after chronic volume overloading produced by a large arteriovenous fistula. These values are compared with the best-fit curve (dashed line) constructed from actual measurements of casts of the left ventricle fixed under differing conditions (closed triangles). (b) Hypothetical representation of changes in sarcomere lengths at the midwall plotted against the average left ventricular volume during changes observed early (closed circles) and late (open circles) after chronic volume overloading by means of an arteriovenous fistula in the dog. Averaged sarcomere lengths observed at the midwall at end-systole after normal ejection were used. (Reproduced from reference 2, by kind permission of authors and publishers.)

are accomplished by a change in left ventricular size and shape within the constraints of a normal extent of sarcomere shortening.

Afterload mismatch and the responses to surgical treatment of mitral regurgitation

In a number of situations, when the preload is either held constant or the limit of preload reserve is reached, as the afterload is then further increased a decrease in the performance of the ventricle is observed; likewise in the presence of chronic left ventricular dilation with depressed inotropic state, afterload (and stress) may be inappropriately high in the resting state and any further increase in afterload will result in a marked decrease in left ventricular performance. All of these situations may be usefully described by the term 'afterload mismatch'[11]. Several frameworks, including the force–velocity–length relation and the standard ventricular function curve can be used to illustrate these phenomena[11], but perhaps the most useful approach is the pressure–volume loop and the linear end-systolic relation between left ventricular pressure and volume[12]. As illustrated in *Figure 12.5*, this end-systolic relation line provides the limits of shortening and end-systolic volume, regardless of the preload and the afterload, so that the entire relation represents a load-independent measure of the level of inotropic state; the linear relation is shifted upward and downward with changes in slope by positive and negative inotropic interventions, respectively[12]. As shown in *Figure 12.5*, if the ventricular end-diastolic volume (preload) is held constant under experimental conditions, when the left ventricular systolic pressure is progressively elevated, there is a progressive reduction of the stroke volume, and an isovolumetric contraction also reaches the linear relation. If the ventricle is forced experimentally to the limit of its preload reserve at a large end-diastolic volume, further increases in loading will then force the ventricle into a descending limb of function, with a progressive drop in the stroke volume and a further rise in end-diastolic pressure[13]; this drop in the stroke volume is related to afterload mismatch, as in the previous example, and can

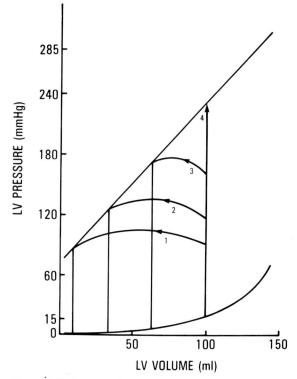

Figure 12.5 Diagrammatic representation of left ventricular (LV) pressure–volume loops, and the linear end-systolic volume–pressure relation, when the preload (end-diastolic volume) is held fixed and the afterload is varied. Beats 1, 2 and 3 show the progressive reductions in stroke volume with increased afterload, and beat 4 represents an isovolumetric contraction.

be attributed to exhaustion of the preload reserve with inability of the left ventricle to compensate for further increases in afterload[11].

The relationship between end-systolic left ventricular volume and peak systolic wall stress in a series of isovolumetric contractions at different preloads has also been shown to be linear[14], and if the instantaneous wall stress is varied *during ejecting* left ventricular beats by varying the inflation of a balloon in the ascending aorta, the ventricle continues to shorten to the same relation at end-systole regardless of the instantaneous loading conditions[14]. This normal linear relation between left ventricular end-systolic volume and end-systolic wall stress is shown diagrammatically in *Figure 12.6* (dashed line), and the relation in the presence of depressed inotropic state or left ventricular failure is also indicated (solid line). The left ventricular diastolic volume-wall stress relation is also indicated. Beat 1 represents a failing ventricle operating in a steady state with sarcomeres extended to the limit of preload reserve; under those conditions any further increase in the afterload must result in a drop in the stroke volume, as the ventricle reaches the linear end-systolic relation at a higher level of systolic wall stress (*see Figure 12.6, beat 2*). Such a response has been documented in the failing ventricle in man during angiotensin infusion[16]. On the other hand, if a vasodilator is given so that the peak systolic pressure and end-diastolic volume change little, but the impedance to ejection early and late in systole is substantially lowered, a considerable improvement in stroke volume can be seen because wall stress is lowered early and late during ejection (*see Figure 12.6, beat 3*).

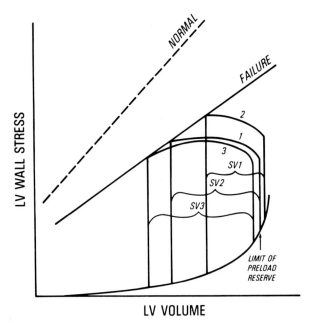

Figure 12.6 Diagrammatic relations between left ventricular (LV) volume and wall stress. The normal end-systolic-volume–wall-stress relation (dashed line) is shifted downward and to the right by myocardial failure. In the failing heart (beat 1) operating at the limit of its preload reserve, further increase in wall stress results in a drop in the stroke volume (beat 2, SV 1) compared with the resting conditions (beat 1, SV 2). Use of a vasodilator lowers the early and late systolic wall stress resulting in a larger stroke volume (beat 3, SV 3) with only a slight fall of end-diastolic volume and peak wall stress. (Reproduced from reference 15, by kind permission of authors and publishers.)

The implications for mitral regurgitation

In compensated chronic mitral regurgitation, the curve relating left ventricular diastolic volume to wall stress is shifted to the right and theoretical considerations imply that the linear end-systolic wall stress-volume relation is also shifted somewhat to the right, even in the presence of normal myocardial contractility[17]. As shown in *Figure 12.7(a)*, the left ventricle, operating at a much larger end-diastolic volume than normal, can maintain a normal level of peak wall stress while shortening

MITRAL REGURGITATION

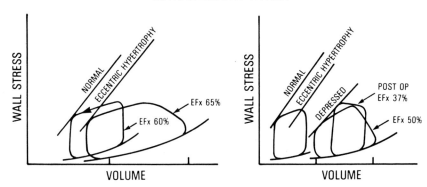

Figure 12.7 Diagrammatic relation between left ventricular volume and wall stress in chronic mitral regurgitation in the compensative state *(a)* and with myocardial depression *(b)*. (Modified from reference 18.)

against a lower afterload early and late in systole (due to the low resistance leak into the left atrium), allowing maintenance of a large total stroke volume and a normal or high ejection fraction. Studies by our group have shown that in such compensated hearts the typical response at 6 months following mitral valve replacement (as studied by echocardiography and radionuclide ejection fraction) is a fall in the end-diastolic dimension, with a slight fall in the ejection fraction within the normal range (*see Figure 12.8*)[19].

In contrast, the response to operation in the patient with chronic mitral regurgitation and a markedly enlarged left ventricular end-diastolic dimension, with an ejection fraction at the lower limit of normal preoperatively, is a marked fall in the left ventricular ejection fraction postoperatively accompanied by little change of the end-diastolic dimension (*see Figure 12.8*)[19]. Thus, in such patients hypertrophy fails to regress and the ejection fraction 6 months postoperatively can be strikingly reduced compared with the preoperative value (*see Figure 12.8*).

This response may be diagrammed within the left ventricular wall-stress–volume diagram as shown in *Figure 12.7(b)*. Preoperative depression of the myocardial inotropic state shifts the linear relation between end-systolic wall stress and volume downward and to the right with reduced slope. In the example shown, prior to operation the ejection fraction was nevertheless maintained at 50% due to reduced afterload early and late during ejection, even though the peak systolic wall stress is somewhat elevated compared with the normal. Thus, marked depression of left ventricular myocardial contractility is not evident preoperatively because of favorable loading conditions produced by the mitral regurgitation. Following surgical correction of the mitral regurgitation, the low impedance leak into the left atrium early and late during ejection is eliminated, and the left ventricle must now

MITRAL REGURGITATION SUBGROUPS

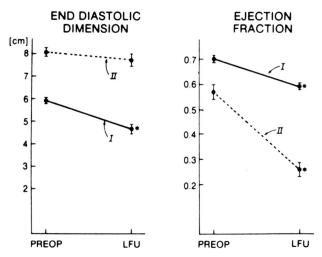

Figure 12.8 Responses of the left ventricle to mitral valve replacement in patients with chronic mitral regurgitation. Preoperative values are shown together with the studies at late followup (LFU) 6 months postoperatively. Group 1 (solid lines) indicates patients with fixed but compensated mitral regurgitation in which the end-diastolic dimension falls and the ejection fraction falls only slightly postoperatively. Group 2 (dashed lines) represents patients with markedly elevated end-diastolic dimension preoperatively who had ejection fractions in the low–normal range and exhibited little change in end-diastolic dimension postoperatively, but a marked drop in the ejection fraction. (Modified from reference 19.)

eject entirely into the high impedance of the aorta. Accordingly, there is a drop of the ejection fraction to 37% postoperatively (*see Figure 12.7(b)*).

It is possible that determination of the entire linear end-systolic-volume–wall-stress relation of left ventricle, which is load independent, can be obtained non-invasively or at cardiac catheterization and will become a useful tool for detecting depressed left ventricular contractility preoperatively. A simplified approach to use of this relation, based end-systolic pressure–volume ratio reported by Sagawa *et al.*[20], has been recently described [21], and is discussed in Chapter 14. From *Figure 12.7(b),* it is apparent that the ratio end-systolic wall stress divided by end-systolic volume will be reduced even in patients with compensated mitral regurgitation because of the shift to the right of this relation and because of the lowered end-systolic wall stress in this condition. It can also be seen from *Figure 12.7(b)* that this ratio should be even lower in patients with a depressed myocardial inotropic state, since the further shift to the right of the end-systolic relation, with maintenance of relatively low end-systolic wall stress, will result in a further reduction of the ratio. In studies on a small number of patients, those who either died or were in Class III postoperatively had end-systolic wall stress–volume ratios (corrected for body surface area) of 2.5 or below[21].

It may be hoped that application of load-independent measures for the assessment of left ventricular contractility in severe chronic mitral regurgitation, together with other measures of left ventricular contractility and diastolic function, will allow detection of depressed contractility at an early phase. This should allow earlier operation in such patients and thereby prevent the occurrence of irreversible left ventricular dysfunction, postoperatively[18].

Summary

Irreversible depression of left ventricular function continues to pose a serious problem following mitral valve replacement for mitral regurgitation. Post-operative survival curves also suggest a higher later attrition than following aortic valve replacement, and such findings suggest that: (1) in the 15–20% of patients who do not respond optimally after operation our methods for detecting depressed myocardial function preoperatively are inadequate; and (2) we are waiting too long to recommend operation in such patients.

The response of the left ventricle to severe chronic volume overload has been studied experimentally. A progressive shift to the right of the diastolic pressure–volume relation has been documented, while sarcomere lengths remain maximum at about 2.2 μm as eccentric left ventricular hypertrophy develops. During the several weeks involved in this response, myocardial contractility shows no change and there is no further use of the Frank–Starling mechanism beyond the acute phase. Such as adaptation allows the dilated ventricle to deliver a greatly enhanced stroke-volume, with normal shortening of each unit of the enlarged circumference.

The reasons why some patients develop irreversible left ventricular dysfunction after long-standing volume overload has not been elucidated. Regardless of the mechanism, the mechanics of left ventricular ejection are now well enough appreciated to describe the response of such ventricles in the pre- and post-operative settings. It is useful to employ for this purpose a framework within which the efforts of altered loading conditions can be understood: the left ventricular pressure–volume loop and the linear end-systolic pressure–volume and wall stress–volume relations.

Mitral regurgitation alters the instantaneous afterload of impedance on the left ventricle throughout systole, particularly the early and late phases (normally isovolumetric). Such favorable loading conditions on the depressed left ventricle can lead to normal fractional shortening and ejection fraction. Under these conditions, when the mitral valve is replaced the instantaneous impedance is markedly altered throughout ejection, and the left ventricle must now inject entirely into the high-impedance aorta. The resulting change in loading conditions, with inability of the depressed ventricular myocardium to unload early and late in ejection, produces a sharp fall in the ejection fraction post-operatively and a poor clinical response.

How can we identify such patients, who often have an ejection fraction within the normal range preoperatively? Approaches using the load-independent end-systolic volume-wall stress framework should be useful, and initial clinical studies suggest that if the ratio of end-systolic wall stress to the end-systolic volume index is low, a poor post-operative result is to be expected. Other non-invasive studies are also useful; thus, echocardiographic and radionuclide angiographic data suggest that when the left ventricular end-diastolic diameter approaches 7.5 cm, the end-systolic diameter exceeds 5.0 cm, and the ejection fraction is 55% or below the lower limit at normal in patients with severe mitral regurgitation, mitral valve replacement should be considered to avoid irreversible left ventricular dysfunction and persistent cardiomegaly post-operatively.

References

1. MCCULLAGH, W.H., COVELL, J.W. and ROSS, J. JR. (1972). Left ventricular dilatation and diastolic compliance changes during chronic volume overloading. *Circulation*, **45**, 943
2. ROSS, J. JR. and MCCULLAGH, W.H. (1972). Nature of enhanced performance of the dilated left ventricle in the dog during chronic volume overloading. *Circ. Res.*, **30**, 549
3. ROSS, J. JR. (1974). Adaptations of the left ventricle to chronic volume overload. *Circ. Res. (Suppl. II)*, **35**, 64
4. ROSS, J. JR., SONNENBLICK, E.H., TAYLOR, R.R. and COVELL, J.W. (1971). Diastolic geometry and sarcomere lengths in the chronically dilated canine left ventricle. *Circ. Res.*, **28**, 49–61
5. SONNENBLICK, E.H., ROSS, J. JR., COVELL, J.W., SPOTNITZ, H.M. and SPIRO, D. (1967). The ultrastructure of the heart in systole and diastole: Changes in sarcomere length. *Circ. Res.*, **21**, 423–431
6. YORAN, C., COVELL, J.W. and ROSS, J. JR. (1973). Structural basis for the ascending limb of left ventricular function. *Circ. Res.*, **32**, 297–303
7. URSCHEL, C.W., COVELL, J.W., SONNENBLICK, E.H., ROSS, J. JR. and BRAUNWALD, E. (1968). Myocardial mechanics in aortic and mitral valvular regurgitation: the concept of instantaneous impedance as a determinant of the performance of the intact heart. *J. Clin. Invest.*, **47**, 867–883
8. GROSSMAN, W., JONES, D. and MCLAURIN, L.P. (1975). Wall stress and patterns of hypertrophy in the human left ventricle. *J. Clin. Invest.*, **56**, 56–64
9. ECKBERG, D.I., GAULT, J.H., BOUCHARD, R.L., KARLINER, J.S. and ROSS, J., JR. (1973). Mechanics of left ventricular contraction in chronic severe mitral regurgitation. *Circulation*, **47**, 1251–1259
10. COOPER, G., PUGA, R.J., ZUJKO, K.J., HARRISON, C.E. and COLEMAN, H.N. (1973). Normal myocardial function and energetics in volume-overload hypertrophy in the cat. *Circ. Res.*, **32**, 140–148
11. ROSS, J. JR. (1976). Afterload mismatch and preload reserve: a conceptual framework for the analysis of ventricular function. *Prog. Cardiovasc. Dis.*, **18**, 255–264
12. SAGAWA, K. (1981). Editorial: The end-systolic pressure-volume relation of the ventricle: definition, modifications and clinical use. *Circulation*, **63**, 1223–1227
13. MCGREGOR, D.C., COVELL, J.W., MAHLER, F., DILLY, R.B. and ROSS. J., JR. (1974). Relations between afterload, stroke volume, and descending limb of Starling's curve. *Am. J. Physiol.*, **227**, 884–890
14. TAYLOR, R.R., COVELL, J.W. and ROSS, J., JR. (1969). Volume-tension diagrams of ejecting and isovolumic contractions in left ventricle. *Am. J. Physiol.*, **216**, 1097–1102
15. ROSS, J. JR. (1984). Mechanisms of cardiac contraction: what roles for preload, afterload and inotropic state in heart failure? *Eur. Heart J.* (in press).
16. ROSS, J., JR. and BRAUNWALD, E. (1964). The study of left ventricular function in man by increasing resistance to ventricular ejection with angiotensin. *Circulation*, **29**, 739–749
17. ROSS, J., JR. (1981). Pathophysiology of the human heart: function of the heart under abnormal loading conditions. In *Kardiologie in Klinik und Praxis* (eds. H.P. Krayenbuehl and W. Kuebler) Vol. **I**, pp. 9–28. Stuggart: Georg Thieme Verlag
18. ROSS, J., JR. (1981). Left ventricular function and the timing of surgical treatment in valvular heart disease. *Ann. Int. Med.*, **94**, 498–504
19. SCHULER, G., PETERSON, K., JOHNSON, A., FRANCIS, G., DENNISH, G., UTLEY, J. DAILY, P., ASHBURN, W. and ROSS, J., JR. (1979). Temporal response of left ventricular performance to mitral valve surgery. *Circulation*, **59**, 1218–1231
20. SUGA, H., SAGAWA, K. and SHOUKAS, A.A. (1973). Load independence of the instantaneous pressure-volume ratio of the canine left ventricle and effects of epinephrine and heart rate on the ratio. *Circ. Res.*, **32**, 314–322
21. CARABELLO, B.A., NOLAN, S.P. and MCGUIRE, L.B. (1981). Assessment of preoperative left ventricular function in patients with mitral regurgitation: value of the end-systolic wall stress-end-systolic volume ratio. *Circulation*, **64**, 1212–1217

13

The timing of surgical intervention in chronic mitral regurgitation

Kirk L. Peterson and Tsukasa Tajimi

Introduction

Over the past 5 years there has been increasing difficulty in establishing widely accepted guidelines for surgical intervention in the patient with isolated, chronic mitral regurgitation[1, 2]. Implantation of a mitral valve prosthesis potentially leads to thromboembolic events, bacterial endocarditis, and/or prosthetic valve dysfunction. Moreover, most patients with chronic mitral regurgitation follow a relatively benign natural course and experience few limiting symptoms until late in their illness, despite a comparatively large hemodynamic burden on the left ventricle[3, 4]. A natural tendency exists, therefore, to delay corrective surgery until the patient is significantly symptomatic. To be weighed against these considerations are recent publications which report a significant decline in operative mortality for mitral valve replacement[5, 6], a relatively high degree of success with mitral valve reconstructive procedures[7–9], and irreversible left ventricular dysfunction postoperatively in some patients if corrective surgery is delayed too long[10].

Survivorship of chronic mitral regurgitation: Surgical versus medical therapy

Assuming that the goals of any therapeutic intervention are improvement in the quality as well as in the duration of life, it is useful to examine the relatively few comparisons of surgical and medical therapy published over the past decade. All such studies, unfortunately, are variably deficient because the patient groups reported:

1. Are non-randomized and generally non-concurrent.
2. Have a variable etiology of mitral regurgitation, e.g. rheumatic versus chordal rupture.
3. Often have coexistent cardiac lesions, including mitral stenosis and coronary heart disease.
4. Generally include more seriously ill patients, i.e. those with more advanced lesions.
5. Have a significant drop-out in follow-up, often as high as 10%.

171

Nevertheless, some insight can be gained by examination of actuarial data where primary emphasis was placed on describing the results of mitral valve replacement yet with some comparisons made either directly, or by implication, with medical therapy (*see Table 13.1*).

In three separate studies the 5-year survival rate for medical therapy of *combined* mitral regurgitation and stenosis is relatively unfavorable, varying between 46% in Munoz's report[11] from Caracas, Venezuala, to 63 and 66% in Rapaport's[4] and Hammermeister's[12] studies compiled in San Francisco and Seattle, respectively. Munoz's comparable surgical cohort exhibited a superior 5-year survival rate of 60%, a figure that included an operative or 1-month mortality rate of 24%; nevertheless, the survival curves for the medical and surgically treated groups were not statistically different. By contrast, in Hammermeister's study, the survival after surgery was 86% at 5 years and 75% at 9–10 years, values that were statistically different from the concurrent medical cohort (p value of 0.006).

TABLE 13.1 Survival rates (%) of patients with mitral regurgitation: Surgical vs. medical therapy

	Munoz[11] (MR + MS)	Rapaport[4] (MR + MS)	Hammermeister[12] (MR + MS)	Rapaport[4] (MR only)	Hammermeister[12] (MR only)
Medical RX:					
5years	46	66	63	80	55
9–10 years	—	33	28	60	22
Surgical RX:					
5 years	60	—	86	—	75
9–10 years	—	—	75	—	62

MS = Mitral stenosis; MR = mitral regurgitation; RX = therapy.

In patients with mitral regurgitation *only*, the Hammermeister analysis[12] revealed nearly significant differences between the medical and surgical cohorts with the surgically treated patients demonstrating improved survival. However, the 62% survival at 9–10 years was no better than the 60% survival reported by Rapaport[4] for a medically treated cohort.

Other series have reported surgical results alone and no effort was made to compare life table results with medical therapy (*see Table 13.2*). For example, Carpenteir[7] and Yacoub[13] have reported 5–year survival rates of 87% and 91%, respectively, and 9–10-year survival rates of 82% and 81%, respectively, in their relatively large cohorts of patients who have undergone mitral valve reconstruction for isolated mitral regurgitation. Duran[8], likewise, has reported a remarkable 96% 5-year survival rate in his surgical cohort undergoing mitral valve reconstruction. The life tables of these cohorts compare very favourably with those reported for patients with mitral regurgitation undergoing a prosthetic valve replacement where 10-year survival rates between 39 and 65% are reported [13–15].

On the basis of these data available in 1982, it seems reasonably safe to conclude that surgical intervention leads to improved survival in the symptomatic patient (late Class II–IV) with hemodynamically significant mitral regurgitation, particularly if a mitral reconstructive procedure rather than a prosthetic valve replacement is performed. There is not sufficient actuarial data, however, to support the notion that mitral valve surgery improves survival in the patient who is asymptomatic or mildly symptomatic (Class I or early Class II). The recent reports that an arteriolar vasodilator, e.g. hydralazine, significantly reduces the regurgitant

TABLE 13.2 Survival rates of patients undergoing mitral valve surgery: Reconstruction *vs.* prosthetic replacement

	Carpentier[7]	Duran[8]	Yacoub[13]	Chaffin[14]	Mcgoon[15]
Reconstruction:					
4–5 years	87%	96%	91%		
9–10 years	82%		81%		
Prosthetic replacement:					
5 years		81%	61%	73%	
8–10 years			39%	65%	50%
16 years					52%

volume and enhances systemic cardiat output with sustained effects for 6 months in patients with chronic mitral regurgitation emphasizes the need for further comparative studies of medical and surgical therapy and their relative effects on survival[16].

Spectrum of etiology of mitral regurgitation: Implication for myocardial function

In the United States today, valve surgery for mitral insuficiency is performed for the following disease processes: (1) rheumatic valvulitis; (2) spontaneous rupture of one or more chordae tendineae; (3) rupture of a papillary muscle after a myocardial infarction; (4) valve or chordal destruction secondary to infective endocarditis; and (5) myxomatous degeneration of the mitral valve with associated annular dilatation. In fact, most surgical candidates are now thought to have insufficiency of the valve related to non-rheumatic causes[17]. Right and left ventricular myocardial function are then generally determined by the adaptations of the myocardium to the left ventricular volume overload rather than to a concomitant myocarditis, be it active or healed.

Right and left ventricular function in chronic mitral regurgitation

Although the right ventricle (RV) is not directly involved in the volume overload imposed by mitral valve leakage, there is evidence that the RV ejection fraction can be depressed in response to pulmonary hypertension. At our institution we have documented by 'first pass' radionuclide angiography (*see Figure 13.1 (a) and (b)*) that the right ventricular ejection fraction preoperatively is inversely related to the systolic pulmonary artery pressure; postoperatively, with a fall in the pulmonary artery pressure, the ejection fraction returns to a near-normal or normal range (*see Figure 13.1 (c)*). These findings suggest that the relatively thin-walled right ventricle is sensitive to the increased afterload imposed by pulmonary hypertension but that irreversible changes in right ventricular myocardial contractility do not occur as a consequence of mitral valve regurgitation, augmented pulmonary arterial systolic pressure, or an elevated pulmonary vascular resistance.

By contrast, assessment of left ventricular myocardial function is a highly complex task in the setting of mitral regurgitation. With this lesion, perhaps like none other, the ejection fraction can be quite misleading as an index of myocardial

174

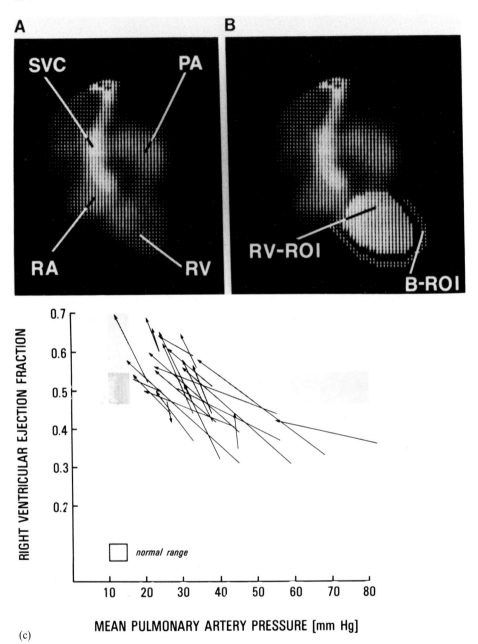

Figure 13.1 Radionuclide angiogram demonstrating visualization of right heart chambers and pulmonary artery in patient with mitral regurgitation. (*a*) Raw image. (*b*) Assigned region of interest (ROI) for background (B) and for right ventricle (RV). Ejection fraction is calculated from the end-diastolic and end-systolic counts, corrected for background. (*c*) Right ventricular ejection fraction plotted against mean pulmonary artery pressure in patients having undergone mitral valve replacement. Preoperative values are represented by the beginning of vector; post-operative values are shown by tip of arrow. Note that ejection fraction returns to near-normal or normal range as pulmonary artery mean pressure declines after mitral valve replacement.

contractility. The low impedance leak early and late during systole allows maintenance of a high normal or augmented ejection fraction when myocardial contractility is normal[18, 19]; and even when contractility seems depressed, a low normal ejection fraction is often noted[10]. In view of this sensitivity of the ejection fraction to afterload, a number of investigators have advocated use of the end-systolic wall stress/end-systolic volume (ESWS/ESV) relation as a preferable approach for assessing myocardial contractile state[20–23]. This construct would seem particularly appealing in volume overload states, such as mitral regurgitation, in view of extensive experimental data in the isolated heart which indicate that the end-systolic pressure/volume (ESP/ESV) and ESWS/ESV relations are independent of alternations in preload.

We have had the opportunity to observe the development of the ESWS/ESV ratio in the chronically instrumented dog over the first 2–7 weeks after creation of *acute* mitral regurgitation (*see Figure 13.2(a)*). While mean and peak stress remain relatively constant, the end-diastolic and end-systolic volumes become progressively larger, thus the ratio becomes incrementally smaller. In these same animals, use of angiotensin to increase, and nitroprusside to decrease, left ventricular afterload has allowed a determination of E_{max} (slope of end-systolic stress-volume relation), and V_0 (theoretical end-systolic volume at end-systolic pressure of zero); the imposition of the acute volume overload decidely shifts the relation to the right, with a coincident lessening of its slope (*see Figure 13.2 (b)*). During this time-frame, the ejection fraction remains essentially unchanged (*see Figure 13.2(c)*).

Thus, it would appear that the left ventricular end-systolic stress/volume relation is sensitive to the myocardial adaptations occurring in response to acutely imposed mitral regurgitation. However, to what extent the rightward shift of the relation reflects a reduction in basal contractility, as opposed to a consequence of the volume overload itself, remains conjectural[24]. For example, serial replication of sarcomeres and myofiber slippage are both thought to occur in eccentric hypertrophy and may themselves cause a shift to the right of the end-systolic relation. Further analysis of myocardial function in the setting of chronic volume overload will be needed to understand the true import of this shift and its value for identifying subtle depression of myocardial contractility in the patient with chronic mitral regurgitation.

Left ventricular function and postoperative course

The important influence of preoperative left ventricular function (and other variables on post-operative survival and quality of life in the patient with chronic mitral regurgitation is now well documented[12, 25]. These variables include:

1. Left atrial enlargement.
2. Age over 60 years.
3. Advanced functional class.
4. Concomitant aortic regurgitation.
5. End-diastolic volume over $140 \, cm^3/m^2$.
6. Ejection fraction under 55%.
7. Cardiac index under $2.5 \, l/min/m^2$.

For example, Phillips *et al.*[26] reported a significant reduction in 5-year survival after 'mitral valve replacement in patients with an ejection fraction below 0.40. A further left ventricular parameter associated with impaired survival after mitral valve replacement is an end-diastolic volume quantitated as greater than 140 cm^3/m^2 by contrast ventriculography[12]. Operative results would clearly seem to be optimized if timed before the left ventricle dilates excessively, myocardial function deterioraters, and a class IV symptomatic status is reached. The task for the cardiologist, therefore, is to find parameter(s) of left ventricular size and function

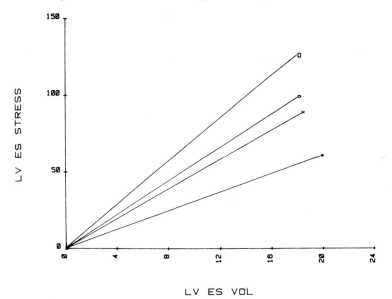

(a)

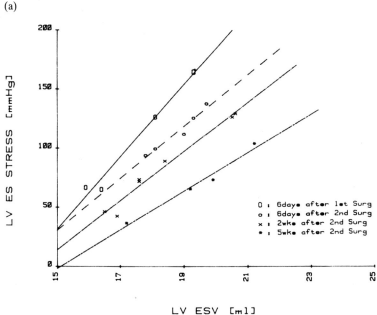

(b)

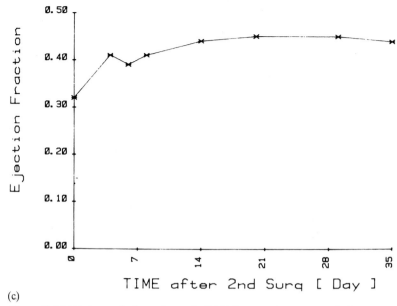

(c)

Figure 13.2 (*a*) Left ventricular end-systolic (LVES) stress plotted against left ventricular end-systolic volume in chronically instrumented dog with acute mitral regurgitation. The animal was instrumented at first surgery; mitral regurgitation was created at second surgical procedure. Note that over a period of 5 weeks, the end-systolic stress to end-systolic volume ratio decreased and shifted to the right. (*b*) LVES stress plotted against LVES volume (LVESV) as determined from increased afterload (angiotensin) and decreased afterload (nitroprusside). E_{max} (slope of end-systolic stress–volume relation) was determined by linear regression of four or more data points for each time period. Note that the relation shifts to the right with decreasing slope as the left ventricle adapts to mitral regurgitation. (*c*) Time course of ejection fraction in animal whose end-systolic stress–volume relation is shown in (*b*) and (*c*).

that allow detection of progressive dilatation and 'silent' depression of myocardial contractility, preferably by techniques that can be performed serially and without risk.

In the mid- late 1970s, development of M-mode and 2-D echocardiography as well as radionuclide angiography provided practical means for multiple, serial assessments of the status of left ventricular function and the temporal response of the left ventricle to correction of mitral valve leakage. Applying these methods serially in patients with pure chronic mitral regurgitation, we have found that end-diastolic and end-systolic left ventricular size, fractional shortening and muscle cross-sectional area are predictive of persistence of symptoms postoperatively and, in some cases, progressive worsening of left ventricular function[10]. Patients with an end-diastolic diameter of 7 cm or greater, as well as an end-systolic diameter of 5 cm or greater, manifested a striking reduction in their ejection fraction over the first 6 months after surgery, a phenomenon that could not be attributed to inadequate myocardial preservation during cardiopulmonary bypass (*see Figure 13.3*). Moreover, there was no detectable regression in myocardial hypertrophy as evidenced by the constancy of the cross-sectional area of the myocardium at the mid-wall out to 18 months postoperatively. We have interpreted the fall in the ejection fraction, as well as the lack of regression of hypertrophy, as indications that left ventricular afterload either increased or at least remained mismatched to

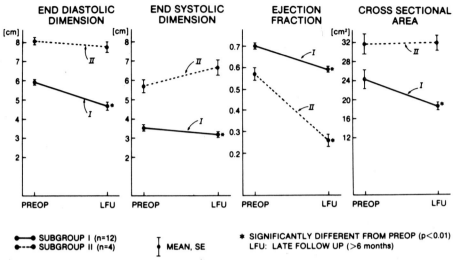

Figure 13.3 Echocardiographic measurements of patients with chronic mitral regurgitation before (PREOP) and at late follow-up greater than 6 months (LFU) after mitral valve replacement. In group I (solid line) there is a decrease in heart size postoperatively, a small fall in ejection fraction, and the cross-sectional area of the minor axis (an index of hypertrophy) declines significantly. By contrast, in group II (dotted line), characterized by end-diastolic diameter greater than 7.0 cm and end-systolic diameter greater than 5.0 cm, there is a marked drop in ejection fraction postoperatively, and myocardial hypertrophy does not regress. (Reproduced from reference 10, by kind permission of authors and publishers.)

the contractile state despite the correction of the mitral valve leakage. By contrast, patients with preoperative end-diastolic and end-systolic diameters of approximately 6 cm and 3.5 cm, respectively, demonstrated a slight reduction in their calculated ejection fraction at 6 months or more postoperatively and exhibited significant regression of hypertrophy (approximately 20% reduction in cross-sectional area) over this time-frame. In this subgroup of patient, any increase in systolic afterload brought about by the closure of the low impedance leak was offset by the concomitant reduction of left ventricular volume.

Carabello *et al.*[27] have applied a measurement of the ratio of end-systolic stress to end-systolic volume index (normalized to body surface area) in 21 patients with *chronic* mitral regurgitation as compared with 20 normal subjects. The ESWS/ESVI ratio in normal persons was 5.6 + 0.9; a smaller ratio indicated progessively worse left ventricular function, reflecting an even larger end-diastolic volume for any given afterload. Four out of five patients with EDWS/ESVI values less than or equal to 2.2 died postoperatively, and the fifth did not improve his clinical or functional status. Interestingly, one of these five patients had a preoperative ejection fraction of 0.81.

Guidelines for timing of mitral valve surgery

In view of these actuarial and pathophysiologic observations, we now look to a constellation of left ventricular function measures as useful for recommendation of valve replacement or reconstruction *in the Class II or greater patient* with significant mitral valve leakage demonstrated by selective contrast ventriculography: (1) an end-diastolic diameter by M-mode echocardiography approaching or greater than 8.0 cm; (2) an end-systolic diameter exceeding 5.5 cm; (3) an ejection fraction of less than 0.55; and (4) an end-systolic stress to end-diastolic volume index ratio of less than 2.2. No patient is presently denied surgery by these criteria because of severely depressed left ventricular function (ejection fraction < 0.40), provided that: the degree of mitral regurgitation is considered large (regurgitant fraction of the total stroke volume greater than 0.50); there is an unsatisfactory response to afterload reduction, digitalis, and diuretics; and the patient understands that further worsening of left ventricular function will probably occur postoperatively thereby limiting his prognosis. Recently, Zile et al.[28] reported on the retrospective application of similar criteria to a group of patients with chronic mitral regurgitation and found that the combination of end-systolic stress and end-systolic dimension measurements segregated four out of 16 patients with poor clinical outcomes and lack of regression of hypertrophy postoperatively. Hopefully, further studies of the predictive value of such preoperative measurements of left ventricular function will provide corroboration of their utility and provide refinement of the criteria for mitral valve surgical intervention.

References

1. BONCHEK, L.I. (1980). Indications for surgery of the mitral valve. *Am. J. Cardiol.*, **46**, 155
2. FOWLER, N.O. and VAN DER BEL-KAHN, J.M. (1980). Operations on the mitral valve: A time for weighing the issues. *Am. J. Cardiol.*, **46**, 159
3. SELZER, A. and KATAYAMA, F. (1972). Mitral regurgitation: Clinical patterns, pathophysiology and natural history. *Medicine*, **51**, 337
4. RAPAPORT, E. (1972). Natural history of aortic and mitral valve disease. *Am. J. Cardiol.*, **35**, 221
5. APPELBAUM. A., KOCHOUKOS, N.T., BLACKSTONE, E.H. and KIRKLIN, J.W. (1976). Early risks of open heart surgery for mitral valve disease. *Am. J. Cardiol.*, **37**, 201–209
6. BONCHEK, L.I., ANDERSON, R.P. and STARR, A. (1974). Mitral valve replacement with cloth-covered composite-seat prostheses. *J. Thorac. Cardiovasc. Surg.*, **67**, 93–109
7. CARPENTIER, A., CHAUVAUD, S., FABIANI, J.N., et al. (1980). Reconstructive surgery of mitral valve incompetence: Ten-year appraisal. *J. Thorac. Cardiovasc. Surg.*, **79**, 338–348
8. DURAN, C.G., POMAR, J.L., REVUELTA, J.M., et al. (1980). Conservative operation for mitral insufficiency: Critical analysis supported by postoperative hemodynamic studies of 72 patients. *J. Thorac. Cardiovasc. Surg.*, **79**, 326–337
9. LESSANA, A., HERREMAN, F., BOFFETY, C., et al. (1981). Hemodynamic and cineangiographic study before and after mitral valvuloplasty (Carpentier's technique). *Circulation*, **64**, (Suppl. II): II–95
10. SCHULER, G., PETERSON, K.L., JOHNSON, A., et al. (1979). Temporal response of left ventricular performance to mitral valve surgery. *Circulation*, **59**, 1218–1231
11. MUNOZ, S., GALLARD, J., DIAZ-GORRIN, J.R. and MEDINA, O. (1975). Influence of surgery on the natural history of rheumatic mitral and aortic valve disease. *Am. J. Cardiol.*, **35**, 234
12. HAMMERMEISTER, K.E., FISHER, L., KENNEDY, J.W., SAMUELS, S. and DODGE, H.T. (1978). Prediction of late survival in patients with mitral valve disease from clinical, hemodynamic, and quantitative variables. *Circulation*, **57**, 341
13. YACOUB, M., HALIM, M., RADLEY-SMITH, R., MCKAY, R., NIJVELD, A. and TOWERS, M. (1981). Surgical treatment of mitral regurgitation caused by floppy valves: Repair versus replacment. *Circulation*, **64** (Suppl. II), 11–210
14. CHAFFIN, J.S. and DAGGETT, W.M. (1978). Mitral valve replacement: A nine-year follow-up of risks and survivals. *Ann. Thor. Surg.*, **37**, 312–319
15. MCGOON, M.D., FUSTER, V., MCGOON, D.C., PLUTH, J.R. and PUMPHREY, C.W. (1982). Long-term survival, symptomatic status and thromboembolism after Starr-Edwards prosthesis for isolated aortic or mitral incompetence. (abstr) *Am. J. Cardiol.*, **49**, 893
16. GREENBERG, B.H., DEMOTO, H., MURPHY, E. and RAHIMTOOLA, S.H. (1982). Arterial dilators in mitral regurgitation: Effects on rest and exercise hemodynamics and long-term clinical follow-up. *Circulation*, **65**, 181

17. FOWLER, N.O. and VAN DER BEL-KAHN, J.M. (1979). Indications for surgical replacement of the mitral valve: With particular reference to common and uncommon causes of mitral regurgitation. *Am. J. Cardiol.*, **44**, 148–157

18. URSCHEL, C.W., COVELL, J.W., SONNENBLICK, E.H., ROSS, J., JR. and BRAUNWALD, E. (1968). Myocardial mechanics in aortic and mitral valvular regurgitation: The concept of instantaneous impedance as a determinant of the performance of the intact heart. *J. Clin. Invest.*, **47**, 867–883

19. BRAUNWALD, E. (1969). Mitral regurgitation: physiologic, clinical, and surgical considerations. *N. Engl. J. Med.*, **281**, 425

20. SAGAWA, K., SUGA, H., SHOUKAS, A.A. and BAKALAR, K.M. (1977). End-systolic pressure-volume ratio: A new index of contractility. *Am. J. Cardiol.*, **40**, 748

21. SAGAWA, K. (1981). The end-systolic pressure-volume relations of the ventricle: Definition, modifications and clinical use. *Circulation*, **63**, 1223

22. GROSSMAN, W., BRAUNWALD, E., MANN, T., MCLAURIN, L.P. and GREEN, L.H. (1977). Contractile state of the left ventricle in man as evaluated from end-systolic pressure-volume relations. *Circulation*, **56**, 845

23. MEHMEL, H.C., STOCKINS, B., RUFMANN, K., OLSHAUSEN, K., SCHULER, G. and KUBLER, W. (1981). The linearity of the end-systolic pressure-volume relationship in man and its sensitivity for assessment of left ventricular function. *Circulation*, **63**, 1216

24. ROSS, JOHN, JR. (1981). Left ventricular function and the timing of surgical treatment in valvular heart disease. *Ann. Int. Med.*, **94**, 498

25. BARNHORST, D.A., OXMAN, H.A., CONNOLLY, D.C., et al. (1975). Long-term follow-up of isolated replacement of the aortic or mitral valve with the Starr-Edwards prosthesis. *Am. J. Cardiol.*, **35**, 228

26. PHILLIPS, H.R., LEVINE, F.H., CARTER, J.E. et al. (1981). Mitral valve replacement for isolated mitral regurgitation: Analysis of clinical course and late postoperative left ventricular ejection fraction. *Am. J. Cardiol.*, **48**, 647–654

27. CARABELLO, B.A., NOLAN, S.P. and LOCKHART, B. (1981). Assessment of preoperative left ventricular function in patients with mitral regurgitation: Value of the end-systolic wall stress to end-systolic volume ratio. *Circulation*, **64**, 1212

28. ZILE, M.R., GAASCH, W.H., CARROLL, J.D. and LEVINE, H.J. (1983). Chronic mitral regurgitation: Predictive value of pre-operative echocardiographic indices of LV function and wall stress: *J. Am. Coll. Cardiol.*, **1**, 625

14

Effects of acute and chronic mitral regurgitation on left ventricular mechanics and contractile muscle function

Blase A. Carabello and William Grossman

Introduction

Patients who present with severe acute mitral regurgitation or severe chronic mitral regurgitation may have similar symptoms of congestive heart failure. However, these symptoms are produced by entirely different pathogenetic mechanisms. In acute mitral regurgitation, heart failure symptoms are produced by the effects of sudden volume overload on an unprepared cardiovascular system. In chronic mitral regurgitation, on the other hand, symptoms of heart failure are usually the result of a progressive decline in left ventricular muscle function. The following is a discussion of contrasting effects of acute versus chronic mitral regurgitation on cardiac mechanics and on left ventricular muscle function.

Acute mitral regurgitation

Acute mitral regurgitation due to chordal rupture, for instance, produces a sudden volume overload upon the left atrium and left ventricle. In the absence of antecedent heart disease, the left atrium will be normal in size and compliance. The obvious consequence of volume overload on a small and relatively non-compliant chamber must be an increase in pressure in that chamber[1]. In such patients there is elevation of mean left atrial pressure together with a large V wave as shown in *Figure 14.1*. The elevation in left atrial pressure is transmitted to the pulmonary venous system with a resultant fall in lung compliance, transudation of alveolar fluid and pulmonary edema. The symptom of dyspnea experienced by most patients with acute mitral regurgitation is in large part due to these changes.

The onset of mitral regurgitation also produced a fall in forward stroke volume, since a significant portion of the total stroke volume pumped by the left ventricle now is delivered into the left atrium instead of forward into the aorta[2]. This fall in forward cadiac output produces symptoms of fatigue and exercise intolerance. Two compensatory mechanisms exist for partially re-establishing forward stroke volume. End diastolic volume increases slightly and end systolic volume falls significantly. These changes obviously increase total stroke volume; a portion of this increase is ejected into the aorta thus tending to increase forward stroke volume back toward normal. These conditions are depicted in *Figure 14.2*. The

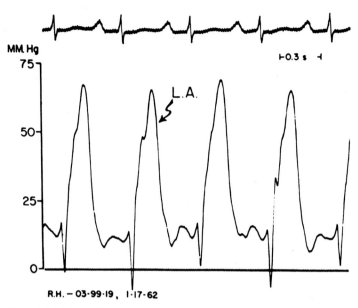

Figure 14.1 A large V wave is present in the pulmonary capillary wedge pressure tracing in a patient with acute mitral regurgitation. (Reproduced from *Circulation* with kind permission of the authors and editors.)

mechanisms producing these changes in ventricular volume are primarily due to alterations in left ventricular loading conditions. The normal cardiac sarcomere operates near its maximum length but allows for a small increase in cardiac end diastolic volume due to volume overload[3, 4], produced by mitral regurgitation. There is thus an increase in preload at a time when eccentric cardiac hypertrophy (replication of sarcomeres in series) has not yet occurred[4].

The regurgitant mitral valve also provides a mechanism by which the ventricle is unloaded during systole. The regurgitant valve allows ejection of a portion of the total left ventricular stroke volume into the relatively low-pressure left atrium. Thus afterload should be reduced by mitral regurgitation. Indeed afterload as quantified by wall tension has been shown to be reduced in the latter part of systole[5] in experimental mitral regurgitation as shown in *Figure 14.3*. A fall in afterload permits more complete left ventricular emptying and thus a reduction in end systolic volume occurs[5–8].

Left ventricular contractile muscle function, on the other hand, is not significantly altered by acute mitral regurgitation. Urschel and his associates have shown normal V_{max} and normal mean velocity of circumferential fiber shortening in experimental acute mitral regurgitation[5].

In summary, acute mitral regurgitation produces sudden volume overload to a small non-compliant left atrium resulting in left atrial hypertension. There is also a fall in forward stroke volume. Alterations in loading conditions permit an increase in total left ventricular stroke volume partially compensating for the loss in forward flow produced by the regurgitation itself. The resultant left atrial hypertension and diminished forward stroke volume produce symptoms of pulmonary congestion and fatigue but occur in the presence of normal left ventricular muscle function.

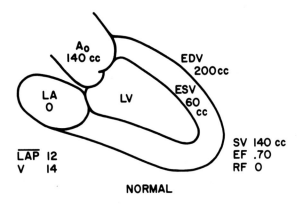

NORMAL

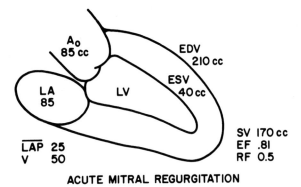

ACUTE MITRAL REGURGITATION

Figure 14.2 Acute mitral regurgitation (MR) is compared with the normal state. Ao = aorta; LA = left atrium; LV = left ventricle; EDV = end diastolic volume; ESV = end systolic volume; SV = stroke volume; EF = ejection fraction; RF = regurgitant fraction; LAP = mean left atrial pressure; and V = V wave. In acute MR, there is an increase in EDV, LAP, V, EF and total SV. There is a fall in ESV. There is also a fall in forward SV as only 50% of total SV is pumped into the aorta.

Chronic compensated mitral regurgitation

If mitral regurgitation occurs more gradually there may be accommodation of the regurgitant volume and the patients may be relatively symptom free for a prolonged period. The relative lack of symptoms in this phase of mitral regurgitation depend upon four basic compensatory mechanisms. These include: (1) enlargement of the left atrium and an increase in its compliance; (2) lymphatic hyperfunction; (3) enlargement (eccentric hypertrophy) of the left ventricle permitting increased stroke volume; and (4) maintenance of relatively normal left ventricular muscle function. Braunwald and Awe described 10 patients with long-standing severe mitral regurgitation in whom the left atria were enlarged but who had normal left atrial pressure[9]. All had atrial fibrillation. They postulated a continuum of increasing atrial compliance in patients with mitral regurgitation. They suggested that with chronicity, left atrial size and compliance increased, permitting accommodation of regurgitant volume at normal or nearly normal left

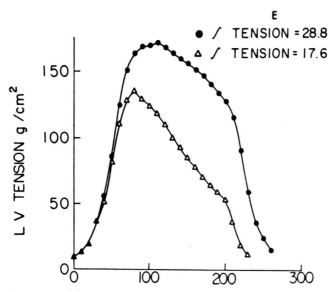

Figure 14.3 Wall tension is plotted against time in systole for a control beat (●) and for a beat evaluated during mitral regurgitation (△) in the dog. There is a significant fall in wall tension during mitral regurgitation. (Reproduced from *J. Clin. Invest.* with kind permission of the authors and editors.)

atrial pressure. In such patients, pulmonary venous hypertension would not be present and symptoms of pulmonary congestion should be diminished or absent.

Additionally, increase in lymphatic flow may aid removal of pulmonary fluid if the changes in left atrial size and compliance do not result in complete normalization of left atrial pressure. Thus in experimental animals, Rabin *et al.* showed an eight-fold increase in pulmonary lymphatic drainage if left atrial pressure was increased acutely to 30 mm Hg[10]. Uhley *et al.* found an even more dramatic increase in pulmonary lymphatic return under conditions of chronic left atrial hypertension[11]. The clinical observation has been made that patients with chronic left atrial hypertension my not experience pulmonary edema even at pulmonary venous pressures that normally would be expected to cause fluid transudation into the alveoli. Increased lymphatic function in such patients may permit increased pulmonary fluid removal and prevent symptoms of pulmonary congestion.

A third important compensatory mechanism in mitral regurgitation is the development of eccentric hypertrophy producing an increase in left ventricular end diastolic volume. The increase in end diastolic volume represents true hypertrophy since left ventricular mass is increased [12]. The increased volume at end diastole permits significant increase in total stroke volume. Although some of this increase is regurgitated into the left atrium, a significant portion is pumped forward into the aorta (*see Figure 14.4*). Thus forward stroke volume is recompensated toward normal. Grossman has postulated that valvular regurgitation, which causes a volume overload on the ventricle, increases end diastolic wall tension which is a stimulus to the laying down of sarcomeres in series[12]. This in turn increases ventricular volume.

Finally, mitral regurgitation may coexist with normal left ventricular muscle function for a prolonged stable period. As noted previously, the incompetent mitral

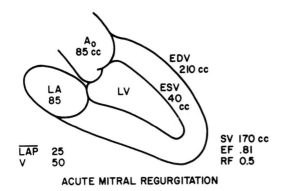

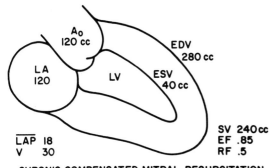

Figure 14.4 Acute mitral regurgitation (MR) is contrasted with chronic compensated MR. Ao = aorta; LA = left atrium; LV = left ventricle; EDV = end diastolic volume; ESV = end systolic volume; EF = ejection fraction; RF = regurgitant fraction; LAP = mean left atrial pressure; V = V wave. In chronic compensated MR, there is an increase in EDV while ESV remains relatively small. This increases total stroke volume. A portion of this increase is pumped forward, thus recompensating forward flow. LAP tends to fall as LA size and compliance increase.

valve diminishes left ventricular afterload. Braunwald has postulated that this reduction in load allows for a large increase in the volume pumped by the left ventricle for a prolonged period without decompensation[13].

In summary, in chronic compensated mitral regurgitation patients may enjoy a prolonged relatively symptom-free period as increased left atrial compliance, increased lymphatic function and increased left ventricular end diastolic volume together with relatively normal muscle function permit compensation for the valvular regurgitation.

Chronic decompensated mitral regurgitation

As is well known clinically, patients with chronic mitral regurgitation eventually develop increasing symptoms of congestive heart failure. In most such cases the cause of this deterioration is decreasing left ventricular contractile muscle function; the left ventricle after an extended period of volume overload begins to fail. Mitral valve replacement is usually contemplated at this time. It is generally accepted that preoperative assessment of left ventricular function is important in assessing operability and operative risk.

Yet a major problem in the evaluation of left ventricular function in patients with mitral regurgitation exists because standard clinical indices of left ventricular function may be misleading in this disease. Changes in afterload and preload affect left ventricular ejection fraction independent of muscle function[14]. As noted above, mitral regurgitation increases end diastolic volume and preload; mitral regurgitation also reduces systolic afterload thus permitting increased left ventricular ejection and reducing end systolic volume. Velocity of circumferential fiber shortening, although relatively independent of changes in preload[15], is still sensitive to afterload changes. These factors present in mitral regurgitation increase standard ejection phase indices of left ventricular performance such as ejection fraction and velocity of circumferential fiber shortening (Vcf). Thus, these indices might remain within the normal range even with significant left ventricular dysfunction. In support of this contention, Schuler and his colleagues described a group of patients with mitral regurgitation with ejection fraction in the low normal range (0.57 ± 0.05) who underwent mitral valve replacement. This group experienced progressive deterioration after surgery and a fall in ejection fraction to 0.26 ± 0.06[16]. Wong and Spotnitz demonstrated a large decrease (24 ± 17%) in echocardiographically determined shortening fraction immediately following mitral valve replacement for mitral regurgitation[17]. A careful analysis of systolic wall stress before and after surgery showed a significant postoperative increase in wall stress (see Figure 14.5). These authors suggested that mitral valve replacement increased afterload by removing the low-impedance pathway of ejection into the left atrium. This increase in afterload in turn induced a significant fall in left ventricular ejection fraction and Vcf. The opposite should have been true prior to surgery.

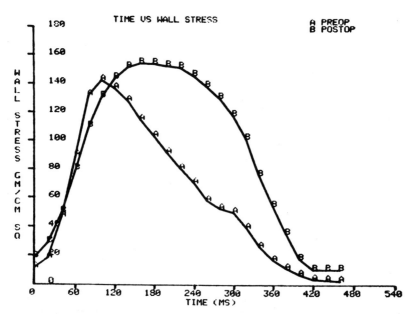

Figure 14.5 Wall stress is plotted against time for a patient with mitral regurgitation before valve replacement (A) and after valve replacement (B). Valve replacement produced a significant increase in stress (afterload) throughout most of systole. (Reproduced from Am. J. Cardiol. with kind permission of the authors and editors.)

Thus in the evaluation of left ventricular muscle function in patients with chronic mitral regurgitation, one must circumvent or take into consideration the effect of altered preload and afterload produced by the lesion. Borow and his colleagues reasoned that end systolic volume might be a better prognosticator of surgical outcome than ejection fraction in patients with mitral regurgitation[18]. Since end systolic volume is largely independent of preload, use of end systolic volume as a measure of ventricular function ought to be a better method of evaluating left ventricular function in a disease affecting preload. Indeed end systolic volume was found to be a better prognostic indicator than ejection fraction in patients with mitral regurgitation in their study. Patients with an end systolic volume index of greater than $60\,cm^3/m^2$ had a particularly bad prognosis.

Since afterload is also altered in mitral regurgitation, an index of ventricular function which is not only preload independent but also afterload independent or corrects for changes in afterload should serve as the best method of evaluation. The relationship of end systolic volume to end systolic left ventricular afterload has been found to be an excellent indicator of left ventricular function, sensitive to changes in inotropic state[6, 8, 19–24]. By manipulating the left ventricle through a range of afterloads using a non-inotropic intervention such as methoxamine infusion or use of a vasodilator, one can obtain end systolic volume at each afterload as shown in *Figure 14.6*. The slope of the line relating these end systolic afterloads (where afterload is quantified as end systolic pressure or wall stress) to the end systolic volume or dimension at that afterload is an accurate measure of ventricular function. It is relatively independent of preload and accounts for afterload. Unfortunately, obtaining the points that describe the line requires

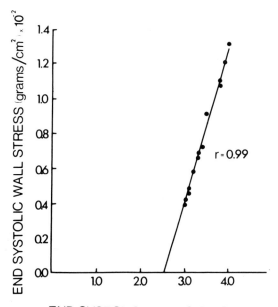

Figure 14.6 Wall stress and echocardiographically determined end systolic dimension were varied using methoxamine in this normal subject. The slope of the line so described is an accurate measure of left ventricular muscle function. (Reproduced from *Am. J. Cardiol.* with kind permission of the authors and editors.)

determination of volume (or dimension if the echocardiogram is used) for at least two different loading conditions. Recently, Pouleur and colleagues examined the slope of the line relating change in volume to changes in afterload (wall stress) in the latter part of systole during a single ventriculogram[25]. They found this method sensitive to changes in inotropic state. In this method, the changes in volume and stress occur naturally as part of the ventricular contraction. It does not require a maneuver to alter loading conditions artificially. This method should be applicable to patients with mitral regurgitation.

It seemed possible that simply correcting end systolic volume index for the afterload present in the ventricle at end systole would also give a good estimate of ventricular function in patients with mitral regurgitation. One of us (B.C.) examined the ratio of end systolic wall stress to end systolic volume index in patients with mitral regurgitation[26]. This ratio was compared with ejection fraction, end systolic volume, cardiac index, pulmonary capillary wedge pressure and pulmonary artery pressure with discriminant multivariate analysis as a predictor of surgical outcome. We found the ratio to be the best prognosticator tested; it provided good separation between patients who had a good surgical outcome and those who did not.

Even those symptomatic patients with chronic mitral regurgitation who did well with surgery had a depressed ratio suggesting that left ventricular dysfunction was already present in these patients.

A summary of the pathophysiologic changes in acute mitral regurgitation, chronic compensated mitral regurgitation and chronic decompensated mitral regurgitation is shown in *Table 14.1*. As noted, alterations in atrial and ventricular volume and compliance are important in producing or ameliorating the patients' symptoms. Assessment of left ventricular function is important with regard to overall prognosis but alterations in loading conditions produced by mitral regurgitation limit the use of standard ejection phase indices. Newer methods of evaluating left ventricular function which account for loading conditions seem particularly applicable in this disease.

Summary

Acute and chronic mitral regurgitation produce symptoms of congestive heart failure by remarkably different pathogenic mechanisms. Abnormalities in left atrial compliance, pulmonary venous pressure, left ventricular pump performance and left ventricular muscle function act in various combinations to produce pulmonary congestion and decreased systemic output.

In acute mitral regurgitation much of left ventricular stroke volume is ejected

TABLE 14.1 Variables in acute and chronic mitral regurgitation

	End diastolic volume	End systolic volume	Forward stroke volume	Ejection fraction	Left atrial compliance	Left atrial pressure	LV muscle function
Acute MR	↑	↓	↓↓	↑	n	↑↑↑	n
Compensated chronic MR	↑↑↑	↓	n	↑	↑	n or ↑	n
Decompensated chronic MR	↑↑↑↑	↑↑	n or ↓	n or ↓	↑	↑↑	↓↓↓

n = normal.

into a non-compliant left atrium resulting in a precipitous rise in pulmonary venous pressure together with a fall in forward stroke volume. The acute volume overload tends to increase preload and end diastolic volume. The incompetent mitral valve provides an avenue for reducing left ventricular ejection and a reduction in end systolic volume. This increase in end diastolic volume and decrease in end systolic volume partially recompensate forward stroke volume. However, forward stroke volume remains depressed until eccentric cardiac hypertrophy produces further enlargement of end diastolic volume. Experimental data show that in acute mitral regurgitation, left ventricular muscle function is normal. Thus in acute mitral regurgitation, symptoms are produced by volume overload to a non-compliant left atrium, together with reduced forward output in the face of normal muscle function.

In chronic mitral regurgitation, on the other hand, the left atrium enlarges and compliance is increased allowing accomodation of the regurgitant volume at relatively normal pulmonary venous pressures. End diastolic volume increases and forward stroke volume is normalized. In this state the patient may be relatively symptom free.

However, if volume overload is prolonged, left ventricular muscle function begins to diminish. Left ventricular emptying becomes less complete and end systolic volume increases. This may in turn lead to a greater increase in end diastolic volume with re-elevation of pulmonary venous pressure. The tendency for end diastolic volume to increase together with the unloading afforded by the incompetent mitral valve tend to maintain ejection phase indices such as ejection fraction in the normal range even in the face of left ventricular dysfunction. Since left ventricular function is of prime importance in evaluating prognosis and surgical risk, an accurate measure of left ventricular function is an obvious need. We have attempted to circumvent problems of interpretation of ejection phase indices imposed by the abnormal loading conditions present in mitral regurgitation by using the end systolic volume index and the afterload-corrected end systolic volume index to assess left ventricular function. End systolic volume is independent of pre-load and is a better prognosticator of surgical outcome than ejection fraction. It was postulated that correction of end systolic volume for end systolic afterload (wall stress) might yield a measure of left ventricular function relatively independent or corrected for both preload and afterload. Thus, the ratio of end systolic stress to end systolic volume index was examined in normals and patients with mitral regurgitation and found to be more useful than ejection fraction and other hemodynamic measurements in predicting outcome of mitral valve replacement.

References

1. ROBERTS, W.C., BRAUNWALD, E. and MURROW, A.G. (1966). Acute severe mitral regurgitation secondary to ruptured chordae tendineae. *Circulation*, **33**, 58
2. ECKBERG, D.L., GAULT, J.H., BOUCHARD, R.L., KARLINER, J.S., ROSS, J., JR. and BRAUNWALD, E. (1973). Mechanics of left ventricular contraction in chronic severe mitral regurgitation. *Circulation*, **47**, 1252
3. LEYTON, R.A., SPOTNITZ, H.M. and SONNENBLICK, E.H. (1971). Cardiac ultrastructure and function: Sarcomeres in the right ventricle. *Am. J. Physiol.*, **221**, 902
4. SONNENBLICK, E.H., ROSS, J., JR., COVELL, J.W., SPOTNITZ, H.M. and SPIRO, D. (1967). Ultrastructure of the heart in systole and diastole. *Circ. Res.*, **21**, 423
5. URSCHEL, C.W., COVELL, J.W., SONNENBLICK, E.H., ROSS, J., JR. and BRAUNWALD, E. (1968).

Myocardial mechanics in aortic and mitral valvular regurgitation. The concept of instantaneous impedance as a determinant of the performance of the intact heart. *J. Clin. Invest.*, **47**, 867

6. MARSH, J.D., GREEN, L.H., WAYNE, J., COHN, P.F. and GROSSMAN, W. (1979). Left ventricular end-systolic pressure-dimension and stress-length relations in normal human subjects. *Am. J. Cardiol.*, **44**, 1311

7. SUGA, H., SAGAWA, K. and SHOUKAS, A.A. (1973). Load independence of the instantaneous pressure-volume ratio of the canine left ventricle and effect of epinephrine and heart rate on the ratio. *Circ. Res.*, **32**, 314

8. GROSSMAN, W., BRAUNWALD, E., MANN, T., MCLAURIN, L.P. and GREEN, L.H. (1977). Contractile state of the left ventricle in man as evaluated from end-systolic pressure-volume relations. *Circulation*, **56**, 845

9. BRAUNWALD, E. and AWE, W.C. (1963). The syndrome of severe mitral regurgitation with normal left atrial pressure. *Circulation*, **27**, 29

10. RABIN, E.R. and MEYER, E.C. (1960). Cardiopulmonary effects of pulmonary venous hypertension with special reference to pulmonary lymphatic flow. *Circ. Res.*, **8**, 324

11. UHLEY, H.N., LEEDS, S.E., SAMPSON, J.J. and FRIEDMAN, M. (1962). Role of pulmonary lymphatics in chronic pulmonary edema. *Circ. Res.*, **11**, 966

12. GROSSMAN, W., JONES, D. and MCLAURIN, P. (1975). Wall stress and patterns of hypertrophy in the human left ventricle. *J. Clin. Invest.*, **56**, 56

13. BRAUNWALD, E. (1969). Mitral regurgitation—physiological, clinical and surgical considerations. *N. Engl. J. Med.*, **282**, 425

14. QUINONES, M.A., GAASCH, W.H. and ALEXANDER, J.K. (1976). Influence of acute changes in preload, afterload, contractile state and heart rate on ejection phase and isovolumic indices of myocardial contractility in man. *Circulation*, **53**, 293

15. NIXON, J.V., MURRAY, G., LEONARD, P.O., MITCHELL, J.H. and BLOMQVIST, C.G. (1982). Effect of large variations in preload on left ventricular performance characteristics in normal subjects. *Circulation*, **65**, 698

16. SCHULER, G., PETERSON, K.L., JOHNSON, A., FRANCIS, G., DENNISH, G., UTELY, J., DAILY, P.O., ASHBURN, W. and ROSS, J., JR. (1979). Temporal response of left ventricular performance to mitral valve surgery. *Circulation*, **59**, 1218

17. WONG, C.Y.H. and SPOTNITZ, H.M. (1981). Systolic and diastolic properties of the human left ventricle during valve replacement for chronic mitral regurgitation. *Am. J. Cardiol.*, **47**, 40

18. BOROW, K.M., GREEN, L.H., MANN, T., SLOSS, L.J., BRAUNWALD, E., COLLINS J.J., JR., COHN, L.H. and GROSSMAN, W. (1980). End-systolic volume as a predictor of postoperative left ventricular function in volume overload of valvular regurgitation. *Am. J. Med.*, **68**, 655

19. IMPERIAL, E.S., LEVY, M.N. and ZIESKE, H., JR. (1961). Outflow resistance as an independent determinant of cardiac performance. *Circ. Res.*, **9**, 1148

20. SAGAWA, K., SUGA, H., SHOUKAS, A.A. and BAKALAR, K.M. (1977). End-systolic pressure/volume ratio: A new index of ventricular contractility. *Am. J. Cardiol.*, **40**, 748

21. WEBER, K.T. and JANICKI, J.S. (1977). Instantaneous force-velocity-length relations: experimental findings and clincial correlates. *Am. J. Cardiol.*, **40**, 740

22. SUGA, H. and SAGAWA, K. (1974). Instantaneous pressure-volume relationships and their ratio in the excised supported canine left ventricle. *Circ. Res.*, **35**, 117

23. WEBER, K.T., JANICKI, J.S. and HEFNER, L.L. (1976). Left ventricular force-length relations of isovolumic and ejecting contractions. *Am. J. Physiol.*, **213**, 337

24. BOROW, K.M., NEUMANN, A. and WYNNE, J. (1982). Sensitivity of end-systolic pressure-dimension and pressure-volume relations to the inotropic state in humans. *Circulation*, **65**, 998

25. POULEUR, H., ROUSSEAU, M.F., VAN EYLL, C., VAN MECHELEN, H., BRASSEUR, L.A. and CHARLIER, A.A. (1982). Assessment of left ventricular contractility from late systolic stress-volume relations. *Circulation*, **65**, 1204

26. CARABELLO, B.A., NOLAN, S.P. and MCGUIRE, L.B. (1981). Assessment of preoperative left ventricular function in patients with mitral regurgitation: Value of the end-systolic wall stress-end systolic volume ratio. *Circulation*, **64**, 1212

Section 5

Surgical treatment using prosthetic valves

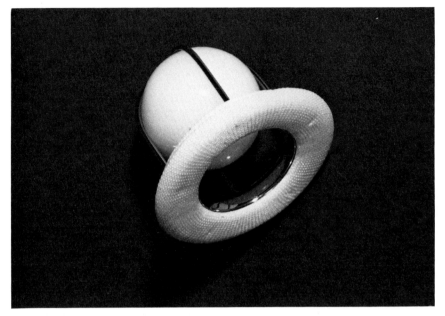

Figure 15.1 Model 6120 Silastic ball valve.

11.   Single casting: no welds or bends.
12.   Amply upholstered sewing ring.
13.   Transparent obdurator cup.
14.   Down-sizing unnecessary.

There is an uncluttered single orifice and a poppet that moves completely out of this orifice during valve function; design features that offer maximum protection against catastrophic thrombosis. The cage configuration protects the poppet from impingement by any intra-cardiac structures that may interfere with valvular function. The spherical poppet itself is capable of rotation on contact and is therefore less likely to be impeded along its pathway. In addition, the spherical shape provides an infinite number of three-dimensional seating possibilities, enhancing the durability of the prosthesis.

In contra-distinction to all bioprostheses and many previous mechanical prostheses, there is no intrinsic materials problem with the 6120 prosthesis. Ball variance or fatty infiltration of the Silastic poppet has not been seen nor has there been any evidence of electrolytic corrosion on the metallic surfaces of the valve. The valve is a single casting without welds; and the metallic parts require no bending to insert the poppet. Since in mitral replacement the cage of the prosthesis is directed away from the surgeon, ease of implantatin is not compromised by this design. The amply upholstered sewing ring obviates the need for pledgeted sutures and provides excellent fixation despite calcific irregularities of the mitral annulus. The transparent obdurator cup for measuring the size of the annulus and the left ventricle is unique and allows confidence in selecting the appropriate sized prosthesis for a particular patient. Since the poppet is so well protected, down sizing is not necessary as it is with so many tilting disc prostheses in the mitral position. The prosthesis is designed so that the secondary orifice (the truncated cone between the ball in the open position and the orifice) is larger in flow area than the primary orifice. This hydrualic safety margin diminishes the possibility that pannus formation in the mitral configuration on the outflow portion of the prosthesis can seriously interfere with adequate hydraulic function.

Fluid dynamics

Laser Doppler anenometry provides a useful tool in examining velocity profiles, turbulence density and sheer forces in pulsatile and non-pulsatile systems for valve testing. In a recent report by Akutsu and Modi utilizing a test chamber characteristic of mitral function, these parameters were measured for the 6120 Silastic ball valve, the St. Jude medical valve and the Björk–Shiley valve[1]. Based on the same annular diameter, the model 6120 had a considerably lower turbulence intensity as well as lower peak velocity compared with the other two valves. In addition, the 6120 is unique in having a uniform circumferential flow pattern with its peak velocity directed laterally, thereby decreasing the possibility of thrombus formation in this vulnerable area.

The medical literature is replete with reports of hemodynamic improvement following mitral valve replacement with the ball valve prosthesis including the model 6120. Indeed, unless there is a valve–patient mismatch, intrinsic prosthetic performance has not been a determinant of poor hemodynamic result. Invasive studies revealed relatively small gradients across the prostheses both at rest and with exercise for size 30–32 mm.[2] The 28 mm prosthesis may be unsatisfactory for large, active individuals under conditions of exercise but it is rarely used under such circumstances.

Clinical material

From 1965 to 1982 there were 259 Model 6120 valves implanted at the Oregon Health Sciences University and affiliated hospitals providing a total follow-up of over 1000 patient years. The mean follow-up was 4.7 years and the maximum follow-up was 17.6 years. The mean age of the patients was 53; 33% were males. Actuarial survival, including operative mortality, was 72% at 5 years and 54% at 10 years. This provides an annualized mortality rate of 5.3% per patient year. Of the late deaths, 48% were cardiac in origin, 19% were clearly delineated non-cardiac in origin and in 12% of the patients there was not enough accurate information with which to categorize the cause of death. In 21% of the patients the cause of late death was clearly related to the presence of an artificial valve. These so-called valve-related deaths included six cerebrovascular accidents assumed to be embolic events, three myocardial infarctions assumed to be embolic events, endocarditis in two cases and hemorrhage possibly related to the use of anticoagulants in one patient.

Valve failure

Using the Stanford definition, valve failure is defined as any valve-related complication such as infection, embolus, bleeding, thrombosis or paravalvular leak causing death or requiring valve removal[3]. It would also include, although it does not pertain to Silastic ball valves, death or reoperation related to a change in the structural integrity of the prosthesis. The percentage of patients who are free of valve failure with the Silastic ball valve is 91% at 5 years, 80% at 10 years and 73% at 15 years. Superimposing four recently reported rates of valve failure for the Hancock bioprosthesis[4-7] on to the valve failure-free curve of the Silastic ball prosthesis reveals in the second 5-year period of follow-up there is a difference most marked by 10 years very much in favor of the Silastic ball valve (*see Figure 15.2*). In another series,[8] in which there is a percentage of Carpentier–Edwards valves, at 5 years there was a difference in valve failure rates in favor of the Silastic ball valve, while in a recent report by Ionescu,[9] the gluteraldehyde-preserved pericardial valve carried with it an extraordinary durability beyond 10 years, but this unusual finding awaits confirmation by other investigators (*see Figure 15.3*).

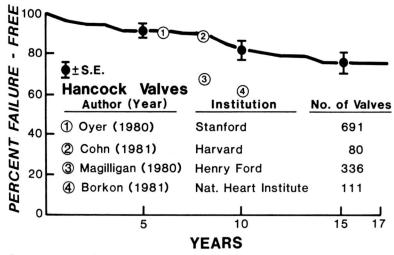

Figure 15.2 Comparative valve failure-free rates of Hancock bioprostheses and Model 6120 valves.

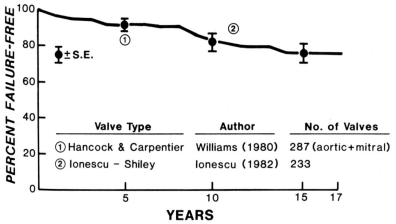

Figure 15.3 Comparative valve failure-free rates of Hancock, Carpentier–Edwards, Ionescu–Shiley bioprostheses and Model 6120 valves.

Thromboembolism and time frame

The Silastic ball valve, model 6120, has been in use since 1965. When the results of early implantations with this model, in terms of percentages of patients free of embolus, were compared with more recently operated patients with cloth-covered ball valves there seemed to be significant improvement in results with the latter. However, when patients operated upon in the same time frame were compared with each other, the embolus-free rates were the same for the Silastic ball valves as for the cloth-covered ball valves. For an accurate presentation of our current experience we considered only those prostheses implanted from 1973 to the present. This is roughly the same period in which other major prostheses have been used in large numbers and is more likely to provide a meaningful comparison. Since 1973, 175 such valves were implanted in patients with a mean age of 55, 33% being male. While the maximum follow-up was 9 years, the mean follow-up was only 2.3 years. A comparison of our experience with thromboembolism by time frame using the 6120 shows 90% of the patients embolus-free at 5 years in the current time frame; the embolus-free curve is compared with various reported embolus-free rates with other prostheses[4, 5, 7–15] as shown in *Figures 15.4* and *15.5*. It is apparent that except for the extraordinary report of Ionescu, there is no significant difference in embolus-free rates between the Silastic ball valve and the Ionescu–Shiley, Björk–Shiley, Angell–Shiley, Hancock and Carpentier–Edwards valves.

Valve thrombosis

The percentage of patients free of thrombotic stenosis of the mitral Silastic ball valve is shown in *Figure 15.6*. Note that 99% of the patients are free of this complication at 5 years and 90% at 15 years. This is compared with 87% free of this complication with the Björk–Shiley valve at 5 years. No patient in our series of Silastic ball valves died of this complication. Since thrombosis in the 6120 is not only rare but occurs very slowly and does not interfere with poppet motion, it thereby allows easy elective reoperation if necessary. This is not the case with the Björk–Shiley valve for which operations for valve thrombosis must be done as an emergency, carrying a higher mortality rate.

Hemorrhagic complications

Hemorrhage from anticoagulant treatment must be considered a valve-related complication and will vary from institution to institution depending upon the ease and precision with which anticoagulant therapy can be managed in a particular population group. Our own experience is shown in *Figure 15.7*. We have only one instance of a fatal bleed in our group of Silastic ball valve patients, and at 15 years the actuarial chance to be free of this complication is 99%. The chance to be free of a fatal or major bleeding episode is 91% and the chance to be free of all bleeding episodes at the end of 15 years is approximately 80%.

    A summary of fatal and non-fatal events following mitral Silastic ball valve replacement on an annualized basis is shown in *Table 15.1*. Of note is that fatal thrombosis did not occur and that the chance of valve removal for thrombosis was 0.5% per year. Fatal infection occurs at a rate of 0.2% per year, and non-fatal

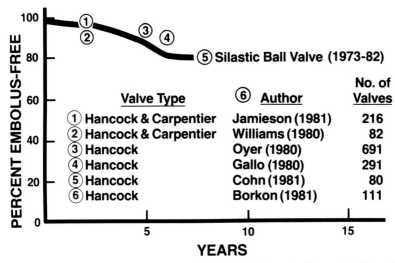

Figure 15.4 Comparative thromboembolus-free rates of Hancock, Carpentier–Edwards bioprostheses and Model 6120 valves.

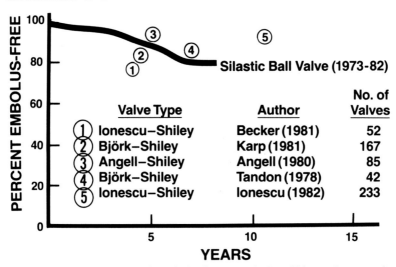

Figure 15.5 Comparative thromboembolus-free rates of selected bioprostheses, mechanical prostheses and model 6120 valves.

infection at a rate of 0.6% per year for an overall incidence of infection of 0.8% per year. The overall incidence of hemorrhagic complications is 1.9% per year. In the current time frame no patient has required removal of the Silastic ball valve because of recurrent embolism and the chance for a fatal embolus is 0.8% per year.

Summary

Based upon its predictable clinical performance over 17 years of use, the Silastic ball valve is our valve of choice for mitral valve replacement except in very elderly patients and those in whom anticoagulation therapy is a considerable risk.

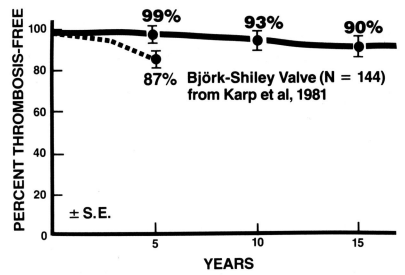

Figure 15.6 Comparative valve thrombosis rates of Björk–Shiley prosthesis and Model 6120 valves.

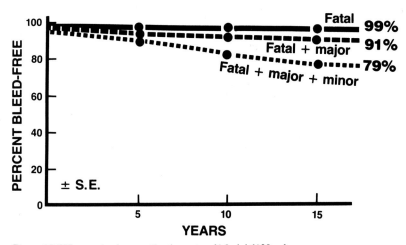

Figure 15.7 Hemorrhagic complication rate of Model 6120 valve.

TABLE 15.1 Fatal and non-fatal events (%/patient-year) associated with mitral valve replacement

Event	Time frame	Fatal	Removal	Other
Embolus	Old	0.8	0.1	5.6
	Current	0.8	0	2.2
Thrombosis	All	0	0.5	—
Infection	All	0.2	0.1	0.5
Hemorrhage	All	0.1	0	1.8

References

1. AKUTSU, T. and MODI, V.J. (1982). *Fluid Dynamics of Several Mechanical Prosthetic Heart Valves Using Laser Doppler Anemometer. Life Support Systems*, pp. 107–14. Proceedings ESAO
2. GLANCY, D.L., O'BRIEN, K.P., REIS, R.L., *et al.* (1969). Hemodynamic studies in patients with 2M and 3M Starr–Edwards prostheses: Evidence of obstruction to left atrial emptying. *Circulation*, **39**, Suppl., 113
3. OYER, P.E., STINSON, E.B., REITZ, B.A., *et al.* (1979). Long-term evaluation of the porcine xenograft bioprosthesis. *J. Thorac. Cardiovasc. Surg.*, **78**, 343
4. OYER, P.E., MILLER, D.C., STINSON, E.B., *et al.* (1980). Clinical curability of the Hancock porcine bioprosthetic valve. *J. Thorac. Cardiovasc. Surg.*, **80**(6), 824–33
5. COHN, L.H., MUDGE, G.H., PRATTLER, F. and COLLINS, J.J. (1981). Five to eight year follow-up of patients undergoing porcine heart valve replacement. *New Eng. J. Med.*, 304(5), 258–262
6. MAGILLIGAN, D.J., LEWIS, J.W., JARA, F.M., *et al.* (1980). Spontaneous degeneration of porcine bioprosthetic valve. *Ann. Thorac. Surg.*, **30**(3), 259–266
7. BORKON, A.M., MCINTOSH, C.L., VON REUDEN, T.J. and MORROW, A.G. (1981). Mitral valve replacement with the Hancock bioprosthesis: Five to ten year follow-up. *Ann. Thorac. Surg.*, **32**(2), 127-37
8. WILLIAMS, J.B., KARP, R.B., KIRKLIN, J.W., *et al.* (1980) Considerations in selection and management of patients undergoing valve replacement with glutaraldehyde-fixed porcine bioprostheses. *Ann. Thorac. Surg.*, **30**(3), 247–258
9. IONESCU, M.I., SMITH, D.R, HASAN, S.S. *et al.* (1982). Clinical durability of the pericardial xenograft valve: Ten years' experience with mitral replacement. *Ann. Thorac. Surg.*, **34**(3), 265–277
10. JAMIESON, W.R., JANUSZ, M.T., MIYAGISHIMA, R.T., *et al.* (1981). Embolic complications of porcine heterograft cardiac valves. *J. Thorac. Cardiovasc. Surg.*, **81**(4), 626–631
11. GALLO, J.I., RUIZ, B., CARRION, M.F., *et al.* (1981). Heart valve replacement with the Hancock bioprosthesis: A 6 year review. *Ann. Thorac. Surg.*, **31**(5), 444–449
12. BECKER, R.M., SANDOR, L., TINDEL, M. and FRATER, R.W. (1981). Medium-term follow-up of the Ionescu–Shiley heterograft valve. *Ann. Thorac. Surg.*, **32**(2), 120–126
13. KARP, R.B., CYRUS, R.J., BLACKSTONE, E.H., *et al.* (1981). The Björk–Shiley valve: Intermediate-term follow-up. *J. Thoracic Cardiovasc. Surg.*, **81**(4), 602–614
14. ANGELL, W.W. and ANGELL, J.D. (1980). Porcine valves. *Prog. Cardiovasc. Dis.*, **23**(2), 141–166
15. TANDON, A.P., SENGUPTA, S.M., LUKACS, L., *et al.* (1978). Long-term clinical and hemodynamic evaluation of the Ionescu–Shiley pericardial xenograft and the Braunwald–Cutter and Björk–Shiley prosthesis in the mitral position. *J. Thorac. Cardiovasc. Surg.*, **76**(6), 763–770

16

Current status of prosthetic valves in the mitral position

V.O. Björk, A. Henze and D. Lindblom

Since the advent of modern antibiotic treatment, rheumatic fever has diminished to such an extent in Sweden that mitral valve preserving operations are performed only on rare occasions. The vast majority of diseased mitral valves are so seriously calcified that conservative surgery is without prospects of success. Many of the cases who once exhibited excellent early results after closed valvulotomy of the rheumatic type mitral stenosis belong to this category when considered for re-operation[1]. In addition, few of the lesions causing mitral incompetence, such as ruptured chordae and 'floppy valve syndrome', are in our opinion suitable for annuloplastic procedures and valvular repair. Over more than one decade, the spectrum of mitral valvular pathology has called for valve replacement as the treatment of choice.

The Delrin disc

The initial model of the Björk–Shiley tilting disc valve for mitral valve replacement, introduced in 1969[2, 3], was equipped with a Delrin disc. The opening angle of this prosthesis was restricted to 50 degrees. Between 1969 and 1971, 51 isolated mitral valve replacements were performed with this early model. After 11 completed years, 27 of the involved patients (53%) were alive.[4]

Design changes

Important design changes of the 'prototype' were made along with the current experience of more than 3000 valve replacements—over 1000 were mitral valve replacements—at the Karolinska Hospital in Stockholm. In 1971, the prosthetic opening angle was increased to 60 degrees and simultaneously Delrin was discarded in favour of pyrolytic carbon, because of the latter's longer durability[5]. In 1976, the shape of the disc was modified from flat to convexoconcave[6], and in 1979 the opening angle was further increased to 70 degrees[7]. At the end of 1981 the continual efforts to obtain optimal durability resulted in the development of the monostrut 70 degree valve prosthesis, in which the entire tilting mechanism with both the smaller and larger struts are integral parts of the Stellite valve ring.

Durability

The main reason for discarding Delrin as disc material was its propensity to absorb water with minor changes in configuration. However, Delrin discs explanted after 6–12 years function in human hearts exhibited minimal wear and a lifespan over 30 years was calculated[8]. Pyrolytic carbon is completely resistant to moisture and therefore the preferred disc material. Its lifespan is considerably extended and should be clearly in excess of a generation, according to calculations from accelerated experimental valve testing[8].

The radiopaque marker

In 1975, the pyrolytic carbon disc was fitted with a ring-shaped radiopaque marker to permit non-invasive functional control of the tilting motion, which can be visualized easily by cineradiography or fluoroscopy. In the event of thrombotic obstruction the motion of the tilting disc is compromised.

The convexoconcave disc

We know today that a prosthetic thrombus probably starts generating along the smaller opening behind the pivot point between the disc and valve ring, where the flow pattern should be stagnant and turbulent[6]. This problem was tackled by the development of the convexoconcave disc valve. The convexoconcave disc is aeroplane-wing-shaped and the prosthetic opening mechanism is designed to add a 2 mm downstream motion when the disc tilts open and, simultaneously, the smaller opening of the prosthesis is enlarged significantly (12%) at the expense of the larger one[6]. This design permits effective washing at the pivot point and prevents stasis at the smaller prosthetic orifice (*see Figure 16.1*). In experimental studies, the resistance to flow is 15% lower for the convexoconcave model than for the standard model Björk–Shiley prosthesis[6]. Lazer Doppler studies in the pulse duplicator indicate that the low flow area behind the disc has diminished by 50% and simultaneously, there is a significant increase in flow through the smaller opening in relation to its enlargement. Diminished opening resistance and reduced regurgitation are further important features of the new design[6].

Carbon-coated Dacron

Our early observation that overgrowth of pannus may be located at the pivot point (*see Figure 16.2*) led to the introduction of the carbon-coated sewing ring. This design change makes neo-intima formation thin and shiny and overgrowth on the Stellite ring has thus far not been observed.

Decline in thromboembolism

The incidence of thromboembolism after aortic valve replacement was acceptably low with the Derlin disc and has remained mainly unchanged (1–2% yearly) with

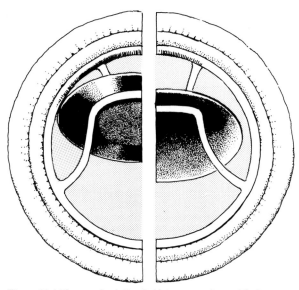

Figure 16.1 The standard disc (left) in comparison with the convexoconcave disc (right). The opening mechanism of the convexoconcave disc creates a clearance at the pivot point when the disc tilts open.

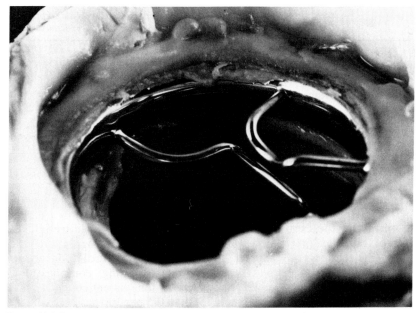

Figure 16.2 Overgrowth of pannus at the pivot point (disc removed)

the further development of the prosthetic valve. However, the design changes have obviously diminished the thromboembolic problems following mitral valve replacement. Early in our experience there was an incidence in the range of 4.1–5.0% yearly. Our recent follow-up showed that this incidence has decreased to 2.1% yearly with the current use of the convexoconcave disc prosthesis (*see Table 16.1* and *Figure 16.3*).

Surgical implications

Since the advent of cold cardioplegia, our surgical mortality associated with mitral valve replacement has decreased from 6% (beating heart) to 2% (cardioplegia). In addition, early neurological complications have markedly decreased in frequency which we believe relates to the greater ease with which air evacuation is performed on the cardioplegic heart. We prefer the double-flanged sewing ring and isolated mattress sutures are always used for valve implantation. Sub-annular fixation of the mitral prosthesis is considered essential, as most strain is exerted on this junction during left ventricular systole. Good fixation is obtained with 20 or more isolated mattress sutures which are passed through the lower ventricular flange of the sewing ring, the mitral annulus from the ventricular aspect and finally tied over the atrial annular portion. The sutures can be reinforced with patches on the atrial side, particularly if the annular tissue is thin and brittle. With this method of fixation, the incidence of paravalvular leakage is kept at acceptable levels (2%). If a leak calls for repair, it is most convenient to place patched mattress sutures from the adjacent atrial wall through the upper atrial flange of the sewing ring. Orientation of the larger downward tilting portion of the disc towards the posterior aspect of the left ventricle should be attempted in order to achieve optimal haemodynamics[9]. This 'posterior orientation' is followed by a lower transprosthetic pressure drop during exercise, in comparison with the reverse or 'anterior orientation'.

Our explanation of this phenomenon is that during diastolic filling of the ventricle there is an inverse movement of the proximal septal position which narrows the 'anterior inflow' but has no influence on the posterior part of the ventricular cavity[10, 11]. A further reason to avoid 'anterior orientation' is that the jet from a slight aortic regurgitation may delay disc closure and thus cause transprosthetic regurgitation (mitral incompetence). It must be emphasized that an absolutely free mobility of the titling disc must have priority over 'ideal orientation' described above. Appropriate orientation in this respect can be achieved even after the prosthesis has been sutured in position, as it can be rotated within its sewing ring. The original valve holder must be used for this purpose, because other instruments, such as forceps or clamps, may damage the prosthesis and cause malfunction or initiate the formation of thrombosis.

References

1. ÅBERG, B., HENZE, A., JONASSON, R., BERGDAHL, L. and BJÖRK, V.O. (1978). Mitral stenosis in association with aortic valvular disease. Closed commissurotomy of mitral valve replacement in addition to aortic valve replacement? *Scand. J. Thor. Cardiovasc. Surg.*, **12**, 1–7
2. BJÖRK, V.O. (1969). A new tilting disc valve prosthesis. *Scand. J. Thor. Cardiovasc. Surg.*, **3**, 1
3. BJÖRK, V.O., BÖÖK, K. and HOLMGREN, A. (1973). The Björk–Shiley tilting disc valve in isolated mitral lesions. *Scand. J. Thor. Cardiovasc. Surg.*, **7**, 131
4. BJÖRK, V.O. (1981). Advantages and long-term results of the Björk–Shiley valve. *Cardiovasc. Med.*, **1**, 293–304
5. BJÖRK, V.O. (1972). The pyrolytic carbon occluder for the Björk–Shiley tilting disc valve prosthesis. *Scand. J. Thor. Cardiovasc. Surg.*, **6**, 109
6. ÅBERG, B. and HENZE, A. (1979). Comparison between the *in vitro* flow dynamics of the standard and the convexo-concave Björk–Shiley tilting disc valve prostheses. *Scand. J. Thor. Cardiovasc. Surg.*, **13**, 177–189
7. BJÖRK, V.O. (1982). Optimal orientation of the 60° and the 70° Björk–Shiley tilting disc valve. *Scand. J. Thor. Cardiovasc. Surg.*, **16**, 113–118
8. BJÖRK, V.O. and HENZE, A. (1979). Ten years experience with the Björk–Shiley tilting disc valve. *Scand. J. Thor. Cardiovasc. Surg.*, **78**, 331–324

9. BJÖRK, V.O., BÖÖK, K. and HOLMGREN, A. (1973). Significance of position and opening angle of the Björk–Shiley tilting disc valve in mitral surgery. *Scand. J. Thor. Cardiovasc. Surg.*, **7**, 187–201

10. BJÖRK, V.O. (1981). The optimal opening angle of the Björk–Shiley tilting disc valve prosthesis. *Scand. J. Thor. Cardiovasc. Surg.*, **15**, 233–227

11. BÖÖK, K. (1974). Mitral valve replacement with the Björk–Shirley tilting disc valve. *Scand. J. Thor. Cardiovasc. Surg.*, **12** (Suppl.), 7–28

Surgical treatment using tissue valves

17

Current status of the pericardial xenograft valve

Marian I. Ionescu, Anand P. Tandon, N. Paul Silverton, Syed S. Hasan and Pierre L. Coulon

Glutaraldehyde–preserved tissue valves have been in clinical use for more than one decade and their performance during this initial period of time has been well documented. The porcine aortic valve and the pericardial xenograft have been introduced almost simultaneously. The pericardial xenograft valve has been used at our institution for mitral replacement since March 1971. Previous publications from this and other centres have described the clinical[1–12] and haemodynamic[4, 5, 8, 10, 12–16] results and have defined the hydraulic, *in-vitro*, characteristics of the valve[8, 17–20].

It is generally considered that tissue valves are subjected to a higher mechanical challenge and associated with a greater propensity for embolic complications when used in the mitral position. As the follow-up of patients with mitral pericardial xenograft valve replacement is now into the twelfth year we have analysed our results and report the data with particular emphasis on clinical and haemodynamic performance, valve durability and embolic risk in the absence of long-term anticoagulant treatment. Clinical and haemodynamic data are also presented from a recent series of patients who received the low-profile pericardial xenograft in the mitral position during 1981 and 1982.

Patient data and methods

Patient data

Since March 1971 a total of 711 patients received 855 pericardial xenografts for heart valve replacement (305 aortic, 272 mitral, 6 tricuspid and 128 multiple replacement).

All 400 patients who have undergone mitral valve replacement with pericardial xenografts between March 1971 and July 1982 were included in this analysis. There were 272 patients with single mitral valve replacement and 128 with multiple replacement (86 mitral and aortic, 26 mitral and tricuspid and 16 mitral, aortic and tricuspid). Details of the patient population are shown in *Table 17.1*. From the total of 152 patients who had concomitant cardiac surgical procedures 49 (32%) were subjected to coronary artery by-pass grafting and 40 (26%) patients to conservative valvular operations.

TABLE 17.1 Preoperative patient data

Variable	Single mitral replacement	Multiple replacement
Number of patients	272	128
Age: range (mean)	14–74 (48.6)	24–75 (51.2)
Male/female	99/173	44/84
Previous cardiac operations (%)	66 (24.3)	45 (35.2)
Concomitant cardiac operations (%)	97 (35.7)	55 (42.9)

The pericardial xenograft

Between March 1971 and March 1976, the valves were constructed in our hospital laboratory and used for single valve replacement only. Since April 1976 all pericardial xenografts have been manufactured by Shiley Inc. (Irvine, Cal., USA) and were used both for single and for multiple replacements.

The technique of valve construction was essentially the same in both 'hospital made' and Shiley valves. However, the 'hospital made' valves did not benefit from the accuracy of standardized production. The thickness and pliability of the pericardium were not assessed and quality control was limited. The glutaraldehyde used in our laboratory was a simple dilution of commercially available glutaraldehyde with an unknown and unstable content of monomers and polymers. Moreover, the pericardial tissue was treated prior to glutaraldehyde fixation with sodium metaperiodate and ethylene glycol, as advocated by Carpentier and Dubost[21].

The Shiley pericardial xenografts are manufactured according to standardized techniques and exacting methods for tissue selection and correct matching of leaflets for uniformity of function. Purified glutaraldehyde[22] is used for tissue fixation without any pressure load[23]. The sodium metaperiodate and ethylene glycol pretreatment is no longer used. The abrasive points in stent design and the quality of Dacron covering have been optimised (Microvel) when compared with the 'hospital made' valves.

In addition to the Standard (ISU) Shiley pericardial valves we have used, since January 1981, the low-profile (LP) pericardial xenograft. The low-profile valve differs in some essential respects from the Standard pericardial xenograft. The support frame is made of Delrin which has a stable molecular memory and therefore is not subjected to 'creep' deformation. This flexible stent carries a radio-opaque marker and is covered with microvel Dacron. The total height of the valve is lower and the implant height is reduced by approximately 30% when compared with the standard pericardial valve. The geometry of the valve is improved by changes in tissue-mounting techniques. 'In-vitro' evaluation of the low-profile pericardial xenograft has shown a reduction in pressure drop of from 10 to 43% and an increase in effective orifice area of from 10 to 32% (depending on size and flow) when compared with the standard pericardial valve. Comparative 'in-vitro' mechanical fatigue testing using the Rowan Ash (Rowan Ash Ltd, P.O. Box 117, Sheffield, UK) life tester[24] has shown the low-profile valve to be twice as durable as the standard pericardial xenograft under identical experimental conditions.

Of the 400 pericardial xenografts implanted in the mitral position 68 were 'hospital-made' valves and 332 Shiley valves (252 Standard–ISU and 80 Low profile valves).

As shown in *Table 17.2* the sizes of pericardial xenografts used in this series varied from 25 to 31 mm diameter. The great majority of valves were of small size: 80 (20%) 25 mm; 240 (60%) 27 mm and 80 (20%) 29 and 31 mm. No effort was made to implant valves larger than could be comfortably accommodated into the left ventricular cavity and the mitral valve annulus.

TABLE 17.2 Sizes of pericardial xenografts implanted in 400 patients

Valve	*Implantation diameter* (mm) *of valve*								
	17	19	21	23	25	27	29	31	Total
Single replacement, mitral					48	175	41	8	272
Multiple replacement:									
Mitral					32	65	28	3	128
Aortic	3	38	34	22	5				102
Tricuspid						16	21	5	52

Surgical technique

The operative technique for valve replacement has remained constant throughout the study period. In the majority of cases (355, 88.7%), one continuous suture was used for valve insertion, while in the remaining 45 patients either interrupted sutures or a mixed technique was employed. Between March 1971 and December 1976 intermittent hypoxia with topical hypothermia was the routine procedure. Since January 1977 total body hypothermia (20–26°C) with cold cardioplegia and additional topical hypothermia were used for all procedures. For the past 6 years, the left auricular appendage was excluded by ligature when accessible.

Definition of valve failure

Pericardial xenograft failure was diagnosed if any of the following criteria were met: (1) postoperative appearance of a new regurgitant murmur, unless proven to be perivalvular in origin; (2) confirmed haemodynamic valvular dysfunction necessitating reoperation or causing death; and (3) thrombotic occulusion of the valve.

Anticoagulant treatment

The initial 68 patients with single mitral valve replacement did not receive any anticoagulation either early or late following the operation. The remaining 332 patients (204 single mitral and 128 with multiple replacement) were treated for 5–6 weeks following valve insertion with warfarin sodium. The prothrombin time of these patients was deliberately maintained at a low level of between 18 and 24 s (hospital laboratory control being 12–13 s). The presence of factors considered to be potentially associated with an increased risk of thromboembolism (*see Table 17.3*) has not influenced our policy and long-term anticoagulants have not been given to any patient.

TABLE 17.3 Factors potentially associated with embolic risk in 400 patients with mitral valve replacement

Variable	Single mitral replacement No.	%	Multiple replacement No.	%
Preoperative systemic emboli (6 years preceding the operation)	28	10.3	11	8.6
Left atrial thrombus	22	8.1	9	7.0
Calcified left atrial wall	2	0.7	2	1.6
Gross left atrial enlargement	95	35.0	49	38.3
Chronic atrial fibrillation	201	74.0	87	68.0
NYHA class III and IV	249	91.6	122	95.3
Exclusion of left atrial appendage	111	40.8	20	15.6

NYHA = New York Heart Association.

Definition of embolism

Embolism is defined as all new focal neurological deficits either transient or permanent as well as all clincally detectable non-cerebral arterial emboli. Early emboli were considered those which occurred within the first 6 postoperative weeks.

Haemodynamic studies

Postoperative haemodynamic investigations at rest and during exercise were undertaken in 53 patients. The criteria for selection were the informed consent of the patient and the availability of preoperative investigations. Long-term postoperative haemodynamic studies were performed in 41 patients with isolated mitral valve replacement (29 patients with standard pericardial valve and 12 with the low-profile valve) and in 12 with multiple valve replacement. Sequential investigations were undertaken in six patients with single mitral valve replacement. In addition to the preoperative investigation these six patients had three postoperative studies performed at mean durations of 11.2, 42.3 and 68.7 months following valve insertion[16]. The methodology of haemodynamic investigations has been previously described[8, 15].

Follow-up data

All patients were seen by the surgeons and the cardiologists at least once every year in the Outpatient Clinic of the hospital. At each visit, in addition to a careful history, various clinical and laboratory parameters of valve performance were evaluated. None of the patients were lost to follow-up. Table 17.4 summarizes current follow-up data for the patient groups analysed.

Data analysis

Patient survival, incidence of embolism and of valve durability are expressed both by actuarial analysis and by linearised occurrence rates[25]. Standard statistical formulae have been used for the analysis of data, as previously described[8, 15].

TABLE 17.4 Patient follow-up data

Variable	Single mitral replacement	Multiple replacement
Number of patients	272	128
Hospital survivors (%)	254 (93.4)	116 (90.6)
Late deaths % per annum	2.6	5.8
Current survivors (%)	229 (84.2)	102 (79.7)
Months of follow-up, range (mean)	3–136 (50.1)	3–62 (28.3)
Cumulative follow-up (years)	961	240

Results

Survival

As shown in *Table 17.4*, 370 (92.5%) patients were alive when discharged from hospital; 254 (93.4%) with single mitral and 116 (90.6%) with multiple valve replacement. The overall late mortality was 3.2% per annum (2.6 for patients with single mitral and 5.8 for those with multiple replacement). The majority of hospital and late deaths were due to cardiac causes. There were three valve-dysfunction related deaths (0.25% per annum). The actuarial survival rate for the whole series is 69.3 ± 15.4% at 12 years of follow-up; 72.4 ± 14.1% for patients with single mitral valve replacement at 12 years and 77.5 ± 8.8% for patients with multiple replacement at 6 years of follow-up (*see Figure 17.1*).

Among long-term survivors there was significant functional improvement in all patients, as shown in *Figure 17.2*.

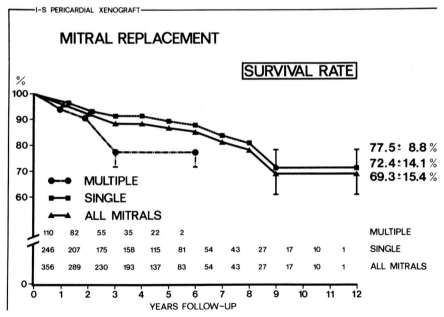

Figure 17.1 Actuarial survival following mitral valve replacment with pericardial xenografts. Individual curves are shown for patients with single and multiple replacement as well as for the entire series of patients with mitral pericardial valves. Numbers above the horizontal axis represent the number of patients at risk.

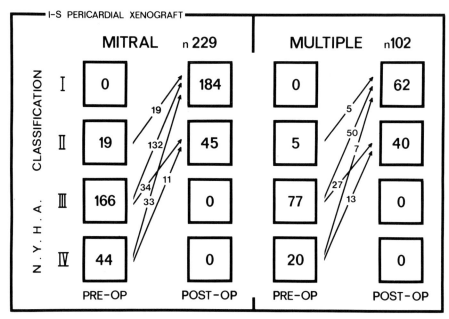

Figure 17.2 Pre-operative and latest post-operative New York Heart Association (NYHA) functional classification of long-term survivors with single mitral and multiple valve replacement with pericardial xenografts

Valve dysfunction

There were eight mitral pericardial xenograft failures in this series (seven in patients with single valve replacement and one in a patient with mitral and tricuspid replacement) (*see Table 17.5*). In three patients one of the valve cusps became partly detached at the suture line. The very first 'hospital made' valves were constructed with a continuous suture along the scallop-shaped outflow border of the support frame in order to secure the pericardium to the frame. The row of perforations acted as a path of least resistance in two of these valves. The third disinsertion of the pericardium from the stent occurred in a Shiley made valve at

TABLE 17.5 Clinical and pathological data of valve failure

No.	Patient age and sex	Cause of valve failure	Duration of implant (months)	Duration of symptoms	Reoperation	Outcome
1	48 M	Cusp disinsertion	13	1 wk	Yes	Alive
2	44 F	Cusp disinsertion	35	3 wk	Yes	Alive
3*	43 F	Cusp disinsertion	38	1 mo	Yes	Alive
4	30 F	Cusp tear	43	6 mo	Yes	Alive
5	52 F	Calcification	60	5 mo	Yes	Alive
6	30 F	Calcification	63	7 mo	No	Dead
7	36 F	Cusp tear	78	6 mo	No	Dead
8	36 F	Calcification	90	6 wk	No	Dead

* Mitral valve failure in a patient with mitral and tricuspid replacement. All valves except from patient No. 3 were 'Hospital made' pericardial valves. M = Male; F = femal; wk = weeks; mo = months.

the level of the suture sewing together two cusps. In two other patients cusp rupture occurred in the form of a vertical tear originating at the free margin of the cusp and extending for 3–4 mm proximally. Light, diffuse calcification of the pericardium occurred in three cases rendering the xenografts rigid. The duration of time for which these eight valves remained *in situ* varied from 13 to 90 months. Five patients underwent reoperation and are alive and well. Three patients died without reoperation. Seven cases of pericardial xenograft failure occurred with 'hospital made' valves and one with a Shiley valve. Thrombotic obstruction of the pericardial xenograft has not occurred in this series.

The linearized rates of valve failure were 0.72% per annum for single mitral valve replacement, 0.42% for multiple replacement and 0.67% for the entire series. The actuarial curves of freedom from valve dysfunction are shown in *Figure 17.3*.

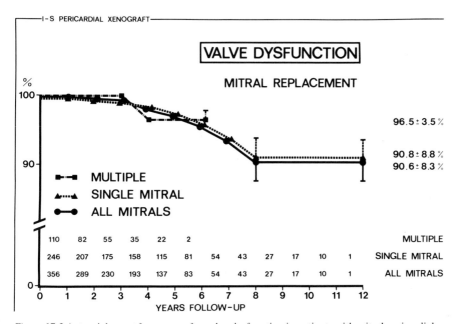

Figure 17.3 Actuarial event free curves for valve dysfunction in patients with mitral pericardial xenograft valve replacement. Individual curves are shown for patients with single and multiple replacement as well as for the entire series of patients with mitral pericardial valves. Numbers above the horizontal axis represent the number of patients at risk.

The freedom from dysfunction for single mitral replacement is $90.8 \pm 8.8\%$ at 12 years, for multiple replacements $96.5 \pm 3.5\%$ at 6 years and for the combined single and multiple series $90.6 \pm 8.3\%$ at 12 years. The actuarial analysis of valve durability is shown in *Figure 17.4*. As only one xenograft failure has occurred with the Shiley valves—used during the past 6.6 years—the acturial figure is $99.1 \pm 0.9\%$. For 63 'hospital made' valves with a follow-up of from 6.6 to 11.7 years the actuarial valve durability is $84.7 \pm 14.1\%$. For the entire series of valves used in the mitral position the projected actuarial figure is $89.5 \pm 9.5\%$ at 12 years of follow-up. Although the number of patients and valves followed up for more than 9 years is small, the actuarial curves remain linear between 8 and 12 years postoperatively.

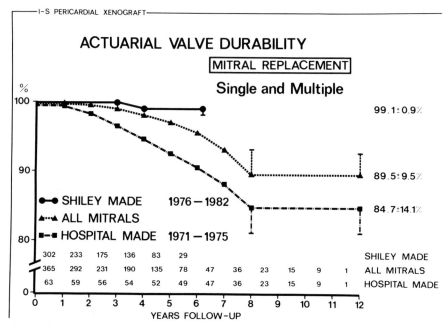

Figure 17.4 Actuarial event free curves for pericardial xenograft valve durability in the mitral position. Individual curves are shown for Shiley-made valves, for the entire series and for the 'hospital made' valves. Numbers above the horizontal axis represent the number of valves at risk.

Other valve related complications

There were seven episodes of perivalvular leak (five in the single mitral group and two in the multiple replacement group). All seven patients were successfully reoperated upon and continue to be well. The linearised rate of perivalvular leak was 0.58% per annum (0.52 for single mitral and 0.83 for multiple replacement). The actuarial freedom from perivalvular leak is 97.8 ± 0.8% at 1 and 12 years postoperatively for the whole series.

Infective endocarditis occurred in 11 patients, five with isolated mitral and six with multiple valve replacement. In the multiple replacement group the mitral valve was affected twice, the aortic three times and both valves once. Five patients survived and six died following reoperation. The linearised rate of endocarditis was 0.92% per annum (0.52 for single mitral and 2.50 for multiple replacement). The actuarial freedom from endocarditis is 95.4 ± 2.5% at 4 and 12 years of follow-up for the entire series.

Embolic complications

Eight episodes of systemic embolization occurred overall; six cerebral and two peripheral arterial. In the single mitral replacement group there were four early (at 3, 17, 30 and 42 days postoperatively) and three late emboli (at 8, 62 and 67 months). In the multiple replacement group, one embolic event occurred on the second postoperative day in a patient with triple valve replacement. With one exception (mild residual paresis) all embolic phenomena were transient (20 minutes to 70 hours).

Table 17.6 shows the subgroups of patients according to the anticoagulant treatment given and the number of embolic complications. The linearised rate of embolism was 0.67% per annum for the entire series (0.72 for single mitral replacement and 0.42 for the multiple replacement group). Actuarially determined rates of

TABLE 17.6 Anticoagulant treatment and embolic complications in patients with mitral and multiple valve replacement

Valves replaced	No. of patients	Anticoagulants Early	Late	Systemic Early	emboli Late
Single mitral	68	No	No	4	1
Single mitral	204	Yes	No	—	2
Multiple replacement	128	Yes	No	1	—
Total	400			5	3

embolism are shown in *Figure 17.5*. For the entire series 95.2 ± 2.8% of patients are expected to be free from emboli at 6 and 12 years postoperatively. For the single mitral replacement group the actuarial figure is 94.8 ± 3.0% at 6 and 12 years and for the multiple replacement group 99.0 ± 1.0% at one and 6 years of follow-up.

Attention has already been drawn in *Table 17.3* to the frequency of the factors potentially associated with thromboembolic risk. In this series there was no signi-

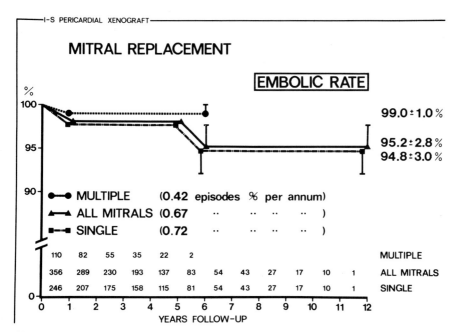

Figure 17.5 Actuarial event free curves for embolic complications in patients with mitral pericardial xenograft valve replacement. Separate curves are shown for patients with single and multiple replacement as well as for the entire series of patients with mitral pericardial valves. Numbers above the horizontal axis denote the number of patients at risk. The figures in parentheses show the embolic rates expressed as episodes percent per annum for each subgroup of patients.

ficant correlation between embolic complications and any of the factors mentioned with the exception of atrial fibrillation. Seven of the eight emboli occurred in patients with atrial fibrillation.

Valve thrombosis has not been encountered in this series.

Haemodynamic data

The results of haemodynamic investigations performed in patients with standard pericardial xenografts (long term and sequential) have been previously reported[8, 12, 14-16]. *Figures 17.6* and *17.7* show in a graphic form the results from cardiac catheterization of patients with single mitral replacement with valve sizes 25, 27, and 29 mm implantation diameter. *Table 17.7* summarizes comparatively the mean values of cardiac index, transvalvular gradients and calculated surface areas (at rest and during exercise) from 29 patients with standard pericardial valves and from 12 patients with low-profile pericardial xenografts.

Discussion

Long-term survival following valve replacement depends on a multitude of factors which are mainly related to the patient pathology and, to a certain extent, to the

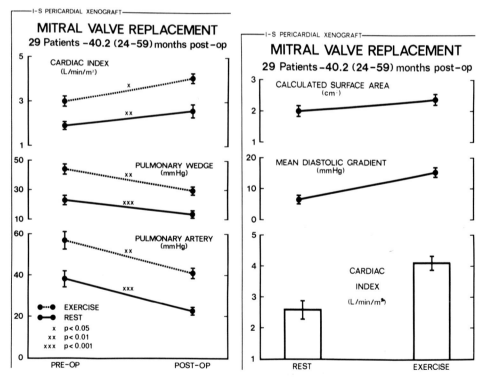

Figure 17.6 (left) Graphic presentation of mean haemodynamic values before and after mitral valve replacement with the standard pericardial xenograft and statistical comparison of the respective data.
Figure 17.7 (right) Graphic presentation of mean haemodynamic values at rest and during exercise in patients having mitral valve replacement with standard pericardial xenografts.

TABLE 17.7 Comparative haemodynamic data (mean values ± SEM) of the standard and low profile pericardial xenografts in patients with mitral valve replacement

Valve	No. of patients	Cardiac index (l/m^2/minute)		Mean diastolic gradient (mm Hg)		Xenograft surface area (cm^2)	
		R	E	R	E	R	E
Standard	29	2.6 ± 0.2	4.1 ± 0.2	6.4 ± 0.5	15.3 ± 0.9	2.0 ± 0.1	2.3 ± 0.1
Low-profile	12	2.9 ± 0.1	4.8 ± 0.1	4.5 ± 0.4	12.8 ± 0.8	2.2 ± 0.2	2.5 ± 0.1

R = Rest; E = exercise.

artificial valve implanted. The actuarial survival rate is therefore a cumulative reflection of these variables. In this series the actuarial survival rate is not different from that reported from other institutions with this or other types of tissue valves at similar durations of follow-up[1, 26–31].

Long-term durability is undoubtedly the most important single determinant in the evaluation of a heart-valve substitute. In our series of 400 patients with mitral valve replacement there were only eight episodes of pericardial xenograft tissue failure (0.67% per annum). In three cases the pericardium became disinserted from the support frame due to poor valve construction. These three cases have been included in the analysis as valve failure. They occurred early postoperatively at 13, 35 and 38 months, respectively. This mode of failure can be eliminated by improved manufacturing techniques. In two other cases cusp tear occurred but due to the very small number of cases and their random appearance (43 and 78 months post-implantation) no significant conclusion can be drawn. Calcification occurred in three patients aged 30, 36 and 52 years and the implant duration averaged 71 months. Reports of sporadic calcification of other tissue valves in adults have been published[27–31]. Ectopic calcification is a general metabolic process of immense complexity which depends on a multitude of biological factors. The artificial valve is only the end point in this hitherto not clearly understood chain of pathological events.

It is important to note that seven out of eight failures occurred with the 'hospital made' valves and that six of them occurred between 13 and 78 months of implantation. The follow-up with the Shiley made valves now extends to a maximum of 78 months and valve failure, as defined earlier, has been encountered in only one instance. A similarly low incidence of pericardial xenograft failure has been reported by other authors[1–6, 10, 11]. The difference in valve failure over the initial 78 months of usage between the 'hospital made' and the Shiley valves can be explained only by the different techniques of tissue treatment and valve manufacture. The Shiley valves are fixed in purified glutaraldehyde without sodium metaperiodate and ethylene glycol pretreatment. Sodium metaperiodate, an oxidizing agent, is now known to be traumatic to the connective tissue. In addition, the general improvement in selection and matching of tissue and the standardization of valve construction have optimised the overall quality of the pericardial xenograft.

Statistical comparison between actuarial data reported from various institutions is very difficult, but a general impression concerning trends can be gained. For tissue valves, the porcine bioprosthesis is a standard against which results can be compared. The Hancock valve has been in use for over 11 years and several reports of long term results have been published[29, 31–33]. *Figure 17.8* compares reported actuarial curves for valve durability. With the exception of Oyer *et al.*[29], who do not include in the actuarial curve failure due to valve thrombosis, intrinsic stenosis and regurgitant murmurs, we and other authors[31–33] have used a very similar definition of valve failure for the actuarial analysis. Despite the variability in patient

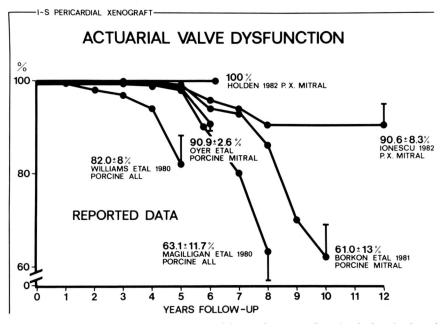

Figure 17.8 Composite graph of reported actuarial event free curves for valve dysfunction in patients with pericardial xenograft (PX) and in patients with porcine valves[6, 29, 31–33].

population and methods for data reporting, the trend in the long-term performance of procine bioprosthesis shows a progressively increasing rate of valve failure after 5 years of follow-up. Although the number of patients at risk beyond 5 years is small in all series, there is an obvious disparity in the performance after 5 years, between the porcine valves on the one hand and the pericardial xenograft on the other.

Our series of mitral replacement with 'hospital made' valves is similar in number of patients, definition of valve failure and duration of follow-up (from 6.6 to 11.7 years) with the porcine mitral series reported by Borkon *et al.* (follow-up from 5 to 10 years)[32]. The actuarial rates of valve failure in these two series follow each other up to 8 years when the curves part and the gap increases significantly (*see Figure 17.9*).

The failure rate in our series with pericardial xenografts has shown an overall incidence of 0.67 episodes % per annum. The actuarial rate of freedom from valve failure of $90.6 \pm 8.3\%$ at 12 years of follow-up for the entire series compares well with reports of porcine valves at similar durations of follow-up[26, 29, 31–34].

The sustained long-term durability of the pericardial xenograft is probably due to the quality of tissue and to the shape of the valve. Both contribute to a smoother opening and closure of the valve without areas of excessive bending or

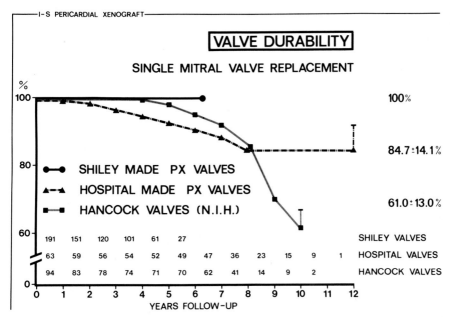

Figure 17.9 Actuarial event free curves for valve durability in patients with single mitral valve replacement. Comparison of Shiley pericardial xenografts with a maximum follow-up of 6.6 years, hospital-made pericardial xenografts followed up from 6.6 to 11.7 years and Hancock porcine valves followed up from 5 to 10 years. Numbers above the horizontal axis denote the number of valves at risk.
PX = Pericardial xenograft; N.I.H. = National Institutes of Health[32].

three-dimensional flexure (*see Figure 17.10*) which are damaging to the connective tissue fibres.

Although both porcine and pericardial valves are collagen structures treated with glutaraldehyde, their shape, technique of mounting, mode of function and hydraulic characteristics are dissimilar and therefore their long-term performance and mode of failure may be different.

The physical, chemical and biological properties of the natural aortic porcine valve have been profoundly altered by various interventions in order to adapt it for therapeutic means. The porcine 'bioprosthesis' has lost all the primordial characteristics of the aortic valve except its shape which remains unchanged and unchangeable. The pericardial valve, on the other hand, has been conceived as an entirely artificial design and therefore its basic shape can be altered in order to optimize its function.

Following extensive *in-vitro* testing, various modifications have been made in the design of the standard valve in order to further increase its durability, reduce its mass and implant height, and improve its overall hydrodynamic performance. All these goals have been attained by the creation of the low-profile valve which has been under clinical evaluation since January 1981. The implant height has been considerably reduced when compared with the standard pericardial valve and with the porcine valves (*see Figure 17.11*). This reduction in height along with the introduction of a flexible stent facilitate surgical insertion. The improved geometry of the low-profile valve has produced further improvement in its haemodynamic performance. The '*in-vitro*' mechanical durability of the valve has been

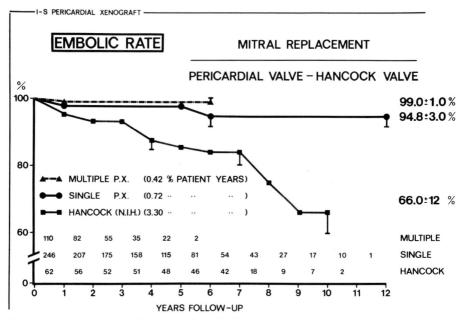

Figure 17.12 Actuarial event free curves for embolic complications in patients with mitral valve replacement. Comparison between the results of multiple and single valve replacement with pericardial xenografts (PX) (upper curves) with those of Hancock porcine valves (lower curve). Numbers along the horizontal axis denote the number of patients at risk. The figure in parentheses show the embolic rates expressed as episodes percent per annum for each group of patients. N.I.H. = National Institues of Health[32].

left atrium with or without thrombus, etc.) are present, patients with porcine valves should be anticoagulated for life[27, 29, 33, 34]. This recommendation, based on clinical results with the porcine bioprosthesis, probably holds true for that type of valve.

Most of the present knowledge of thromboembolic phenomena in the context of heart valve replacement is based only on clinical experience and general impression. There is no scientific evidence available concerning the exact nature or the anatomical origin of emboli. The patient's cardiovascular and general pathology are certainly responsible for emboli, but only to a certain extent and probably less so following the improvement achieved in cardiac and circulatory performance by valve surgery. *Table 17.8* outlines the incidence of systemic embolism in three well-documented series of medically treated patients with chronic rheumatic mitral valve disease. In these series, the embolic rate without anticoagulant treatment varied between 1.5 and 3.7 episodes % per annum.

Table 17.9 displays data from six reported series of patients with mitral valve disease subjected to conservative operative procedures (closed mitral valvotomy, open mitral commissurotomy and mitral annuloplasty). Although there is variation in the number of patients receiving long-term anticoagulation there is a striking similarity in the low rates of systemic embolism (0.34–1.1% per annum) following such conservative mitral valve operations. A comparison of embolic incidence between these two groups of patients with mitral valve disease, those medically treated and those with conservative mitral valve operations, necessarily

TABLE 17.8 Embolic complications in medically treated patients with mitral valve disease (without anti-coagulant treatment)

Sources	No. of patients	Follow-up (years) Max.	Mean	Emboli % per annum
Rowe *et al.* (38)	250	10	—	2.0
Szekeley (39)	754	22	7.7	1.5
Coulshed *et al.* (40)	166	17	3.9	3.7

incriminates more the diseased mitral valve than the remainder of cardiac pathology (atrial fibrillation, size of left atrium, etc.) as a cause of embolisation.

Many recent reports concerned with heart valve replacement, embolic risk and anticoagulant treatment imply that patients with mitral valve disease and mitral replacement carry a higher risk of embolisation if one or several of the following factors are present: atrial fibrillation, a history of emboli, advanced age or advanced stage of disease, large left atrium, clot in the left atrium or appendage and calcified valve or atrial wall. On the basis of these criteria a decision is made by many to give long-term anticoagulant treatment to patients with mitral valve replacement with tissue valves. A careful scrutiny of several reports concerned with this matter has shown that with the exception of atrial fibrillation none of the presumed factors has demonstrated to be statistically significantly related to systemic embolisation (*see Table 17.10*). It is against the background of this data that one must consider the embolic propensity of tissue valves.

The implanted artificial valve introduces an additional hazard of embolism in patients with mitral valve disease and atrial fibrillation. The risk, however, varies with each type of valve substitute.

Clinical studies have shown that the risk of thromboembolism is higher in patients with mechanical prostheses than in those with porcine valves[7, 49-51].

Among groups of patients with porcine valves the embolic risk is not significantly different whether a small proportion of patients (2.3% to 6.4%) receive anticoagulants[31, 32], or whether more than half of the patients (50% to 100%) are given long term anticoagulants[48, 52-54]. *Tables 17.11* and *17.12* show the reported incidence of embolism in patients with porcine valves treated in various proportions with anticoagulants. Despite the differences in long-term anticoagulation among the reported series there is a marked similarity in the incidence of embolism of about three episodes % per annum. This incidence is considerably greater than that seen after conservative mitral valve procedures and than that reported with the pericardial valve. These observations suggest that each type of tissue valve has a specific propensity for embolism which cannot be reduced below a certain level even under 'ideal' conditions of anticoagulation.

An additional element of risk in this equation lies in the use of long-term anticoagulants. *Table 17.13* summarizes the incidence of severe and fatal haemorrhage associated with anticoagulant treatment. This varies from 0.5 to 6.3% per annum in the reported series.

In view of this risk of haemorrhage and because the reported incidence of embolism with the pericardial xenograft is extremely low, even in the absence of long-term anticoagulation[2-6, 37], we are not using prothrombin depressants in our patients at any stage for routine prophylaxis of systemic emboli. Since June of 1982 we have discontinued the use of early postoperative treatment with warfarin

TABLE 17.9 Embolic complications following conservative mitral valve operations

Source	No. of patients	Atrial fibrillation (%)	Years follow-up Max.	Years follow-up Mean	Operations	Anticoagulant treatment (%)	Emboli (% per annum)
Ellis and Harken (41)	1390	51.6	11.0	6.0	Closed mitral valvotomy	None	0.46
Ellis et al. (42)	913	?	15–20	—	Closed mitral valvotomy	?	1.1
Kalseth et al. (43)	191	28.8	10.0	4.5	Open mitral commissurotomy	14	0.36
Gross et al. (44)	197	'common'	10.1	3.5	Open mitral commissurotomy	20.3	0.34
Vega et al. (45)	159	40.0	5.3	3.0	Open mitral commissurotomy and/or mitral repair	?	0.61
Tandon et al. (46)	113	72.5	19.0	9.0	Mitral valve repair	20	0.61

TABLE 17.10 Factors considered to be related to systemic embolism in patients with mitral valve disease

Source and treatment	No. of patients	History of embolism	Age	AF	NYHA class	CTR (LA size)	Clot in LA–LAA	Calcified valve
Medical treatment[40]	839	N/A	+	+	+	-	-	-
Medical treatment[47]	500	N/A	+	+	-	-	-	-
Closed mitral valvotomy[41]	1500	?	-	+	-	-	-	-
Open mitral commissurotomy[45]	159	?	-	+	-	-	?	-
MVR (Hancock)[32]	62	-	-	+	-	-	-	-
MVR (Hancock)[48]	124	-	-	+	-	-	-	-
MVR (Hancock)[28]	125	-	-	+	-	?	-	-
MVR (Hancock)[27]	80	-	-	+	-	?	-	-
MVR (Pericardium)	400	-	-	+	-	-	-	-

AF = Atrial fibrillation; NYHA = New York Heart Association; CTR = cardiothoracic ratio; LA = left atrium; LAA = left atrial appendage; N/A = not applicable; MVR = mitral valve replacement; Hancock = Hancock porcine valve; Pericardium = pericardial xenograft valve (present study).

TABLE 17.11 Embolism in patients having mitral valve replacement with Hancock porcine valves

Institution	Years of valve usage	No. of patients	Emboli (% per annum)	Long-term anticoagulation
Kansas University[50]	1970–75	104	4.8	If LA thrombus
Henry Ford Hospital[52]	1971–75	228	4.7	54% of patients
Henry Ford Hospital[53]	1971–75	125	2.9	75% of patients
Stanford University[51]	1971–75	243	5.2	15% of patients
Stanford University[36]	1971–78	561	3.1	31% of patients
Brigham Hospital[27]	1972–77	131	3.8	If AF of large LA

LA = Left atrium; AF = atrial fibrillation.

TABLE 17.12 Embolism in patients having mitral valve replacement with tissue valves

Institution	Valve	Years of valve usage	No. of patients	Emboli (% per annum)	Long-term anticoagulation
Pacific Medical Center[54]	Hancock	1974–77	126	5.3	50 % of patients
Pacific Medical Center[48]	Hancock	1974–79	124	3.12	62 % of patients
Pacific Medical Center[48]	Hancock	1974–79	72	3.16	100 % of patients
British Columbia University[34]	Carpetier– Edwards	1975–78	261	3.5	45 % of patients
NIH Bethesda[32]	Hancock	1970–75	62	3.3	6.4% of patients
Good Samaritan Hospital[26]	Angell– Shiley	1975–80	103	3.4	If AF, history of T/E, LA thrombus, giant LA, intimal disruption
Leeds University*	Ionescu– Shiley	1971–82	400	0.67	NONE

* Present study.
AF = Atrial fibrillation; T/E = thrombo-embolism; LA = left atrium; NIH = National Institutes of Health.

sodium and replaced it with the administration of dipyridamole for the first 6 postoperative weeks in all patients having mitral or multiple valve replacement with the pericardial xenograft.

Previously reported results of haemodynamic studies in patients with pericardial xenograft valve replacement from this and other institutions have shown that the performance of the pericardial valve is superior to that of porcine valves[4, 5, 10, 12, 13–16]. The results of the sequential studies have demonstrated that the initial circulatory improvement was maintained and that there was no change in the essential haemodynamic parameters up to 73 months following the operation[14, 16]. Postoperative haemodynamic investigations performed in patients with low-profile valves have shown an improvement in both transvalvular pressure gradient and calculated valve surface area when compared with results from patients with the standard pericardial xenograft.

TABLE 17.13 Serious and fatal bleeding complications in patients with mitral valve disease treated with anticoagulants

Sources	Year of publication	No. of patients	Follow-up (years) Max.	Follow-up (years) Mean	Treatment	Episodes (% per annum)
Fleming and Bailey (47)	1971	217	9	—	Medical	2.3
Gross et al. (44)	1981	40	10.1	3.5	Open mitral valvotomy	0.79
Hill et al. (48)	1982	72	—	2.2	Mitral Hancock	6.32
Angell et al. (26)	1982	103	5	—	Mitral Angell–Shiley	2.1
Borkon et al. (32)	1981	32	10	5.4	Mitral Hancock, Aortic Starr	4.9
Bjork and Henze (49)	1979	413	10	4.8	Mitral Björk–Shiley	6.3
Edmunds (55)	1982	21.550 patient years from 9 reports			Various mitral prostheses	0.5–6.3 (2.19)

The superior haemodynamic performance of the pericardial xenograft allows the selection and implantation of valve sizes that comfortably match the left ventricular and mitral annular dimensions without the necessity of oversizing in order to obtain lower transvalvular pressure gradients.

Conclusions

The analysis of our results with the pericardial xenograft has demonstrated that mitral valve replacement can be performed without long-term anticoagulation and with only a minimal risk of embolic complications. Moreover, valve thrombosis or lethal emboli have not been encountered in this series and the potential hazard of anticoagulant related haemorrhage was eliminated.

The superior haemodynamic performance of the pericardial xenograft, further improved with the low-profile valve, represents an additional advantage especially in patients with small left ventricular cavity.

The incidence of valve failure during a period of more than 11 years of follow-up was very low and the results with the Shiley-made valves showed an even lower incidence of valve dysfunction.

For these reasons we consider the pericardial xenograft to be the valve of choice for mitral replacement.

References

1. BECKER, R.M., SANDOR, L., TINDEL, M. and FRATER, R.W.M. (1981). Medium term follow-up of the Ionescu–Shiley heterograft valve. *Ann. Thorac. Surg.*, **32**, 120
2. COLES, J.G., DEVINERI, R., BUTLIN, G.M., GOLDBACH, M.M. and COLES, J.C. (1982). The Ionescu-Shiley valve—A clinical and pathological assessment. Presented at *The Cardiac Prostheses Symposium, Pebble Beach, California, 30–31 August*
3. DEAC, R., LIEBHART, M., BRATU, D., BRADISTEANU, S. and BENEDEK, J. (1981). Cardiac valve replacement with pericardial xenograft. In *Cardiovascular Surgery 1980* (eds. W. Bircks, J. Ostermeyer, J.D. Schulte), pp. 640–644. Berlin, Heidelberg, New York, Springer
4. GARCIA-BENGOCHEA, J.B. (1982). Valve replacement with the Ionescu-Shiley xenograft: Results at 5 years of follow-up. Presented at *The Cardiac Prostheses Symposium, Pebble Beach, California, 30—31 August*
5. GARCIA-BENGOCHEA, J.B., ALVAREZ, J.R., CARRENO, C.I. and CENDON, A.A. (1981). Resultados clinicos y hemodinamicos a medio plazo con el xenoinjerto de pericardio Ionescu-Shiley. *Rev. Espanola Cardiol.*, **34**, 283
6. HOLDEN, M.P. and BEHL, P.R. (1982). Six years of pleasure with the Ionescu-Shiley pericardial valve. Presented at *The Cardiac Prostheses Symposium, Pebble Beach, California, 30–31 August*
7. IONESCU, M.I., SMITH, D.R., HASAN, S.S., CHIDAMBARAM, M. and TANDON, A.P. (1982). Clinical durability of the pericardial xenograft valve: Ten years experience with mitral replacement. *Ann. Thorac. Surg.*, **34**, 265
8. IONESCU, M.I. and TANDON, A.P. (1979). The Ionescu-Shiley pericardial xenograft heart valve. In *Tissue Heart Valves* (ed. M.I. Ionescu), pp. 201–252. London: Butterworths
9. IONESCU, M.I., TANDON, A.P., MARY, D.A.S. and ABID, A. (1977). Heart valve replacement with the Ionescu-Shiley pericardial xenograft. *J. Thorac. Cardiovasc. Surg.*, **73**, 71
10. OTT, D.A., COELHO, A.T., COOLEY, D.J. and REUL, G.J. (1980). Ionescu–Shiley pericardial xenograft valve: Hemodynamic evaluation and early clinical follow-up of 326 patients. *Cardiovasc. Dis. (Bull Texas Heart Ins.)*, **7**, 137
11. OTT, D.A., COOLEY, D.A., REUL, G.J., FRAZIER, O.H., DUNCAN, J.M. and LIVESAY, J.J. (1982). Ionescu–Shiley pericardial xenograft: 3 year follow-up from a data base of 2247 patients. Presented at *The Cardiac Prostheses Symposium, Pebble Beach, California, 30–31 August*
12. TANDON, A.P., WHITAKER, W. and IONESCU, M.I. (1980). Multiple valve replacement with pericardial xenograft. Clinical and haemodynamic study. *Brit. Heart J.*, **44**, 534

13. BECKER, R.M., STROM, J., FRISHMAN, W., OKA, Y., LIN, Y.T., YELLIN, E.L. and FRATER, R.W.M. (1980). Hemodynamic performance of the Ionescu–Shiley valve prosthesis. *J. Thorac. Cardiovasc. Surg.*, **80**, 613

14. SMITH, D.R., TANDON, A.P., HASAN, S.S. and IONESCU, M.I. (1981). Long term and sequential haemodynamic investigations in patients with Ionescu–Shiley pericardial xenograft. In *Cardiovascular Surgery 1980* (eds. W. Bircks, J. Ostermeyer, H.D. Schulte), pp. 43–49. Berlin: Springer

15. TANDON, A.P., SMITH, D.R. and IONESCU, M.I. (1978). Hemodynamic evaluation of the Ionescu–Shiley pericardial xeongraft in the mitral position. *Am. Heart J.*, **95**, 595

16. TANDON, A.P., SMITH, D.R. and IONESCU, M.I. (1979). Sequential hemodynamic studies of the Ionescu–Shiley pericardial xenograft valve up to six years after implantation. *Cardiovasc. Dis. (Bull Texas Heart Inst.)*, **6**, 271

17. GABBAY, S., MCQUEEN, D.M., YELLIN, E.L., BECKER, R.M. and FRATER, R.W.M. (1978). *In vitro* hydrodynamic comparison of mitral valve bioprostheses at high flow rates. *J. Thorac. Cardiovasc. Surg.*, **76**, 771

18. RAINER, W.G., CHRISTOPHER, R.A., SADLER, T.R. and HILGENBERG, A.D. (1979). Dynamic behaviour of prosthetic aortic tissue valves as viewed by high-speed cinematography. *Ann. Thorac. Surg.*, **28**, 274

19. WALKER, D.K., SCOTTEN, L.N., MODI, V.J. and BROWNLEE, R.T. (1980). *In vitro* assessment of mitral valve prostheses. *J. Thorac. Cardiovasc. Surg.*, **79**, 680

20. WRIGHT, J.T.M. (1979). Hydrodynamic evaluation of tissue valves. In *Tissue Heart Valves* (ed. M.I. Ionescu). pp. 29–88. London: Butterworths

21. CARPENTIER, A. and DUBOST, C. (1972). From xenograft to bioprosthesis: Evolution of concepts and techniques of valvular xenografts. In *Biological Tissue in Heart Valve Replacement* (eds. M.I. Ionescu, D.N. Ross and G.H. Wooler), pp. 515. London: Butterworths

22. WOODROOF E.A. (1979). The chemistry and biology of aldehyde treated tissue heart valve xenografts. In *Tissue Heart Valves* (ed. M.I. Ionescu), pp. 347–362. London: Butterworths

23. BROOM, N.D. and THOMOSON, F.J. (1979). Influence of fixation conditions on the performance of glutaraldehyde treated porcine aortic valves. Towards a more scientific basis. *Thorax*, **34**, 166

24. MARTIN, T.R.P., VAN NOORT, R., BLACK, M.M. and MORGAN, J. (1980). Accelerated fatigue testing of biological tissue heart valves. In *Proceedings European Society of Artificial Organs (ESAO)* (ed. E.S. Bucherl), vol. 7, pp. 315–319. Geneva

25. ANDERSON, R.P., BONCHECK, L.I., GRUNKEMEIER, G.L., LAMBERT, L.E. and STARR, A. (1974). The analysis and presentation of surgical results by actuarial methods. *J. Surg. Res.*, **16**, 224

26. ANGELL, W.W., ANGELL, J.D. and KOSEK, J.C. (1982). Twelve-year experience with glutaraldehyde preserved porcine xenografts. *J. Thorac. Cardiovasc. Surg.*, **83**, 493

27. COHN, L.H. and COLLINS, J.J. (1979). The glutaraldehyde stabilized porcine xenograft valve. In *Tissue Heart Valves* (ed. M.I. Ionescu), pp. 173–200. London: Butterworths

28. LAKIER, J.B., KHAJA, F., MAGILLIGAN, D.J. and GOLDSTEIN, S. (1980). Porcine xenograft valves. Long-term (60–89 months) follow-up. *Circulation*, **62**, 313

29. OYER, P.E., MILLER, D.C., STINSON, E.B., REITZ, B.A., MORENO-CABRAL, R.J. and SHUMWAY, N.E. (1980). Clinical durability of the Hancock porcine bioprosthetic valve. *J. Thorac. Cardiovasc. Surg.*, **80**, 824

30. THIENE, G., BORTOLOTTI, U., PANIZZON, G., MILANO, A. and GALLUCCI, V. (1980). Pathological substrates of thrombus formation after heart valve replacement with the Hancock bioprosthesis. *J. Thorac. Cardiovasc. Surg.*, **80**, 414

31. WILLIAMS, J.B., KARP, R.B., KIRKLIN, J.W., KOUCHOUKOS, N.T., PACIFICO, A.D., ZORN, G.L., BLACKSTONE, E.H., BROWN, R.N., PIANTADOSI, S. and BRADLEY, E.L. (1980). Considerations in selection and management of patients undergoing valve replacement with glutaraldehyde-fixed porcine bioprosthesis. *Ann. Thorac. Surg.*, **30**, 247

32. BORKON, A.M., MCINTOSH, C.L., VON RUEDEN, T.J. and MORROW, A.G. (1981). Mitral valve replacement with the Hancock bioprosthesis: Five to ten year follow-up. *Ann. Thorac. Surg.*, **32**, 127

33. MAGILLIGAN, D.J., LEWIS, J.W., JARA, F.M., LEE, M.W., ALAM, M., RIDDLE, J.M. and STEIN, P.D. (1980). Spontaneous degeneration of procine bioprosthetic valves. *Ann. Thorac. Surg.*, **30**, 259

34. JAMIESON, W.R.E., JANUSZ, M.T., MIYAGISHIMA, R.T., MUNRO, A.I., TUTASSURA, H., GEREIN, A.N., BURR, L.H. and ALLEN, P. (1981). Embolic complications of porcine heterograft cardiac valves. *J. Thorac. Cardiovasc. Surg.*, **81**, 626

35. OYER, P.E., STINSON, E.B., GRIEPP, E.B. and SHUMWAY, N.E. (1977). Valve replacement with the Starr–Edwards and Hancock prostheses. Comparative analysis of late morbidity and mortality. *Ann. Thorac. Surg.*, **186**, 301

36. OYER, P.E., STINSON, E.B., REITZ, B.A., MILLER, D.C., ROSSITER, S. and SHUMWAY, N.E. (1979). Long term evaluation of porcine xenograft bioprosthesis. *J. Thorac. Cardiovasc. Surg.*, **78**, 343

37. COOLEY, D.A. Discussion of paper by Becker, R.M., Sandor, L. Tindel, M. and Frater, R.W.M.

(1981). Medium-term follow-up of the Ionescu–Shiley heterograft valve. *Ann. Thorac. Surg.*, **32,** 120

38. ROWE, J.C., BLAND, E.J., SPRAGUE, H.B. and WHITE, P.D. (1960). The course of mitral stenosis without surgery: Ten and twenty year perspectives. *Ann. Intern. Med.*, **52,** 741
39. SZEKELY, P. (1964). Systemic embolism and anticoagulant prophylaxis in rheumatic heart disease. *Brit. Med. J.*, **1,** 1209
40. COULSHED, N., EPSTEIN, E.J., MCKENDRICK, C.S., GALLOWAY, R.W. and WALKER, E. (1970). Systemic embolism in mitral valve disease. *Brit. Heart J.*, **32,** 26
41. ELLIS, L.B. and HARKEN, D.E. (1961). Arterial embolization in relation to mitral valvuloplasty. *Am. Heart J.*, **62,** 611
42. ELLIS, L.B., SINGH, J.B., MORALES, D.D. and HARKEN, D.E. (1973). Fifteen to twenty year study of one thousand patients undergoing closed mitral valvuloplasty. *Circulation*, **68,** 357
43. HALSETH, W.L., ELLIOT, D.P., WALKER, E.L. and SMITH, E.A. (1980). Open mitral commissurotomy. *J. Thorac. Cardiovasc. Surg.*, **80,** 842
44. GROSS, R.I., CUNNINGHAM, J.N. JR., SNIVELY, S.L., CATINELLA, F.P., NATHAN, I.M., ADAMS, P.X. and SPENCER, F.C. (1981). Long-term results of open radical mitral commissurotomy: Ten year follow-up study of 202 patients. *Am. J. Cardiol.*, **47,** 821
45. VEGA, J.L., FLEITAS, M., MARTINEZ, R., GALLO, J.I., GUTIERREZ, J.A., COLMAN, T. and DURAN, C.M.G. (1981). Open mitral commissurotomy. *Ann. Thorac. Surg.*, **31,** 266
46. TANDON, A.P., LUKACS, L.I., SMITH, D.R. and IONESCU, M.I. (1979). Mitral annuloplasty—A long term clinical and haemodynamic study. *Thorac. Cardiovasc. Surg.*, **27,** 39
47. FLEMING, H.A. and BAILEY, S.M. (1971). Mitral valve disease, systemic embolism and anticoagulants. *Post Med. J.*, **47,** 599
48. HILL, J.D., LAFOLLETTE, L., SZARNICKI, R.J., AVERY, G.J. II, WILSON, R.M., GERBODE, F., KERTH, W.J. and RODVIEN, R. (1982). Risk-benefit analysis of warfarin therapy in Hancock mitral valve replacement. *J. Thorac. Cardiovasc. Surg.*, **83,** 718
49. BJORK, V.O. and HENZE, A. (1979). Prosthetic heart valve replacement. Nine years' experience with the Bjork–Shiley tilting disc valve. In *Tissue Heart Valves* (ed. M. I. Ionescu), pp. 1–28. London: Butterworths
50. HANNAH, H. III and REIS, R.L. (1976). Current status of porcine heterograft prosthesis: A 5 year appraisal. *Circulation*, **54,** Suppl 3, III–27
51. STINSON, E.B., GRIEPP, R.B., OYER, P.E. and SHUMWAY, N.E. (1977). Long term experience with porcine aortic valve xenografts. *J. Thorac. Cardiovasc. Surg.*, **73,** 54
52. DAVILA, J.C. and MAGILLIGAN, D.J. (1977). Experience with the Hancock porcine xenograft for mitral valve replacement. In *Second Henry Ford Hospital International Symposium on Cardiac Surgery* (ed. J.C. Davila), pp. 485–491. New York: Appleton-Century-Crofts
53. DAVILA, J.C., MAGILLIGAN, D.J. and LEWIS, J.W. (1978). Is the Hancock porcine valve the best cardiac valve substitute today? *Ann. Thorac. Surg.*, **26,** 303
54. HETZER, R., HILL, J.D., KERTH, W.J., ANSBRO, J., ADAPPA, M.G., RODVIEN, R., KAMM, B. and GERBODE, F. (1978). Thrombo-embolic complications after mitral valve replacement with Hancock xenograft. *J. Thorac. Cardiovasc. Surg.*, **75,** 651
55. EDMUNDS, L.H. JR. (1982). Thromboembolic complications of current cardiac valvular prosthesis. *Ann. Thorac, Surg.*, **34,** 96

18

Current status and the future of tissue valves

Alain Carpentier

'Tissue valve' is a generic term which serves to design cardiac valves made from tissues explanted either from human (allogenic tissues) or from animal (xenogenic tissues).

Allogenic tissues, the so-called valvular homografts, are still used with excellent results by scattered surgical groups, particularly in the correction of congenital heart diseases; but problems of procurement size and sterility have been and still are serious limitations to their widespread use.

Xenogenic tissues are either porcine valves or bovine pericardium, which have been confronted in the past with problems of immunological rejection and tissue degeneration. The introduction in 1968 of the technique of tissue preservation using glutaraldehyde[1] and the development of the concept of the bioprosthesis[2, 3] minimized these drawbacks and made possible the development of valvular bioprostheses on an industrial scale. Their clinical use has markedly increased in the last 10 years and valvular bioprostheses today represent approximately half of the total production of valvular prostheses. The reasons for this development are the specific advantages associated with biological valves when compared with mechanical valves: absence of hemolysis, lower risk of thromboembolism, avoidance of anticoagulants and progressive onset of occasional failures.

Currently available bioprosthetic valves

There are approximately 10 different types of valvular bioprostheses commercially available. They are all made of xenogenic biological tissues preserved in buffered glutaraldehyde of which the concentration is almost identical, varying from 0.2 to 0.8%. The additional use of formalin either during one stage of the procedure of preservation or in the solution storage is intended to improve the sterility of the biological tissue. Differences between the various valves include the type of tissues (porcine valve or bovine pericardium), the stent design and the method of mounting (*see Table 18.1 and Figure 18.1*).

Bioprosthetic valve performances

Since valvular bioprostheses have been introduced in clinical experimentation since 1968[1] and in clinical practice since 1971[2], long-term results over 10 years are

TABLE 18.1 Characteristic features of currently commercially available valves

Valve	Tissue (% glutaraldehyde)	Stent	Orifice	Cloth
Carpentier–Edwards	Porcine (0.625)	Eligiloy: flexible	Flexible	Teflon
Hancock	Porcine (0.2–0.1)	Polypropylene: flexible	Rigid	Dacron
Ionescu–Shiley	Bovine pericardium (0.5)	Titanium: rigid	Rigid	Dacron
Carpentier–Edwards pericardial	Bovine pericardium (0.6)	Elgiloy: flexible	Flexible	Teflon

available in the literature. Although it is questionable to compare different series of patients operated on by different groups of surgeons, a review of the literature may give some insight into the performance of the valves currently available (*see Table 18.2*)[2–13].

Hemodynamics

Numerous studies have been published on the hemodynamics of valvular bioprostheses. They mainly concern valves in the aortic position. This because any artificial valves, whether biological or mechanical, give rise to less severe problems of gradient in the mitral position since the average valve size is 31 mm in women and 33 mm in men. Below 31 mm, any mitral valve may lead to some degree of transvalvular gradient, particularly during exercise. A specific advantage of the porcine valve bioprostheses is the possibility of using a valve larger than a mechanical valve for a given mitral orifice, since the opening mechanism of the valve is not impaired by the ventricular contraction. Because of their rather sharp and protruding struts the pericardial valves do not offer the same advantage. Because of the hemodynamics of valvular bioprostheses, pericardial valves in particular may change with time as a result of fibrin deposition on the tissue[14].

Thromboembolism

Tissue valves are not totally free from thromboembolic complications. During the first 3 months after surgery, the risk of thromboembolism is similar to that of mechanical valves because the synthetic material of the valve is exposed to blood before fibrin covering occurs. Hence anticoagulants must be systematically given for 3 months to patients with a bioprosthesis. After 3 months the risk of thromboembolism is reduced and anticoagulants can be discontinued, except in those patients having one or several of the following risk factors: (1) poor myocardial function; (2) enlarged, calcified, or thrombosed left atrium; (3) persistent atrial fibrillation; and (4) a small prosthesis. Data from the literature indicate an incidence of 83–92% emboli-free patients 5 years postoperatively in the mitral position, despite the fact that 55% of the patients were not taking long-term anticoagulants (*see Table 18.2*). This low incidence of thromboembolic complications can be further reduced by minimizing the risk factors—i.e. operation at an earlier stage, prevention of low cardiac output, partial resection of the left atrium to reduce its size, electrical conversion to sinus rhythm, and use of large prostheses.

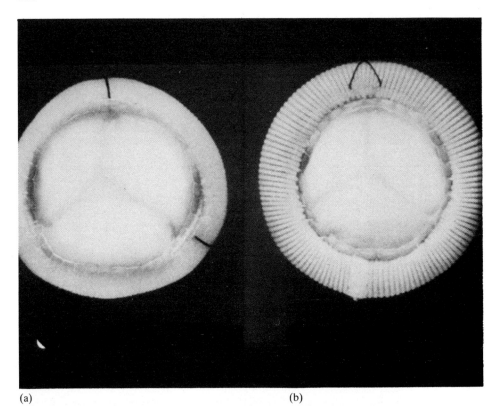

(a)   (b)

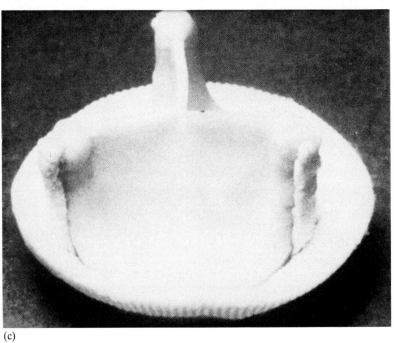

(c)

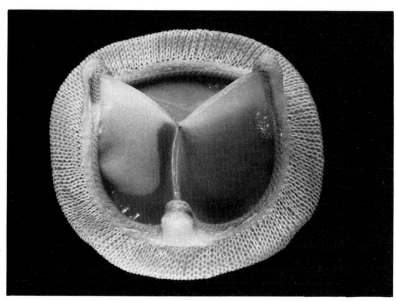

(d)

Figure 18.1 Currently available tissue valves. (*a*) Carpentier–Edwards porcine valve. (*b*) Hancock porcine valve. (*c*) Ionescu–Shiley pericardial valve.
(*d*) Carpentier–Edwards pericardial valve.

Anticoagulant related complications

Systematic long-term postoperative anticoagulation has been advised in patients with atrial fibrillation and we have been following this policy for several years. However, the iatrogenic risks associated with anticoagulation seem at least similar and may even be greater than the risk of thromboembolism in patients with a mitral valvular bioprosthesis. One per cent per patient year mortality versus 0.8% and 4.% per patient year morbidity, versus 2–3%. For this reason, we don't anticoagulate patients in atrial fibrillation any more except for patients with a low cardiac ouput or whenever the endothelium of the left atrium is calcified or severely altered as observed during the operation.

TABLE 18.2 Risks associated with the various techniques of mitral valve surgery (average values from references 2–13)

Valve	Mortality (%/patient/year)	Thromboembolism (%/patient/year)	Anticoagulant–related complications (%/patient/year)	Valve failure (%/patient/year)
Starr 6120	4–5	4–6	2–4	2
Björk	3–5	3–6	2–4	2
Bioprostheses	3–4	2–3	*	2–3

*Varies between 0 and 4% depending on whether the patients are taking anticoagulatants.

Valve durability

Limited durability is the main concern associated with tissue valves. According to the most recent reports, actuarial valve survival at 8 years is 94% in the mitral position for the currently available porcine valves[5]. There are discrepancies in the results from the literature which may be explained by the large variations in histological structure and *in-vitro* durability observed with the currently available tissue valves before implantation (*see Figure 18.2*). Investigations in our laboratory with fatigue testers have shown that valve durability varied from 11×10^6 cycles to 650×10^6 cycles: an equivalent time difference of 17 years in the same valve series[12]. As we will see below these variations were proved to be the result of valve preparation and therefore could be reduced by improved preservation methods. Other factors that may explain discrepancies in the results involve hazards of surgical implantation, insufficient valve irrigation to prevent drying out of the tissue during valve implantation, and excess intravenous injections of calcium postoperatively. It is too early to recognize differences in durability between different types of porcine valve or pericardial valve bioprostheses.

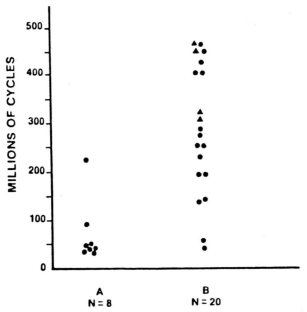

Figure 18.2 Fatigue testing of commercially available valves from two laboratories, showed large variations in durability from 1 to 15 year equivalent time. ▲ = continuing; ● = fatigue failure.

The mode of tissue valve failures is of three types: (1) bacterial endocarditis the incidence of which is similar to that of mechanical prostheses; (2) tissue damage (holes or tears) by fatigue lesions or inflammatory reaction or both; and (3) calcification. The incidence of valve calcification is of particular concern in children. Several publications have reported an incidence calcification between 20 and 50% at 5 years, depending on the age of the patient. The younger the patient the higher the risk of calcification[15, 16]. The risk of calcification is also higher in patients with chronic renal failure because of abnormal calcium metabolism.

Limited valve survival should be regarded as the normal fate of any biological tissue implanted within the body. It is the price to pay for the advantages associated with this method of valvular replacement, particularly a better quality of life and a lower incidence of catastrophic events whether valve related, thromboembolism related, or anticoagulant related. Reoperation for tissue valve failure does not imply the death of the patient, whereas a complication affecting a mechanical prosthesis is often fatal.

Patient survival

Duration of life after valve replacement is one of the basic criteria for assessing the value of the type of valve used. Actuarial survivals at 8 and 10 years are now available from several groups. Actuarial survival with porcine bioprostheses in the mitral position ranged from 65 to 85% at 8 years. This rather low mortality may be explained by a risk of acute complications, particularly thromboembolism and anticoagulant-related complications, lower than with mechanical valves. However, this must be confirmed by longer follow-ups.

Future developments of tissue valve

The future of tissue valves depends on our ability to solve the pending problems associated either with porcine valve bioprostheses—i.e., transvalvular gradients, limited durability and calcification—or with pericardial valves—i.e., excess protrusion and rigidity of the stent, transvalvular gradients in the mitral position, limited durability, and calcification.

Transvalvular gradient

Since transvalvular gradients result mainly from the impedence caused by the stent and the aortic remnant supporting the cusps, valve design is important. Hemodynamics through the valve can be improved by reducing the amount of synthetic material by optimizing valve design and by reducing the protrusion of the struts into the ventricular cavity (*see Figure 18.3*). The Edwards Laboratories supra-annular valve (SAV) was developed according to these specifications and its hemodynamic performance was evaluated *in vitro*. At a steady flow rate of 15 *l*/min, the SAV was compared with the current Edwards valve and the Hancock modified orifice valve. Gradient through the SAV was found to be lower than that of the latter two valves. Transvalvular gradients of pericardial bioprostheses in the mitral position may be explained by several factors: rigid stent, excess protrusion of the stent within the ventricle, geometry and insufficient excursion of the cusps, excess fibrin deposition and fibrous proliferation. The following features should minimize these drawbacks: total flexible support, improved mounting and fixation avoiding the suture of the commissures to maintain leaflet coaptation, improved sewing ring to reduce the risk of periprosthetic leak, and reduced height of the stent to diminish intraventricular protrusion (*see Figure 18.1(d)*).

Tissue failure

Histological and electron microscopic analysis of non-implanted commercially available valves showed several lesions before implantation, i.e. cellular alteration,

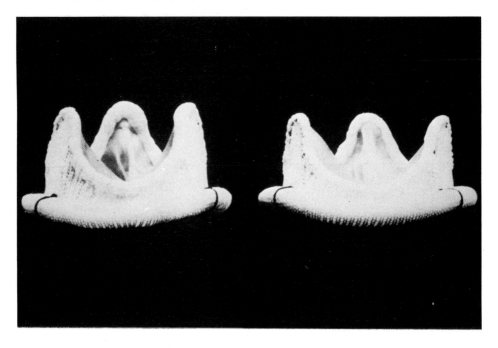

Figure 18.3 Improvement in valve design. *Left*: Current Carpentier–Edwards valve. *Right*: Supra-annular valve (SAV).

collagen bundle splitting, and loss of elastic fiber crimp, which correlated well with large variations in durability as assessed by *in-vitro* testing (*see Figure 18.4*).

An extensive review of the entire process of valve preparation revealed that the alterations in histologic structure resulted from large variations in intervals from 10 to 120 hours between harvesting and glutaraldehyde treatment and high pressure during fixation. The first two factors led to cellular alterations and early tissue degeneration and the third led to splitting of collagen bundles and loss of elastic fiber crimp. Several modifications in the handling and fixation of the valves were initiated to eliminate the histologic alterations and increased valve longevity, i.e. reduced shipping time, preservation of the valve in a shipping medium before fixation and glutaraldehyde fixation at 4 mm Hg.

Histologic and electron microscopic studies performed on valves that were shipped and processed according to the new specificiations showed that the natural structure of the valvular tissue was better preserved when compared with previous techniques. There was no alteration of cells or components of the tissue, and the crimp of the collagen bundles was preserved. This preservation of histologic structures resulted in improved durability averaging 350×10^6 cycles with limited variations.

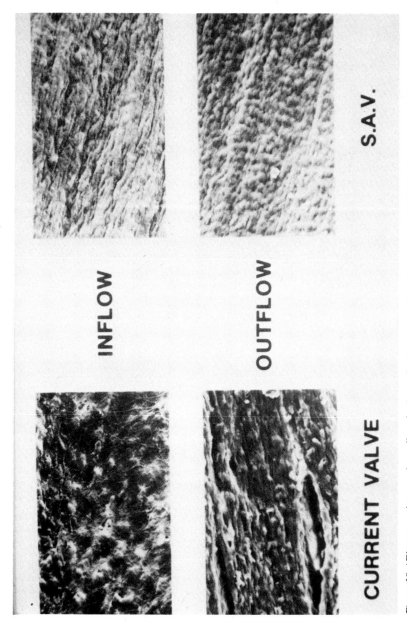

Figure 18.4 Electron-microscopic studies of valves prior to implantation. Current valve (left) displays alteration. The SAV which benefits from an improved tissue preservation (right) shows no alteration. (Top) Inflow; (bottom) outflow.

Calcification

Tissue calcification in children is a considerable challenge. The incidence of calcification is as high as 30–50% at 5 years in children younger than 12 years. The incidence of calcification is lower between 12 and 20 years but still much higher than in the adult population. Early calcification may occur occasionally in adults. We have observed calcification of a valvular bioprosthesis 1 month post-operatively in a patient who died of cardiac failure after having received repeated intravenous injections of calcium gluconate for 15 days. The influence of calcium intake—i.e. intravenous calcium or a high-calcium diet—was further demonstrated by experiments carried out in our laboratory[17]. From these experiments we derived the following recommendations: repeated intravenous injections of calcium should be avoided in the postoperative period as they may lead to early calcification and excessive calcium intake through increased consumption of milk or dairy products should be avoided in children. On the other hand drying out of the leaflet tissue during surgical implantation must be prevented by permanent irrigation, because tissue dehydration following exposure of leaflet tissue to air led to early calcification in the animal model[17].

These precautions added to the supravalvular configuration that reduces turbulence and the improved preservation, which eliminates preimplantation tissue alterations, should minimize but will probably not eliminate the risk of calcification in children. The solution to this problem depends on our ability to influence the other factors involved, whether they are valve related or patient related. Improved techniques of preservation may represent an important step forward: we have experimentally demonstrated that a non-hepes buffer, magnesium chloride solution added to the glutaraldehyde reduces the incidence of calcification in the animal model. Another alternative is the use of surfactant in association with glutaraldehyde[18].

It is too early to assess the effects, if any, that these modifications may have on the long-term durability of these valves and on the process of calcification. Several clinical series are currently under investigation to answer this question.

References

1. CARPENTIER, A., LEMAIGRE, G., ROBERT, L., CARPENTIER, S. and DUBOST, CH. (1969). Biological factors affecting long term results of valvular heterografts. *J. Thor. Cardiovasc. Surg.*, **58**, 467
2. CARPENTIER, A., DELOCHE, A., FABIANI, J.N., FORMAN, J., CAMILLERI, J.P., SOYER, R. and DUBOST, CH. (1974). Six-year follow-up of glutaraldehyde-preserved heterografts. *J. Thor. Cardiovasc. Surg.*, **58**, 771–782
3. CARPENTIER, A. (1977). From valvular xenograft to valvular bioprosthesis (1965–1977). *Medical Instrumentation*, **II**, pp. 98–101
4. LEE, G., GREHL, T.M., JOYCE, J.A. *et al.* (1978). Hemodynamic assessment of the new aortic Carpentier–Edwards bioprosthesis. *Cathet. Cardiovasc. Diagn.*, **4**, 373
5. OYER, P.E., STINSON, E.B., REITZ, B.A., MILLER, D.C., ROSSITER, S.L. and SHUMWAY, N.E. (1979). Long term evaluation of the porcine xenograft bioprosthesis. *J. Thor. Cardiovasc. Surg.*, **78**, 343–50
6. MILLER, D.C. (1981). Rational favouring the use of the porcine xenograft bioprosthesis in patient with acquired valvular heart disease. *Presented at American College of Cardiology*. San Francisco: Minicourse
7. HERTZER, R., HILL, J.D., KERTH, W.J., ANSBRO, J., ADAPPA, M.G., RODVIEN, R., KAMM, B. and GERBODE. F. (1978). Thromboembolic complications after mitral valve replacement with Hancock xenograft. *J. Thor. Cardiovasc. Surg.*, **75**, 651–8
8. CEVESE, P.G., GALLUCCI, V., MOREA, M., VOLDA, S.D., FASOLI, G. and CASAROTTO, D. (1977) Heart valve replacement with the Hancock bioprosthesis. Analysis of long-term results. *Circulation*, **56** (Suppl.) **3**, 111–6

9. LAKIER, J.B., KHAJA, F., MAGILLIGAN, D.J. and GOLDSTEIN, S. (1980). Porcine xenograft valves, long term (60–89 month) follow-up. *Circulation*, **62**, 313–8

10. SPRAY, T.L. and ROBERTS, W.C. (1977). Structural changes in porcine xenografts used as substitute cardiac valves. *Am. J. Cardiol.*, **40**, 319–30

11. FERRANS, V.J., SPRAY, T.L., BILLINGHAM, M.E. and ROBERTS, W.C. (1978). Structural changes in glutaraldehyde treated porcine heterografts used as substitute cardiac valves. *Am. J. Cardiol.*, **41**, 1159-83

12. CARPENTIER, A., DUBOST, CH., LANE, E., NASHREF, A., CARPENTEIR, S., RELLAND, J., DELOCHE, A., FABIANI, J.N., CHAUVAUD, S., PERIER, P. and MAXWELL, S. (1982) Continuing improvements in valvular bioprosthesis. *J. Thor. Cardiovasc. Surg.*, **83**, 27–42

13. IONESCU, M.I. and TANDON, A.P. (1979). Long term clinical and hemodynamic evaluation of the Ionescu–Shiley pericardial heart valve. In *Bioprosthetic Cardiac Valves* (ed. F. Sebening), Munchen: Deutsches Herzzentrum

14. STROM, J., BECKER, R.M., FISHMAN, W., SALAZAR, C., OKA, Y., BASSELL, G., LIN, Y.T. and FRATER, R.W. (1978). Hemodynamics evaluation of the Ionescu Shiley bovine heterograft valve. *Am. J. Cardiol.*, **41**, 221

15. SILVER, M.M., POLLOCK, J., SILVER, M.D., WILLIAMS, W.G. and TRUSSLER, G.A. (1980). Calcification in porcine xenograft in children. *Am. J. Cardiol.*, **45**, 685–9

16. ROSE, A.G., FORMAN, R. and BOWEN, R.M. (1978). Calcification of glutaraldehyde fixed porcine xenografts. *Thorax*, **33**, 111–4

17. CARPENTIER, A., CARPENTIER, S., GOUSSEF, N., PAILLET, C., FISHBEIN, M.C., LEVY, R. and NASHEF, A. (1981) Calcification intake as a factor affecting calcification in glutaraldehyde treated biological tissue. *Artificial Organs*, **5** (Suppl.)

18. CARPENTIER, A., NASHEF, A., CARPENTIER, S., GOUSSEF, N., RELLAND, J., LEVY, R., FISHBEIN, M.C., EL ASMAR, B., BENOMAR, M. and EL SAYED, S. (1984). Prevention of tissue valve calcification by chemical techniques. In *Proceedings of the International Symposium on Cardiac Bioprostheses 1982* (ed. L.H. Cohn) (in press)

'Primary tissue failure' (spontaneous tissue degeneration) was assigned either at reoperation or at post-mortem examination if the valve leaflets exhibited gross calcification and/or perforation or disruption in the absence of an antecedent history of infective endocarditis involving the prosthesis.

Thromboembolism was defined as the occurrence of any new focal neurologic deficit, whether transient or permanent. This included patients who failed to regain consciousness after operation or who awoke with a focal neurologic deficit. In addition, all episodes of peripheral embolization were considered to be valve related.

The term 'intrinsic stenosis' was used to describe valves in patients who exhibited large transvalvular gradients and required bioprosthesis replacement, but in whom the valve leaflet tissue appeared to have full mobility and integrity at the time of rereplacement.

Standard actuarial analysis according to the product-limit method of Kaplan and Meier[4] was used to express the occurrence rates of various events. Linearized rates were computed for each yearly follow-up interval to describe more clearly the varying risks of valve-related complications as a function of time.

Anticoagulation with warfarin sodium was prescribed for a period of 3 months following operation, after which warfarin was discontinued unless anatomical findings at operation suggested an increased propensity for late thromboembolic complications. All patients who developed thromboemboli were thereafter given anticoagulant therapy. Atrial fibrillation alone was not considered sufficient cause for long-term anticoagulation.

Results

The specific modes of valve failure observed in this analysis, according to the definitions given above, are listed in *Table 19.1*, along with the relative frequencies of their occurrence. A total of 78 failures occurred in 76 patients. Two patients suffered two independent failures of their valves, the first failure in each case was a bland periprosthetic leak requiring reoperation and simple resuturing of the leak; the second failure in each was primary tissue failure occurring several years later. An actuarial analysis of the occurrence of overall valve failure in these 76 patients is given in *Figure 19.3*, with the number of failures that occurred in each yearly postoperative interval. Also shown are the interval linearized rates of valve failure. A constant, low risk of valve failure from all causes is clearly shown by the interval rates through 5 years of follow-up, with a substantial increase in the probability of failure notable during the eighth and ninth years of follow-up.

TABLE 19.1 Modes of mitral valve failure in 786 adult patients

Failure mode	No. of events (%)
Primary tissue failure	37 (47.4)
New murmur	10 (12.8)
Prosthesis infection	10 (12.8)
Thromboembolism	8 (10.3)
Thrombosis/tissue occlusion	4 (5.1)
Bland periprosthetic leak	6 (7.7)
Anticoagulant hemorrhage	2 (2.6)
Intrinsic stenosis	1 (1.3)

MITRAL VALVE REPLACEMENT
OVERALL VALVE FAILURE
(Adult Patients, n=786)

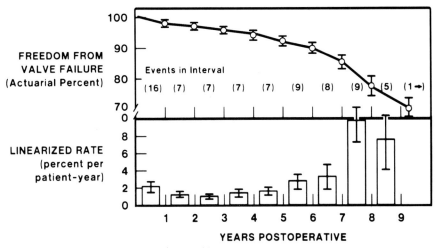

Figure 19.3 Actuarial freedom from valve failure from all causes is shown in the upper panel. Linearized occurrence rates during each interval are shown below. Brackets denote standard errors of the mean. The actual number of events that occurred in each interval are shown.

The principal failure mode contributing to this acceleration in the overall valve failure rate was primary tissue failure, as shown in *Figure 19.4*. Both actuarial and interval linearized rates are shown, clearly documenting the previously reported slight increase in spontaneous degeneration rates during the sixth follow-up year, and the further increasing risk of tissue failure during the ninth and tenth years of observation. Eighty per cent ($\pm 3.7\%$ SE) of patients were free of spontaneous degeneration through 9 years of follow-up. A total of 37 instances of primary tissue failure occurred; 33 patients underwent reoperation for this complication (with four operative deaths) while four others died without reoperation, the diagnosis being established at post-mortem examination.

Thromboembolic episodes occurred in a total of 69 of the 786 patients. As shown in *Figure 19.5*, the risk of such complications was highest during the first postoperative year, with most of these occurring during the initial 3 months after operation. Subsequently, a small, constant risk of embolic episodes was observed, as shown on the lower panel of the figure. Analysis of the risk of thromboembolism as a function of heart rhythm in patients with bioprosthetic valves, confirms a significantly higher probability of this complication in patients with irregular rhythms; a more detailed assessment of this relationship will be included in a future report. Eighty-seven per cent ($\pm 1.7\%$ SE) of all patients in the analysis were free of any embolic episodes. A total of eight thromboembolic episodes resulted in death; these were included in the calculation of 'overall valve failure' rates according to the definition previously outlined.

The frequencies of other modes of valve failure observed are included in *Table 19.2*, expressed as linearized rates computed over the entire 3408 patient-year follow-up period. Although such overall linearized rates do not fully describe the

248

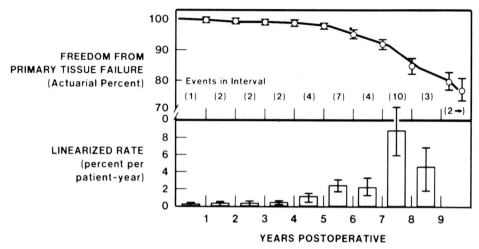

MITRAL VALVE REPLACEMENT
PRIMARY TISSUE FAILURE
(Adult Patients, n=786)

Figure 19.4 Actuarial and linearized interval rates of primary tissue failure are depicted, with the number of events that occurred in each yearly interval.

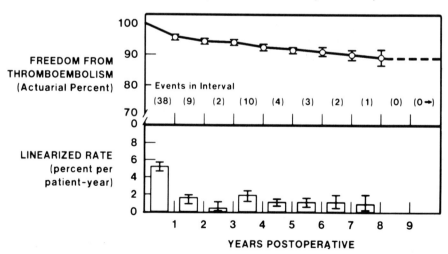

MITRAL VALVE REPLACEMENT
THROMBOEMBOLISM
(Adult Patients, n=786)

Figure 19.5 Actuarial and linearized rates of thromboembolism are shown. The number of patients in each year who exhibited such complications are also given.

TABLE 19.2 Valve-related morbidity rates in 786 adult patients (%/patient-year)

Cause	Rate
Thromboembolism	2.3
Prosthesis infection	0.5
Anticoagulant-related hemorrhage	1.1
Periprosthetic leak	0.2
Overall valve failure	2.3
Primary tissue failure	1.1
Reoperation	1.4

risk of given events at intermediate times during the follow-up period, they do serve as benchmark figures for comparison with data from other centers (and for comparison with other valve types) so long as cumulative and mean follow-up durations are similar.

It is noteworthy that the overall rate of reoperation in this patient group was 1.4% per patient year, a figure similar to that reported for two of the most widely used mechanical valves after periods of follow-up shorter than those reported herein. Forty-eight reoperations were required among patients in this series, the reasons for which are given in *Table 19.3*. As shown in *Figure 19.6*, the probability of reoperation increased during the sixth postoperative year. Seventy-six per cent (±4.6% SE) of patients were free of reoperation through 9.5 years postoperatively. Reoperation was performed in 33 patients for primary tissue failure; four operative deaths occurred among this group, resulting in a reoperative mortality of 12.1% for this indication.

TABLE 19.3 Conditions mandating reoperation in 786 adult patients

Condition	No. of events
Primary tissue failure	33
Prosthesis infection	7
Periprosthetic leak	6
Thrombosis/tissue occlusion	1
Intrinsic stenosis	1
Total	48

Discussion

Data presented in this report represent an extension of experience with the Hancock mitral bioprosthesis to a maximum of 11.5 years, with sufficient numbers of patients to assess its performance on a statistically-firm basis through 9.5 years. Previous observations regarding a number of valve-related complications—including the frequencies of thromboembolism, endocarditis, anticoagulant-related hemorrhage and bland periprosthetic leak—are confirmed in this extended experience. More importantly, late clinical durability of the bioprosthesis is now more fully defined. Spontaneous degeneration of leaflet tissue clearly becomes manifest during the eighth and ninth postoperative year, resulting in a probability of reoperation or death from this complication of 22.4% (±4.3% SE) after 9.5 years. Nevertheless, the rate of failure of the bioprosthetic valve from

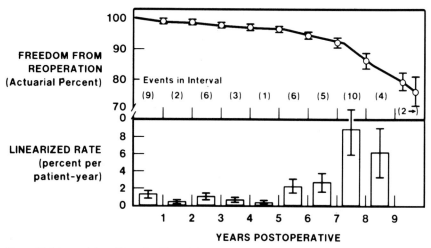

Figure 19.6 Actuarial and linearized interval rates of reoperation are given, along with the actual number of such events that occurred in each interval. Brackets denote standard errors of the mean.

all causes, including spontaneous degeneration, after this extended follow-up interval (70.3 ± 4%) is virtually identical with that observed with the Starr—Edwards mechanical valve after a similar postoperative interval (71 ± 2%) in a recently published report from this institution using similar criteria to define overall failure of the valve. Moreover, the rate of reoperation observed in these two series of patients did not differ significantly within the 9.5 year postoperative time frame for which firm data are available. Thus, the argument that use of mechanical valves may reduce the necessity for reoperation does not appear valid, at least within the constraints of the current follow-up period.

In summary, the Hancock bioprosthesis continues to perform satisfactorily through at least 9.5 years postoperatively. Clearly, the rate of spontaneous degeneration becomes important during the latter portion of this period, emphasizing the necessity for close surveillance of patients with this valve throughout this later time frame so that reoperation can be performed prior to the development of important myocardial damage. Notwithstanding the probability that reoperation will eventually be needed in these patients, it appears that the bioprosthetic valve continues to offer substantial benefit in terms of relative freedom from devastating thromboembolic and anticoagulant-related complications throughout its useful lifetime and may thereby, in spite of the eventual necessity for rereplacement, reduce overall long-term morbidity and mortality sustained by those who require new cardiac valves.

Bibliography

1. OYER, P.E., MILLER, D.C., STINSON, E.B., REITZ, E.A., MORENO—CABROL, R.J. and SHUMWAY, N.E. (1980). Clinical durability of the Hancock porcine bioprosthetic valve. *J. Thorac. Cardiovasc. Surg.*, **80**, 824

Mitral reconstruction in predominant mitral stenosis

Carlos M.G. Duran

The surgeon's approach to mitral surgery fortunately has not remained static. Early closed commissurotomies were followed by valve replacement when cardiopulmonary bypass became safe. Simultaneously a variety of techniques for valve repair were being described, remaining usually confined to the domain of a particular surgeon. Their difficulty and lack of standardization impaired the transmission of these skills to other surgical groups.

Today, the awareness of the many problems related to mitral prosthesis together with the availability of a safe myocardial protection has awaken a new interest in this conservative surgery. Early and more recent surgical techniques are contributing towards a new radically different approach to reconstructive surgery. No longer a single technique but a variety of manoeuvres must be applied to the specific pathology of each valve.

Patient selection

In our opinion, mitral surgery must be considered a continuum which extends from a simple commissural splitting to total replacement, passing through more or less complex reconstructive manoeuvres determined by the individual characteristics of each patient and not of each surgeon. For our purpose—besides age, sex, geographic and socioeconomic factors—our attention must focus on three essential levels: atrial, mitral and ventricular.

At left atrial level the presence of a thrombus must be sought preoperatively as, in our opinion, it constitutes an absolute indication for surgery and will determine a long-term anticoagulation therapy. This thrombus is diagnosed not only by the typical contrast defect in recirculation but also by the presence of neovascularization and fistulae arising usually from the circumflex coronary artery in the angiogram (*see Figure 20.1*)[1]. If present, our surgical technique consists in passing a Foley catheter through the mitral orifice to avoid, once inflated, the risk of embolization. The thrombus is dissected subendocardially and often extracted *in toto* (*see Figure 20.2*)[2].

Secondly, left atrial compliance. The influence of the atrial pump on cardiac output is well known. In the presence of mitral stenosis and atrial fibrillation, atrial

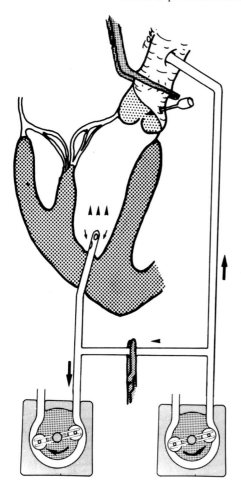

Figure 20.3 Mitral valve closure check. A side branch connects the arterial line to the apical left vent. When competence is to be checked the side branch is unclamped and the left vent sump stopped. Arterial blood fills the ventricle and closes the mitral valve. The aorta remains cross clamped and vented.

Reconstructive techniques available

A number of reconstructive techniques have already sufficient follow-up to consider them established (*see Table 20.1*). Sectioning of the fused commissures, section of thickened secondary chordae, splitting of matted chordae and longitudinal incision of the papillary muscles, increase remarkably the mobility of the mitral apparatus. Calcific nodules can be excised with or without complete section of the leaflet. The leaflets can be deinserted and resutured. The chordae can be shortened by pulling them downward into a split papillary muscle. Selective and measured annulus reduction can be performed with the help of prosthetic rings. This is indicated whenever a disproportionate leaflet/orifice ratio is present either because of an enlargement of the annulus or a reduction in leaflet tissue. Several models, all based on the same principle, are commercially available at present.[6-9] All these techniques have been described in detail in the literature.[10] Their relative merits and disadvantages are mostly theoretical and outside the scope of this work.

presented. The mean age was 42
There were 61 males and 216 fe
class of these patients was: Class
(52%); and Class IV, 28 (10.5%
our indications for this surger
preoperatively. All patients had
diagnosis of pure mitral stenosis
15% and a mixed lesion in 55%.
are performed on predominantl
was performed in 133 patients (5(
on another valve: 102 patients
commissurotomy was performed
only on 2% of insufficiencies. The
of the cases. Chordal shortenings
in 12% of cases.

The hospital mortality was o
three have been lost to follow
12 616.5 months or 1051 years.]
close to 8 years (93 months).
thromboembolism (4 patients),
unknown (1). The linearized rat

Most patients improved dram
Class II, 21%) and only 3% in (
have been detected in 34 patie
thrombi were anticoagulated pe
anticoagulants for the first 3 j
thromboembolism was of 3.7%

Fifteen patients required
dehiscence of the ring in eigh
repair in four. There were 13
and 4 years postoperatively.

TABLE 20.3 Reoperation on mitral flex

Cause	Time (months
Unsatisfactory repair	1
Ring dehiscence	2
Ring dehiscence	2
Ring dehiscence	3
Unsatisfactory repair	4
Unsatisfactory repair	4
Ring dehiscence	5
Ring dehiscence	9
Unsatisfactory repair	9
Ring dehiscence	16
Ring dehiscence	18
Restenosis	55
Ring dehiscence	58
Restenosis	63
Restenosis	71

Hck = Hancock valve; SJ = St Jude medical va

TABLE 20.1 Established surgical techniques for mitral valve reconstruction

Annulus	Ring annuloplasty
	Partial plicature
Leaflet	Local resection
	Decalcification
	Deinsertion
Commissure	Splitting
	Decalcification
Chords	Primary—splitting, shortening
	Secondary—section
Papillary muscle	Splitting

We favour a totally flexible ring (Duran Flexible Ring, Hancock Laboratories, Anaheim, Cal., USA) (*see Figure 20.4*)[8] which adapts to the continuous changes of the mitral annulus during the cardiac cycle. This 3 mm thick Dacron ring contains a radiopaque thread to make it radiologically visible and comes in different sizes to accomodate each mitral (or tricuspid) orifice. Sizes are identified by the distance between any two of the three equidistant markers present in the ring and should correspond with the measured distance between the right and left fibrous trigones of the heart (*see Figure 20.5*).

Other techniques such as cusp extension[11] and chordal replacement[12], although promising, still lack either the availability of the correct material or sufficient experience to consider them established.

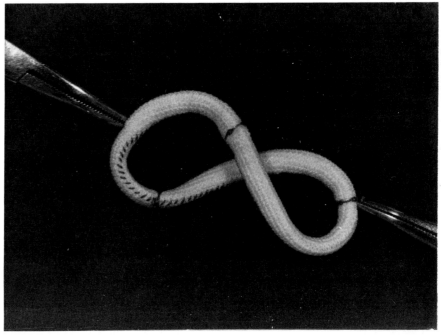

Figure 20.4 The Duran flexible ring showing how it flexes in any direction. Note the three equidistant markers for sizing and to simplify its placement.

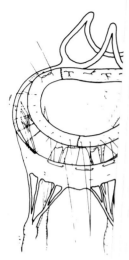

Figure 20.5 Duran flexible
and through the ring. (B) (
leaflet areas.

Clinical experienc

From May 1974 until
at our Institution. Th
time (*see Table 20.2*
III–IV. Patients in
showed a good qua
absolute indication f
recently, the onset c
an indication for su

TABLE 20.2 Surgical in

Functional class	V
I	(
II	
III	
IV	

AF = Atrial fibrillation. This

These 1522 o
reconstructions w
74 mechanical va
the use of an an
performed.

Two types of
and, since Janua
reviewing a hom

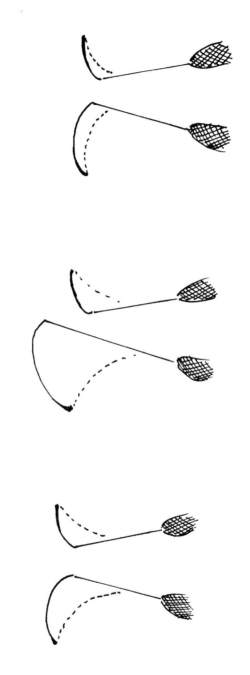

Figure 21.1 Functional classification of mitral valve incompetence. Left: Normal leaflet motion; centre: prolapse leaflet; right: restricted leaflet motion.

TABLE 23.1 Indications for reoperation

Patient	Years after operation	NYHA class	PA Syst-Pr.	Cardiac index	Ejection fraction	Preoperative stroke
			Mechanical valve dysfunction			
1	3	III	50	2	Normal	Yes
2	10	IV	45	2.5	Normal	No
3	8	IV	70	2.3	64%	No
4	8	IV	48	2.3	52%	No
5	8	IV	75	3.0		No
6	2	IV	45	2.1	Normal	No
7	5	IV	75	1.8	30%	No
8	5	IV	65	2.0	48%	No
			Biological valve dysfunction			
9	3	IV	49	4.0	—	No

NYHA = New York Heart Association; PA = pulmonary artery systolic pressure.

TABLE 23.2 Clinical conditions at time of surgery for mitral valve re-replacement

Patient	Years after operation	NYHA class
10	2	Cardiac arrest
11	2	IV
12	2	IV
13	3	IV
		Valve infections
14	1	I
15	6 weeks	II
		Multiple emboli
16	9	I

failure. Emobolism occurred in one. Abnormal disc motion was seen both on angiography and two-dimensional echocardiography in one. Three patients with ball valves with cloth covered struts had either inappropriate and excessive fibrous tissue ingrowth with jamming of the metal balls, or disintegration of the cloth. The presentation in this group was recurrent congestive cardiac failure with an embolic episode in addition in one. Fluoroscopy or angiography showed improper ball motion in two but echocardiography was equivocal. The interval between first and second operations averaged 7 years with a range of 2–10 years. One patient with a tanned xenograft bioprosthesis had premature rupture of a cusp at 3 years, which produced pulmonary edema and severe congestive heart failure. Two-dimensional echocardiography defined the nature of the valve dysfunction precisely.[14]

Valve thrombosis

In four patients valve thrombosis was the indication for re-replacement. The valves were non-tilting disc valves in each case. Coumadin anticoagulation appeared deficient in two patients but adequate in the other two. All had experienced return of dyspnea on exertion, progressing quite rapidly over a few weeks to episodes of pulmonary edema. The prosthetic opening click was muffled in one case but the closing clicks were always well heard. Despite marked pulmonary edema as judged by the chest X-rays in all, and very high pulmonary capillary pressure in the three in whom it was measured, these patients commonly were not orthopneic but instead lay flat in bed. All, however, had tachypnea and a sense of difficulty in breathing. Commonly, they presented with evidence of poor peripheral blood flow in the form of cold, cyanosed extremities with small peripheral pulses and slow capillary filling. One patient had a cardiac arrest shortly after admission. She was revived by external cardiac message and intubation, taken straight to the operating room and put on femoro-femoral cardiopulmonary bypass, before proceeding to median sternotomy and successful prosthetic valve replacement. This was also the only patient of these four to have had a cerebral embolus preoperatively. The interval between first and second operations was from 2 to 3 years.

Infected valves

Two patients had infected valves. One presented evidence of infection 6 weeks after primary valve replacement. At the original operation extensive cultures during and after surgery and including the pump blood had been negative for the α-hemolytic streptococcus that was the organism that caused the valve infection. During the third week after the start of appropriate antibiotic therapy he had two emboli, one benign and one causing hemoplegia. He was given another 5 days for some presumed stabilization of the fresh cerebral infarction to occur, in an attempt to lower the risk of hemorrhage when heparinized for cardiopulmonary bypass, and, hopefully, to prevent aggravation of the lesion by any of several possible mechanisms associated with major cardiac surgery. He then underwent successful valve replacement and made an excellent recovery from his hemiplegia. The other patient was a relapsed addict who returned to hospital 1 year after mitral valve replacement for endocarditis. Cultures were initially negative but despite massive antibiotic therapy there was no resolution of the signs of infection and small peripheral emboli typical of endocarditis were occurring. Fungal infection was suspected and *Candida albicans* was in fact growing luxuriantly on the valve. The valve replacement surgery was quite uneventful and was followed by six weeks of amphotericin therapy. Although gross perivalvular leaks or obstruction by large vegetations can occur in mitral prosthetic endocarditis, it was not seen in these two patients and neither case had congestive cardiac failure.

Contemporaneously with this series other cases were seen in which organisms were found in blood cultures taken in the first week after a primary valve replacement, generally because of a postoperative fever higher, or slower to resolve, than normal. No other evidence of valve infection existed and no further positive cultures were obtained. Antibiotic treatment was immediately instituted and was continued for 3–4 weeks; no case was subsequently seen to develop prosthetic valve infection. There is, of course, no proof that the prosthetic valves were ever infected.

Multiple emboli

One patient had valve replacement at the age of 19, with a University of Cape Town Prosthesis that had a Silastic occluder meeting bare steel in the orifice. On coumadin anticoagulation she had a successful pregnancy with delivery of a normal infant and no problems until the beginning of the ninth year, when she had two episodes, 2 months apart, of aphasia lasting several hours. She was started on aspirin and persantine in addition to the coumadin, but 9 months later while driving her car developed slurred speech and right hemiparesis, which took over a week to resolve. At valve replacement small thrombi were seen on the ventricular side of the prosthesis, attached to the junction of cloth and steel, but not, of course, adherent to the latter. They were in a position to have been knocked off by the impact of occluder with ring. After removal of the densely adherent prosthesis a 1.5 cm length of the circumflex coronary artery was seen to be attached to it. There was no suitable marginal artery for grafting and the ends were ligated from inside. The atrium and ventricle were reattached and a biological prosthesis was successfully inserted. The postoperative course was uneventful.

Cardiac catheterization data

Cardiac catheterization with or without angiography was available preoperatively in 11 patients. The data served to confirm in all the valve dysfunctin cases that the recurrent symptoms had a definite hemodynamic correlate and that the mitral valve was at least a substantial cause for this. Left ventricular function was satisfactory in eight patients, but depressed in two. Occluder motion was seen to be abnormal in two ball valves and one caged disc valve.

Echocardiography

M mode and two-dimensional echocardiography was performed in nine patients. Abnormal occluder motion was suspected in the same patients in which it was observed roentgenographically, but definitively abnormal motion was seen in only one of three cases. In the single case of bioprosthetic disruption the two-dimensional echocardiogram was definitively diagnostic. On the other hand cloth wear, thrombi and vegetations appeared to be hidden by the metal and plastic of the rings, struts and occluders.

Surgical technique

The surgical technique used during these 12 years was relatively constant, having developed during secondary operations in patients who had previously had closed or palliative valve surgery.

Preoperative information

The presence of a right ventricular parasternal lift, observation of right ventricular contact with the sternum on the lateral chest X-ray and knowledge of previous right ventricular enlargement and present right ventricular pressure, combined with information on the previous incision and whether or not the pericardium was closed all help to determine the degree of danger of entering the right ventricle on making the median sternotomy.

Incisions

In all patients the thorax was entered by a median sternotomy. In all 11 patients judged to be at some risk of right ventricular damage, the femoral artery and vein on one side were exposed and made ready for cannulation prior to thoracotomy and in the patient already mentioned, who presented with a cardiac arrest, cardiopulmonary bypass was actually instituted before sternotomy (*see Figure 23.1*).

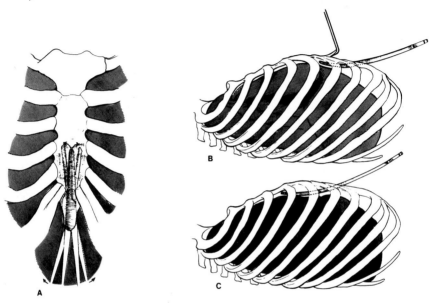

Figurer 23.1 Technique for avoiding ventricular injury. A curved clamp is passed without force behind the sternum, opened, closed, removed and passed behind again (*a, b, c*). Separation of adhesions is achieved by lateral action only. When the manubrium is reached the saw is used.

The sternotomy was and is made in the following way. The scar is excised. The wires are exposed, cut and removed. The suprasternal notch is dissected out and the linea alba divided. The lower end of the sternum is then pulled forward by pulling on the adjacent ribs. Fibrous tissue attached to the back of the lower sternum is then cut, using a curved Mayo scissors with the points against the bone. A wide enough plane is developed so as to be able to introduce a curved Kelly clamp with its concave surface forward and its tips always in contact with the bone. The Kelly clamp is then gently spread so as to separate the tips by 1–2 cm, removed, reintroduced, spread and removed repeatedly. After each spreading with the tips in contact with the posterior table of the bone it is found that the clamp can be introduced further and further behind the sternum. Eventually, by laying the length of clamp that has passed up behind the inner table against the outer table, it is seen that the manubrium has been reached. A similar but much less extensive development of a plane behind the manubrium is made from the suprasternal notch with a larger right angled clamp. After that the sternal saw is used from below upwards in the usual way.

As soon as the sternum has been cut the two halves are in turn very gently pulled forward, commonly with vein retractors, so that the fibrous tissue connecting the bone with the heart can be cut at the level of the bone. It is convenient to do this with the electrocautery since these connnections are often vascular. Blunt dissection is never used since the adhesions are stronger than the bare epicardium and myocardium or innominate vein to which they may be attached.

Dissection of the heart

Epicardium and pericardium are separated over: (a) the diaphragmatic surface of the right ventricle; (b) the lateral wall of the right atrium; (c) the inferior and superior venae cavae; and (d) the right superior pulmonary vein, and the aorta. This dissection is clearly limited but it allows defibrillation with one paddle directly beneath the right ventricle, one in contact with the undissected pericardium over the left ventricle. It also allows the passage of tapes around the venae cavae and aorta (*see Figure 23.2*).

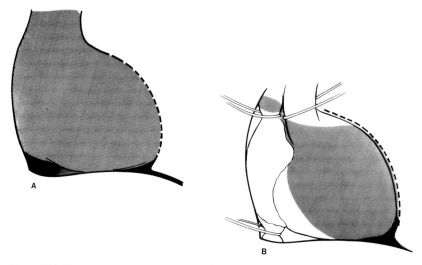

Figure 23.2 (*a*) The heart prior to dissection. (*b*) The limited extent of dissection needed for successful re-replacement surgery.

Cannulation

In the patient who needs cardiopulmonary bypass before starting anesthesia the initial cannulation is of the common femoral artery and of the right atrium via the common femoral vein. The venous cannulation is completed by cannulating the superior vena cava once the chest is open. Most often, however, the ascending aorta and venae cavae can be cannulated electively after making the sternotomy. Purse-string sutures for the caval cannulae are placed posteriorly and quite close to the cavae so that the cannulae are sufficiently separated to allow the surgeon access to the septum via the right atrial wall.

   A left atrial pressure catheter is inserted into the left atrium via the right superior pulmonary vein, leaving room for a vent to be placed at the junction of the vein and left atrium. The pressure catheter is positioned with the aid of ink markers so that it is just 2 cm inside the left atrium and secured with a purse string in the atrial wall, catgut sutures holding it against the pericardium and a heavy silk stitch at the skin.

The vent is placed prior to opening the left atrium if after going on bypass the left atrial pressure is high, but it is not advanced further than the 4 cm needed for all its distal holes to be within the atrium. It is allowed to drain by siphonage to the oxygenator or placed on low-vacuum section if necessary to lower the left atrial pressure. Before clamping the aorta two large plastic cannulae, each with a side hole close to the tip, are inserted between 1 and 2 cm through the anterior wall of the aorta. One is for the infusion of fluid into the aortic root and the other for clearing air from it. The latter cannula is connected by intravenous tubing to a stopcock and the Y connector in the main venous line (*see Figure 23.3*).

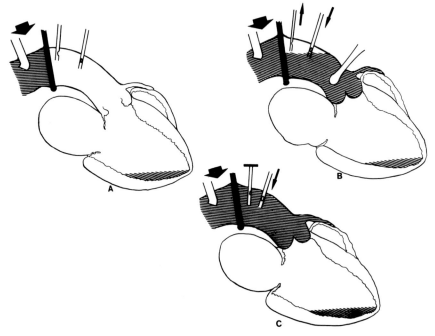

Figure 23.3 The aorta to venous line shunt. (*a*) Siphonage by the action of the venous return to the oxygenator. (*b*) Left to right shunt from aorta to right atrium after discontinuation of bypass and clamping the venous line.

Conduct of cardiopulmonary bypass

In all of these cases a bubble oxygenator was used. Flow was set at $3\,l/m^2$ of body surface area with some reduction at lower temperatures, if reduced return of blood to the heart was desired. During the first 6 years (i.e. seven cases), moderate systemic hypothermia to 30°C was used. The heart was allowed to beat except for short 5–15 minute periods of aortic clamping used to achieve the better exposure provided by a flaccid heart. With each declamping a specific routine was followed to diminish the possibility of air embolism (*see* below).

For the last 8 years hypothermia hyperkalemic hypothermic cardioplegic arrest has been used. Since the pericadial adhesions are not divided it is not possible to insulate the heart from the rest of the body and it is presumed that these will provide extracoronary sources of myocardial blood supply. For these reasons the general body temperature is dropped initially to 20°C. Extra doses of cardioplegic solution are given through the ascending aorta every 30 minutes, or more often, if the constantly monitored septal temperature rises to 20°C. The exposed right ventricle is bathed continuously in electrolyte solution at 8°C

Approach to the mitral valve

This was in every case via a horizontal right atriotomy back to the right superior pulmonary vein and an incision through the septum, starting from the latter point and extending forward and inferiorly to the coronary sinus. If this approach was not used before, the incision is made through the fossa ovalis just below the thick limbus of the annulus ovalis (*see Figure 23.4(a)*). It does not extend beyond the coronary sinus and does not pass anterior to it. If more length is necessary the incision is extended posteriorly and laterally into the right superior pulmonary vein. This incision avoids at least one if not two internodal atrial pathways as well as the atrioventricular node and also keeps clear of the aortic root. The old atrial incision is reopened in cases in which this approach has been used before.

Two heavy, buttressed mattress sutures are placed in the two edges of this incision 1–2 cm back from the coronary sinus. The upper is anchored to the left side of the sternal retractor and the other to its cross bar inferiorly. Commonly, no extra traction is then needed to see the valve. The operating table is tilted to the left as necessary to aid exposure. The mitral valve is made incompetent if necessary as soon as the atrium is opened, care being taken not to dislodge thrombus.

Excision of the mitral valve

Traction on the valve is obtained by passing a stitch through the cloth close to the rim of the prosthesis along the subaortic curtain. The incision is started with a No. 15 blade along this margin of the suture line, keeping either right on the tissue fabric interface or within the fabric leaving some of it, at least temporarily, on the heart. As the commissures are reached the possibility of stent adherence to the ventricular endocardium is looked for and dealt with by incision of the fibrous ingrowth right on the strut involved. A heavy curved scissors is generally the best instrument for the excision around the mural part of the mitral orifice. Here particularly the incision is made without hesitation through the cloth. Each cut is made under direct vision with the curve of the blades matching the curve of the ring and the tips staying close to the frame of the sewing ring (*see Figure 23.4(b)*).

All of this is most important when going around the corner at the lateral commissural end where the natural tendency is for the tip of the scissors to stray towards the atrioventricular groove and the circumflex coronary vessels. The atrial and ventricular cavities and the atrioventricular junction are then carefully inspected for loose particles. Wet gauze sponges, passed into the ventricle and retrieved, occasionally will pick up loose pieces of tissue or material.

The atrioventricular junction is debrided as necessary, but firmly adherent cloth is left unless infection was the indication for surgery. The new valve is sutured in

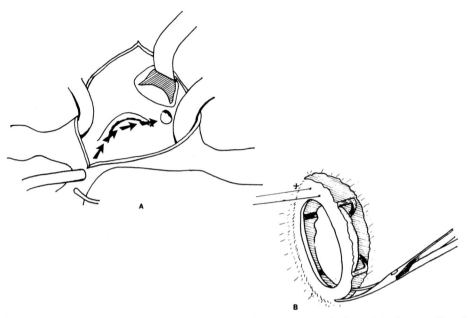

Figure 23.4 (*a*) Septotomy incision from the right superior pulmonary vein through the fossa ovalis to the coronary sinus. It does not go above the limbus or in front of the coronary sinus. (*b*) Excision of a valve starting at the subaortic area and cutting with curved blades parallel to the axis of the valve and through the fabric to avoid damage to the heart. The dangerous arterio lateral corner is marked.

with 15–18 interrupted mattress sutures, some with bolsters and others in a figure of eight form. If necessary, shallow surfaces in greater numbers than usual will be used if there is fear of catching the circumflex vessels or the conducting tissue. Once the valve is securely in, the vent is advanced through it into the ventricle and the first few sutures are placed in the septotomy before declamping the aorta.

Clearing air from the ascending aorta, atrium and ventricle

This is a concern both when a repeat dose of cardioplegic solution needs to be injected and on declamping the aorta preparatory to restarting the heart. Almost inevitably the aortic valve opens during the manipulations of mitral valve re-replacement so that either unclamping the aorta or injecting cardioplegic fluid will result in closure of the aortic valve with some air being trapped between the fluid and the anterior wall of the aorta. In the earlier cases a large, angled clamp was passed through the mitral orifice back up the aortic valve so as to hold the aortic valve incompetent during the first few seconds after declamping or starting an aortic root infusion. Athough the patients in this series did not apparently suffer serious cerebral embolism, bubbles or air were seen in the right coronary artery or would appear in the aortic root cannula quite often. A more sophisticated technique has evolved and is used whenever the left heart has been opened. The steps are as follows (*see Figures 23.3, 23.5*):

1.   Pinch off the aorta just distal to the orifice of the right coronary artery.
2.   Start the cardioplegia infusion.

3. As soon as it has started flowing open the stopcock on the venous line; there will be suction on the air clearing cannula as a result of this. The cardioplegic delivery system uses a pump so that it is possible for the surgeon to then pinch off the aorta with one hand and control the siphonage by opening and closing the stopcock with the other (*see Figure 23.3*). All that is needed at this stage is a few brief periods of suction and then the air clearing line can be closed and the right coronary orifice allowed to receive fluid. With this method air is not seen in the right coronary system (*see Figure 23.5*).

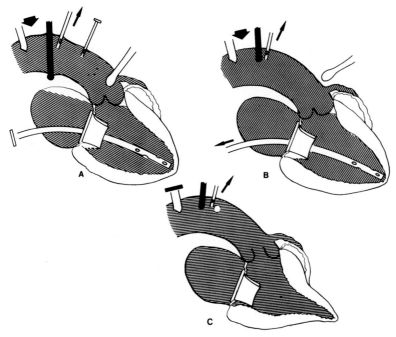

Figure 23.5 Technique for clearing air from the ascending aorta for repeat infusion of cardioplegic solution. *See* text.

A similar but slightly different routine is followed on declamping the aorta (*see Figure 23.6*)[19].

1. The perfusion temperature is brought up to 30°C so that the heart has the best possible chance of early resumption of beating after declamping.
2. The vent is taken off suction and the cardiotomy reservoir to which it is connected is opened to the atmopsphere.
3. The perfusion pressure is brought down temporarily by lowering the flow.
4. The aorta is pinched closed just distal to the right coronary orifice.
5. The stopcock on the air removal line is opened as the aortic clamp is slowly released. The venous drainage produces a constant left to right shunt from the aorta to the venous side of the oxygenator (*see Figure 23.3*).
6. After a few seconds, and the observation that a clear stream of blood is passing through the air clearing line, the right coronary artery is allowed to take flow.

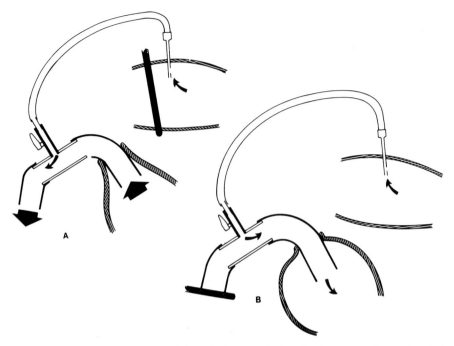

Figure 23.6 Technique for clearing air from the heart on declamping the aorta and restarting the heart. *See* text.

7. The aortic clamp is now used to clamp the aorta partially so as to produce a small cul-de-sac between the air clearing cannula and the aortic perfusion cannula. If air is ejected from the ventricle it will be trapped there and sucked out via the air removal cannula.
8. The vent is maintaining an incompetent mitral valve at this point as well as allowing blood to overflow from the left ventricle back to the oxygenator. As the septotomy closure is completed the level in the atrium is watched for any tendency to fall; if this happens the vent is clamped. Generally, coronary sinus return flows over into the left atrium and the pump suckers must be judiciously used to make suture placement possible. Before tying this suture blood is allowed to leak from left atrium to right and needle aspiration of the highest part of the left atrium is used to confirm the absence of air.
9. In the minute or two that have elapsed since aortic declamping the heart has either restarted spontaneously or can be defibrillated. Air trapped between ventricular trabeculae, behind the cusps of biological valves or in the outflow tract behind a closed aortic valve is now liable to be ejected into the aorta as soon as the ventricular pressure rises. The air cul-de-sac and removal cannula are therefore maintained.
10. Because reintroduction of the vent may be difficult or impossible across a prosthesis and with a bound-down ventricle, it is left in place while the right atriotomy is closed and rewarming is completed. It is then pulled back into the atrium and clamped to be removed completely as soon as the left ventricle has demonstrated its capacity to take over the circulation by producing phasic blood pressure.

11. As bypass is discontinued the likelihood that previously trapped air will be ejected is high and the air cul-de-sac is maintained for another few minutes, care being taken to see that the clamp is not producing aortic obstruction. The air clearing line is now functioning as a left to right shunt from aorta to right atrium since the venous line is now clamped between patient and oxygenator and at least one venous cannula is still in place. After the clamp producing the cul-de-sac is removed, the aorto-right atrial shunt is allowed to function for a while longer to catch any late-appearing air.

Management of patient and aortic insufficiency

The presence of mild aortic insufficiency, not severe enough to warrant valve replacement, was handled in two patients in the following way:

1. The patient was cooled slowly to 20°C.
2. As soon as the heart fibrillated (26°C), the aorta was clamped and opened and the coronary arteries were infused with cardioplegic solution.
3. After the valve insertion was completed the systemic temperature was brought up to 30°C while the aortotomy was being closed.
4. With the air-evacuating needle in the ascending aorta, the right coronary orifice pinched off, and the vent through the valve in the ventricle, the perfusion pressure was brought down and the aortic clamp removed as usual. However, in these cases the perfusion pressure was kept at 40 mm Hg for several minutes and the vent kept on suction to avoid ventricular distension until the heart was ready to resume active contractions. By declamping with the systemic blood already warm the time after resuming flow to being ready for defibrillation was reduced to a minimum.

Poll

An informal poll was taken of 25 surgeons experienced in valvular surgery. The questions asked were:

1. Is prosthetic valve infection an automatic indication for surgery?
2. (a) Do you distinguish between mechanical and biological prosthetic valve infections?
   (b) If Yes, which kind of infected valve needs replacement more urgently: biological, or mechanical?
3. What is your preferred thoracic approach for isolated native mitral valve replacement? Median sternotomy, right thoracotomy, or left thoracotomy?
4. (a) What is your preferred thoracic approach to replacement of a mitral valve prosthesis? Median sternotomy, right thoracotomy, or left thoracotomy?
   (b) Do you deliberately try to approach the heart by a previously unused route?
5. What is your preferred cardiac access to the mitral valve for primary isolated mitral valve replacement? Left atrial anterior to left or right pulmonic veins, superior left atrial (Dome), trans-septal (including duBost)?
6. (a) What is your preferred access to a mitral valve prosthesis for replacement? Left atrial anterior to left or right pulmonic veins, superior left atrial (Dome), or trans-septal (including duBost)?

(b) Do you deliberately try to gain access to the prosthetic valve via a previously unused route?
7. Do you divide all the adhesions between epicardium and pericardium? Routinely? Only when easy? Never?
8. (a) At what level do you keep the systemic temperature during cardiopulmonary bypass? Normal; 28–32°C; 22°C; 22°C or less?
(b) Do you arrest the heart?
(c) If you arrest the heart do you use: induced fibrillation, ischemia alone, ischemia and clear cardioplegia, or ischemia and blood cardioplegia?
(d) If you use cardioplegia, do you use multiple doses?
(e) If you use multiple doses, do you use any specific techniques to clear air from the ascending aorta before each injection?
9. Have you had trouble with clearing air from the heart:
(a) with the heart incompletely freed?
(b) with the heart completely freed?

Results of surgery

Mortality—There was no 30-day hospital mortality.

Injury during sternotomy—No serious injury occurred during sternotomy and exposure of the heart.

Injury during valve removal—The patient who was operated on for multiple embolism lost a portion of her circumflex coronary artery without ill effect. No other injuries occurred in removing the valves.

Heart block—No patient developed heart block.

Air embolism and cerebrovascular accident—No patient developed evidence of a cerebrovascular accident.

Impaired myocardial performance—Seven patients needed inotropic support postoperatively. One patient following a cardiac arrest was on inotropic agents pre-operatively. Of two patients with seriously impaired ventricular function preoperatively one needed inotropes before cardiopulmonary bypass and both afterwards. The other four patients had dysfunctional valves and had severely disordered hemodynamics preoperatively. For seven of the 16 valve re-replacement operations, ventricular function and clinical state was probably better than it had been before the first operation. The remaining nine patients were as bad or worse and the need for postoperative inotropic support was directly related to the preoperative condition.

Postoperative bleeding—Two patients were reopened for bleeding. This is more than expected for primary operations but the numbers were too small for significance.

Prolonged respirator support—Three patients needed prolonged ventilator support. These patients were in the group with Class IV symptoms and severely disordered hemodynamics. Two had depressed pulmonary function preoperatively. One developed adult respiratory distress syndrome, pneumonia and a disrupted sternum. All were eventually successfully weaned from the respirator.

Sternal disruption—This occurred in two patients, one mentioned above and the other a cachectic female with prosthetic valve dysfunction. Both healed.

Late mortality—Late mortality has occurred from 2 months to 4 years postoperatively. Of the nine patients with valve dysfunction five have died, two of cerebrovascular accidents (one post-traumatic) in the first 6 months after surgery, one of spinal meningitis 2 yearts postoperatively, and two with ventricular failure (one with chronic obstructive pulmonary disease) 4 years postoperatively. Four are alive 1½–10 years following the second valve replacement and 8–13 years after the first valve replacement. One of the four patients with valve thrombosis died suddenly of unknown cause in the first 6 months postoperatively. One came for a second valve re-replacement 8 years after the first, this time for prosthetic valve dysfunction. The three survivors have listed 1½–10 years following their second operations and 8–12 years following their first. Of the two patients with valve infection, the addict died with a combination of Gram-negative sepsis and valve thrombosis 6 months after his second operation. At autopsy cultures and histology of the thrombus were negative for bacteria or fungi. The surviving patient has lived 8 years after his two replacements. The patient operated on for multiple emboli has now lived 6 and 15 years following her second and first operations, respectively. Thus, seven out of 15 patients have died late following secondary mitral valve replacements. Nevertheless, the duration and quality of survival of the remainder has been excellent.

Poll results

The 25 respondents were in agreement on most of the questions but there were interesting minority opinions.

Infection—One-third regarded prosthetic valve infection as a mandatory indication for surgery and over 1/3 regarded mechanical valve infection as more urgent than bioprosthetic infection.

Surgical approach—All used medium sternotomy for the primary operation but a small minority opted for choosing a different approach for the second operation. The most popular access route to the mitral valve was through the left atrial wall anterior to the pulmonary vein. However, a few used the transatrial approach for re-replacement.

Dividing adhesions—The great majority did not divide all adhesions.

Systemic temperature—All used hypothermia, most keeping the temperature between 22 and 28°C.

Cardiac arrest—All arrested the heart with a majority using ischemia and crystalloid cardioplegia. Two thirds used multiple injections but only a minority of these used any special techniques to clear air from the ascending aorta.

Clearing air—Despite the failure to use special techniques to clear air only a small minority admitted to any difficulty in clearing air from their cases.

Mortality—Only a few respondents reported mortality figures and these ranged from 4% to 15%.

Discussion

Indications for surgery, thrombosis and dysfunction

Although the patients in this series survived their second operations there were delays that could have resulted in surgical failure. There were other patients during the course of this series who died before surgery because of failures of diagnosis or failure to understand the potential lethality of failure of artificial heart valves. Any hint of a change in either the patient's or the valve's status demands urgent investigation and simultaneous surgical referral since it may be appropriate to proceed straight to surgery. The surgeon is likely to have a more concentrated experience of the behavior of a particular device than most individual cardiologists and therefore be in a better position to make an urgent decision to act on clinical information.

The valve dysfunction patients form a rather special group. Cloth and occluder wear producing combinations of stenosis and insufficiency, with embolism in some cases, was regarded by some physicians as representing a perivalvular leak, the 'normal' tendency for mechanical valves to embolize and a reflection of the failure of valve replacement to help the cardiac status of some patients. The answer, again, lies in early and aggressive investigations for any change in the status of patient or valve. Nuclear ventricular function studies can eliminate ventricular failure as a cause for the change. Echocardiography is excellent for diagnosing calcification or leaflet disruption of bioprosthesis, but, because of the highly reflective nature of the materials used in mechanical valves, and because parts of some valves interfere with observation of other parts, it is only sometimes successful in detecting valve dysfunction[15, 16]. Cardiac catheterization and angiography remains the best method for confirming dysfunction of mechanical valves.

Infection

In infected cases the question is whether surgery is indicated on diagnosis. As the poll results show, a significant proportion of cardiac surgeons think so. In my experience there are patients very early after primary valve replacement with a possible diagnosis of infection who respond well to antibiotics. There are others who present late with fever and positive blood cultures who, with either mechanical or biological valves, immediately become afebrile and do not develop any complications. It seems reasonable to accept that these patients do not need surgery. While some surgeons regard the presence of all infected mechanical valves as an urgent indication for surgery it seems more appropriate to say that, if embolism or heart failure occur, or if the response to antibiotics is not immediate, urgent surgery is indicated. The critical point is that if infection in any valve spreads outside the prosthetic ring the surgical problems are increased and the chance for successful replacement is inevitably reduced. It is difficult to show that this is going on until the process is quite advanced and it is far better to assume that it is likely if the response to treatment is not immediate. With biological valves, once infection extends through the cusp, early valve disruption or late calcification are highly likely. The presence or development of insufficiency implies valve dehiscence due to perivalvular infection or, even if it was present before, a vulnerability to such infection. Alternatively with a bioprosthesis it may indicate cusp disruption. Distinction between these possibilities is irrelevant. The lesser risk is to regard them as an immediate indication for re-replacement. Vegetations, which have important implications for surgery in natural valve infections,[17] are poorly seen on artificial valves because they are obscured by struts and rings and occluders.

Multiple embolism

There can be no dogmatism on this indication but in the one case in this series the source of the small cerebral emboli that were occurring was apparent on the removed valve and these ceased with a change to a bioprosthesis. In patients having multiple small emboli of the kind likely to be coming from the valve, and without atrial wall disease, giant atrial enlargement or atrial fibrillation, an excellent case can be made for changing from a mechanical to a biological valve.

Surgical technique

The techniques described in this paper have worked for one surgeon. A minority of surgeons polled opted for choosing a previously unused route for the re-replacement operation. Lesser danger in reopening is gained thereby but at the cost of some difficulties in cannulation and less access to other valves and other parts of the heart. In the patient with previous surgery and extensive adhesions, this may limit the technical options available—e.g. perfusing the coronaries in the presence of minor aortic insufficiency, access to the aorta for clamping, cardioplegic injection and air evacuation. However, these strictures have less force when the left or right thoracic approach is used for primary mitral valve surgery; it may be a good idea to do more primary mitral valve replacements by left or right thoracotomies. Median sternotomy in patients having open or closed mitral commissurotomies by a lateral route is generally easier than it is when the previous approach was also a median sternotomy. The key to this is that, since the pericardium was opened laterally, even when not closed it remains as a barrier between sternum and right heart anteriorly. This, in turn, emphasizes the importance of closing the pericardium or using pericardial substitutes whenever this is not possible.[18]

The trans-septal approach has, when made in this manner described, not resulted in permanent alterations of cardiac rhythm and not produced heart block at any time. It produces excellent exposure of the mitral valve even when the heart is bound down by adhesions. However, most other surgeons seem to manage well enough without it.

Minimal dissection of adhesions reduces the operated area that will be prone to bleed postoperatively. It does make the removal of air somewhat more difficult but with the method described for removing air this has not been a problem.

There is much agreement on the necessity for systemic hypothermia and cardiac arrest for this operation. In the ideal case the operation is achieved with one injection of cardioplegic solution. Surprisingly, the majority of surgeons polled said that they used no special techniques to clear air from the aorta with multiple cardioplegic doses and stated also that they experienced no difficulty in clearing air from the heart with or without freeing the adhesions. However, two of the best-known, most experienced mitral valve surgeons did acknowledge that special methods to clear air are appropriate and that clearing air may be a problem.

Morbidity and mortality of re-replacement

Morbidity was high, but was confined to the patients with valve dysfunction who had been allowed to become very sick preoperatively. The hospital mortality was highly satisfactory in this series and may be attributable to the methods used. Much higher mortalities have been reported in the past, although lower figures are now being recorded, except in the patients with Class IV disease.

Conclusions

Mitral valve re-replacement is a potentially hazardous operation. Failure to act vigorously on the suspicion of imperfect function results in surgery being performed on unnecessarily sick patients. Despite this it is possible to perform this surgery with low hospital mortality using the techniques for entering the chest, gaining access to the valve and avoiding intraoperative embolism described in this chapter.

Summary

The techniques used for mitral valve re-replacement in 16 instances are described in detail. There was no hospital mortality, although morbidity was high in the patients allowed to deteriorate excessively before surgery. The techniques used are designed to avoid injury to the heart on opening the chest and exposing and removing the artificial valve, and to protecting the heart and avoiding air embolism during the operation.

References

1. IBEN, A.B., HURLEY, E.J. and ANGELL, W.W. (1966). Repeat open-heart surgery. *Ann. Thorac. Surg.*, **2**, 334
2. MARY, D.S., BARTEK, I.T., ELMUFTI, M.E., *et al.* (1974). Analysis of risk factors involved in reoperation for mitral and tricuspid valve disease. *J. Thorac. Cardiovasc. Surg.*, **67**, 333
3. LONDE, S. and SUGG, W.L. (1974). The challenge of reoperation in cardiac surgery. *Ann. Thorac. Surg.*, **17**, 157
4. SANDZA, J.G., JR., CLARK, R.E., FERGUSON, T.B., CONNORS, J.P. and WELDON, C.S. (1977). Replacement of prosthetic heart valves: a 15 year experience. *J. Thorac. Cardiovasc. Surg.*, **74**, 864
5. MAGILLIGAN, D.J., LAM, C.R., LEWIS, J.W. and DAVILA, J.C. (1978). Mitral valve—The third time around. *Circulation* **58**, Suppl I, 1–36
6. STEWART, S. and DEWEESE, J.A. (1978). The determinants of survival following reoperation of prosthetic cardiac valves. *Ann. Thorac. Surg.*, **25**, 555
7. ENGLISH, T.A.H. and MILSTEIN, B.B. (1978). Repeat open intracardiac operation: Analysis of 50 operations. *J. Thorac. Cardiovasc. Surg.*, **76**, 56
8. ROSSITER, S.J., MILLER, D.C., STINSON, E.B., OYER, P.E., REITZ, B.A. and SHUMWAY, N.E. (1979). Aortic and mitral prosthetic valve reoperations: early and late results. *Arch. Surg.*, **114**, 1279
9. MAGILLIGAN, D.J., JR., LEWIS, J.W., JR., ALAM, M. and LAKIER, J.B. (1981). Surgery for intrinsic dysfunction of prosthetic cardiac valves. (abstr) *Circulation* **64**, Suppl IV, IV–76
10. COHN, L.H., KOSTER, J.K., JR., VANDEVANTER, S. and COLLINS, J.J., JR. (1982). The in-hospital risk of rereplacement of dysfunctional mitral and aortic valves. *Circulation* **66**, Suppl I, 1–153
11. DIAZ, D.C., VIGIL, G., RODRIGUEZ, G.F., MARTINEZ, B.R. and PALACIOUS, M.X. (1982). Infectious endocarditis of the heart valves and valvular prostheses. *Arch. Inst. Cardiol. Mex.*, **52**(2), 169–74
12. WILSON, W.R., DANIELSON, G.K., GIULIANI, E.R. and GERACI, J.E. (1982). Prosthetic valve endocarditis. *Mayo Clin. Proc.*, **57**, 155
13. HOLTZK, FELLER A.M. and SEYBOLD, EPTING W. (1982). Thrombotic obstruction of tilting disc valves. *Dtschr. Med. Wochenschr.*, **107**, 494
14. GABBAY, S., FACTOR, S.M., STROM, J. and FRATER, R.W.M. (1982). Sudden death due to cuspal dehiscence of the Ionescu–Shiley valve in the mitral position. *J. Thorac. Cardiovasc. Surg.*, **84**, 313
15. MINTZ, G.S., CARSLON, E.B. and KOTLER, M.N. (1982). Comparison of noninvasive techniques in evaluation of the nontissue cardiac valve prosthesis. *Am. J. Cardiol.*, **49**, 39
16. DEPACE, N.L., KOTLER, M.N., MINTZ, G.S., LICHTENBERG, R., GOEL, I.P. and SEGAL, B.L. (1980). Echocardiographic and phonocardiographic assessment of the St. Jude cardiac valve prosthesis. *Chest* (3), 272–7
17. STROM, J., BECKER, R.M., DAVIS, R., MATSUMOTO, M., FRISHMAN, W., SONNENBLICK, E. and FRATER,

R.W.M. (1980). Echocardiographic and surgical correlations in bacterial endocarditis. *Circulation*, **62**, I–164

18. GALLO, J.I., POMAR, J.L., ARTINANO, E., VAL, F. and DURAN, C.M.G. (1978). Heterologous pericardium for the closure of pericardial defects. *Ann. Thorac. Surg.*, **26**, 149–154

24

Mitral valve replacement with coronary artery disease

Lawrence Czer, Jack Matloff, Richard Gray, Timothy Bateman and Aurelio Chaux

Introduction

Mitral valve replacement in the United States is being performed with increasing frequency in older patients[1-3]. The incidence of coronary artery disease increases with age[4-9]. Therefore it is not surprising that patients undergoing both mitral valve replacement and coronary artery bypass grafting are being encountered more commonly.

A wide spectrum of pathologic conditions affecting the mitral valve is seen in association with coronary artery disease. Some of these conditions represent separate and distinct entities aside from coronary disease. However, a significant proportion of patients have mitral valve disease as a consequence of and etiologically related to coronary atherosclerosis. Although much has been made of the role of papillary muscle dysfunction, we have observed that the underlying pathophysiologic mechanism is less often reversible papillary muscle ischemia, and more frequently is a fixed papillary muscle infarction, rupture of the chordae tendineae and/or papillary muscle head, or annular dilation associated with left ventricular dilation. Given this variety of pathologic entities involving the mitral valve, we have found that mitral valve replacement, rather than repair, results in a more predictable outcome, except in minor degrees of regurgitation where annuloplasty suffices. Mitral repair for mitral stenosis in advanced age populations is unusual since these patients commonly have heavily scarred and calcified valves that are not amenable to repair. An additional reason favoring replacement over repair is the progressive nature of coronary disease, making the long-term results of repair less certain in patients whose mitral valve disease is etiologically related to coronary disease.

It has been our impression that this increasing experience with concomitant valve and coronary surgery has indicated that there are two separate and distinct populations, each with a different severity of illness and a different prognosis. We have therefore reviewed our most recent results with mitral valve replacement and concomitant coronary artery bypass grafting. As a clinical control, we have also reviewed our experience with isolated mitral valve replacement during this same period of time.

Methods

Patient selection

From January 1976 to June 1982, 380 patients underwent mitral valve replacement at Cedars–Sinai Medical Center. The 131 patients who had additional procedures involving more than the mitral valve and coronary arteries (double valve replacement, tricuspid annuloplasty, aneurysmectomy, ventricular septal repair, atrial septal repair) were excluded from this analysis. The remaining 249 patients form the basis of this report: 131 had mitral valve replacement with concomitant coronary artery bypass grafting (MVR + CABG), and 118 had mitral valve replacement alone (MVR).

The etiology of the mitral valve disease was determined from the clinical history, cardiac catheterization data, the surgical findings, and the gross and microscopic pathology. Patients were considered to have *rheumatic* mitral valve disease if typical rheumatic scarring of the mitral valve and chordae were described by the surgeon and the pathologist. A history of rheumatic fever was confirmatory evidence for this diagnosis. *Ischemic* mitral valve disease was considered present if the patient had coronary artery disease on coronary angiography, and a clinical history consistent with and angiographic findings of mitral regurgitation. Surgical findings were confirmatory when papillary muscle infarction, rupture of the chordae or papillary muscle head, or mitral annular dilation associated with left ventricular dilation were found in the absence of rheumatic or other types of mitral valve disease. Included in this third cagetory of *'other'* were mitral valve prolapse, infective endocarditis, prosthetic dysfunction, Marfan's syndrome, congenital and degenerative causes of mitral regurgitation. Prolapse was considered present when angiographic and surgical findings of redundant mitral leaflet tissue or elongated chordae, or both, were present. A diagnosis of endocarditis was based on the typical microbiologic and pathologic findings. Prosthetic valve dysfunction was identified on the basis of a prior history of mitral valve replacement, with subsequent angiographic evidence of regurgitation. A congenital cause of mitral valve disease occurred in one patient, and Marfan's syndrome in two patients. If none of these causes of mitral valve disease was identified, then the mitral valve disease was classified as 'degenerative'.

The patients' hospital charts were reviewed for the following preoperative information: age, sex, symptoms (heart failure, angina, embolus, arrhythmias); New York Heart Association class; mitral valve lesion (mitral stenosis, mitral regurgitation, or mixed); etiology of the mitral valve disease (rheumatic, ischemic, or other causes as outlined above); the presence of coronary artery disease; and the left ventricular ejection fraction.

Cardiac catheterization

All patients underwent cardiac catheterization prior to the operative procedure. All patients with MVR + CABG had coronary artery disease, defined as 50% or greater diameter narrowing in at least one coronary artery. The left ventricular ejection fraction (LVEF) was calculated in 179 patients by the area–length method from the right anterior oblique left ventricular cineangiogram. Mitral regurgitation was considered to be present if more than trace opacification of the left atrium occurred during left ventriculography. Mitral stenosis was considered to be present if the mitral valve area calculated from the Gorlin formula was less than $1.5\,cm^2$.

Surgical techniques

Mitral valve replacement was performed under general endotracheal anesthesia, with hemodynamic monitoring by means of radial artery and pulmonary arterial thermodilution catheters. Cardiopulmonary bypass was performed with a bubble oxygenator. Prior to April 1978, intermittent ischemic cardiac arrest was performed in 71 patients. After April 1978 (178 patients), myocardial protection consisted of moderate systemic hypothermia (20–25°C) and intermittent multidose potassium cardioplegia with either a crystalloid (St Thomas solution) or modified blood solution at 4°C infused into the aortic root or coronary ostia. The mitral valve was replaced with a porcine heterograft (Hancock or Carpentier–Edwards) in 175 patients, with a St Jude mechanical prosthesis in 71 patients, and with a Harken Surgitool valve in three patients. If concomitant coronary artery bypass was performed (131 patients), it was accomplished utilizing autologous reversed saphenous vein. Distal bypass anastomoses were performed first, followed by mitral valve excision and replacement, and finally the proximal anastomoses. Hemodynamic instability in spite of pharmacologic therapy with vasoactive drugs necessitated placement of an intraaortic balloon pump (IABP) in 24 patients. All patients received long-term anticoagulation therapy with sodium warfarin, unless contraindicated by other medical problems.

Follow-up

Postoperative follow-up information was obtained by means of a questionnaire mailed to each patient every 6 months, patient examination by one of the authors, or by telephone conversation with the patient. Duration of follow-up ranged from 3 to 81 months, and averaged 29 months. Only six patients (2.4%) were lost to follow-up. Postoperative NYHA classsification was determined on the basis of symptoms reported.

Mortality

Operative mortality was defined as death within 24 hours of the operation. Early mortality was defined as death between 24 hours and 30 days after the operation. Deaths occurring after 30 days postoperatively were classified as late mortalities.

Causes of death were classified into three broad groups: cardiac non-valve-related (pump failure including inability to wean from cardiopulmonary bypass, chronic congestive heart failure, myocardial infarction, arrhythmia, sudden death); cardiac valve-related (thromboembolism, coumadin-related hemorrhage, prosthetic dysfunction, prosthetic infection); and non-cardiac causes (pulmonary failure, renal failure, cancer, trauma, and other causes). The precise causes of death could not be determined in 4 patients (6% of all deaths).

Statistical methods

Values of continuous variables are expressed as mean ± SD. Comparison between two continuous variables was made using the unpaired t-test. Discrete variables were compared by means of Fisher's exact test (for 2×2 tables) or by χ^2 analysis (tables larger than 2×2). Survival curves were constructed using the life table method, and all mortalities (operative, early, and late) were included in the analysis. Differences between survival curves were analyzed by the generalized Wilcoxon test. Values of p less than 0.05 were considered statistically significant. Two models for prediction of outcome were utilized: binary logistic regression, and discriminant analysis. Both models predicted the same variables as important determinants of outcome. All statistical analyses were performed utilizing BMDP Statistical Software[10].

Results

Preoperative variables

The 249 mitral valve recipients forming the basis of this report were stratified into two groups of MVR alone (n = 118), and MVR + CABG (n = 131) and were compared with respect to a number of preoperative variables. The results of this comparison are listed in *Table 24.1* and *Figure 24.1*. Patients with the combined

TABLE 24.1 Preoperative and intraoperative variables examined in 249 patients with mitral valve replacement alone (MVR) and with coronary artery bypass (MVR + CABG)

	MVR (n = 118)	MVR + CABG (n = 131)	Total (n = 249)
Age (years)*			
Mean ± SD	58.2 ± 12.8	64.0 ± 9.3	61.2 ± 11.5
< 60	55 (47%)	36 (27%)	91 (37%)
⩾ 60	63 (53%)	95 (73%)	158 (63%)
Sex*:			
Male	38 (32%)	75 (57%)	113 (45%)
Female	80 (68%)	56 (43%)	136 (55%)
Symptoms*:			
Failure	112 (95%)	66 (50%)	178 (72%)
Angina	1 (1%)	21 (16%)	22 (9%)
Angina + failure	2 (2%)	44 (34%)	46 (18%)
Other	3 (2%)	0	3 (1%)
NYHA class*:			
I	3 (2%)	1 (1%)	4 (1%)
II	6 (5%)	4 (3%)	10 (4%)
III	69 (59%)	54 (41%)	123 (50%)
IV	40 (34%)	71 (55%)	111 (45%)
Use of IABP*	2 (2%)	22 (17%)	24 (10%)
Valve lesion*:			
Mitral stenosis	25 (22%)	13 (10%)	38 (16%)
Mitral regurgitation	43 (39%)	89 (71%)	132 (56%)
Mixed	43 (39%)	24 (19%)	67 (28%)
Etiology*:			
Rheumatic	81 (69%)	43 (33%)	124 (50%)
Ischemic	3 (2%)	68 (52%)	71 (29%)
Prolapse, degenerative	25 (21%)	18 (14%)	43 (17%)
SBE, congenital	6 (5%)	0	6 (2%)
Prosthetic	3 (2%)	2 (1%)	5 (2%)
Valve substitute:			
Porcine	85 (72%)	90 (69%)	175 (70%)
St Jude	31 (26%)	40 (30%)	71 (29%)
Other	2 (2%)	1 (1%)	3 (1%)

IABP = Intra-aortic balloon pump.
*Difference between MVR and MVR + CABG groups statistically significant (p < 0.05).

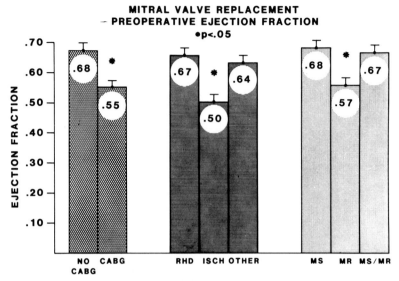

Figure 24.1 Preoperative ejection fraction. CABG = Coronary artery bypass grafting; RHD = rheumatic heart disease; ISCH = ischemic etiology of mitral valve disease; Other = other etiology of mitral valve disease; MS = mitral stenosis; MR = mitral regurgitation. MS/MR = mixed lesions. Data represented as means ± SE.

procedure (MVR + CABG) were older (64.0 *vs.* 58.2 years for the patients with MVR alone); were more often males (57% *vs.* 32%); had a lower incidence of congestive heart failure alone as an indication for surgery (50% *vs.* 95%) but a higher incidence of angina alone or in combination with heart failure (50% *vs.* 3%); a higher proportion of preoperative NYHA class IV patients (55% *vs.* 34%); and a higher utilization rate of the IABP preoperatively or intraoperatively (17% *vs.* 2%). In addition, patients with MVR + CABG had a higher proportion with mitral regurgitation alone as the mitral valve lesion (71% *vs.* 39%), and a lower proportion with either mitral stenosis (10% *vs.* 22%) or mixed lesions (19% *vs.* 39%). The etiology of the mitral valvular disease in these patients was more often ischemic (52% *vs.* 2%), and less often rheumatic (33% *vs.* 69%) or due to other causes (15% *vs.* 28%). All of these differences were statistically significant.

The preoperative LVEF (*see Figure 24.1*) was lower in the patients with MVR + CABG (0.55 ± 0.18 *vs.* 0.68 ± 0.15). In addition, the LVEF was lower in those whose mitral disease etiology was ischemic (0.50 ± 0.18 with ischemic etiology, 0.67 ± 0.14 with rheumatic, and 0.64 ± 0.18 with other etiologies), and lower in those whose valve lesion was regurgitation (0.57 ± 0.18 in mitral regurgitation, 0.68 ± 0.14 in mitral stenosis, and 0.67 ± 0.13 in mixed lesions). All of these differences were statistically significant.

Mortality and causes of death

Operative, early, and late mortalities are shown in *Table 24.2*. Patients with MVR + CABG had higher operative (3.1% *vs.* 0.8%) and early mortality (9.9% *vs.* 1.7%) compared to patients with MVR alone. Causes of death (*see Table 24.3*) were determined from autopsy report whenever possible (75% of the deaths).

TABLE 24.2 Operative, early, and late mortality in patients with MVR alone (MVR) and with coronary artery bypass (MVR + CABG)

	Operative (24 hours)	*Early* (30 days)	*Late* (>1 month)
MVR (n = 118; 5 lost)	0.8% (1/118)	1.7% (2/118)	16.8% (19/113)
MVR + CABG (n = 131; 1 lost)	3.1% (4/131)	9.9% (13/131)	18.5% (24/130)

TABLE 24.3 Causes of death in patients with MVR alone (MVR) and with concomitant coronary artery bypass (MVR + CABG)*

Cause	*MVR* (n = 22)	*MVR + CABG* (n = 41)	*Overall* (n = 63)
Cardiac non-valve	8 (36)	33 (81)	41 (65)
Cardiac valve-related	4 (18)	2 (5)	6 (10)
Non-cardiac	9 (41)	3 (7)	12 (19)
Unknown	1 (5)	3 (7)	4 (6)

*Results are given as numbers of patients, with percentages in parentheses.

Autopsy reports were not obtained in some patients who clearly died from non-cardiac causes, such as motor vehicle accidents, murder, suicide, or disseminated cancer.

Prediction of survival

All of the variables listed in *Table 24.1* and *Figure 24.1* were analyzed in order to determine which were significant determinants of outcome. Two models of prediction (discriminant analysis and logistic regression) gave similar results, listing the same four variables in the same rank order: (1) use of the IABP ($p < 0.001$); (2) LVEF ($p < 0.001$); (3) age ($p < 0.01$); and (4) preoperative NYHA class ($p < 0.05$). Using the logistic regression model, these four variables alone correctly predicted 93% of the survivors and 44% of the deaths, with an overall accuracy of 79%.

Life tables

CABG—Patients with MVR + CABG demonstrated a significantly lower survival than those with MVR alone (*see Figure 24.2*; $p < 0.05$). All patients with MVR + CABG had coronary artery disease ($\geq 50\%$ stenosis). All patients with MVR alone were free of coronary artery disease except for 12 patients who had coronary disease that was not amenable to bypass either because the involved arteries supplied an infarcted area, or were too diffusely diseased distally. When stratified by presence of coronary artery disease rather than CABG, survival curves were nearly identical with those in *Figure 24.2*. The lower survival of patients with coronary artery disease is a composite of two very different groups (*see Figure 24.3*): those with single-vessel and double-vessel coronary artery disease whose probability of survival at 6 years is 80%; and those with triple-vessel and left main coronary artery disease, whose probability of survival at 6 years is under 40%.

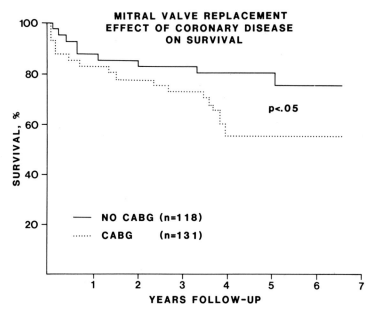

Figure 24.2 Survival after mitral valve replacement alone (No CABG) and after mitral valve replacement with concomitant coronary artery bypass grafting (CABG).

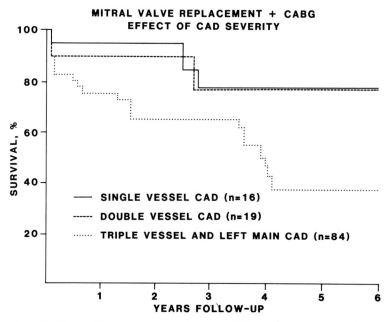

Figure 24.3 Survival by coronary artery disease (CAD) severity in patients with mitral valve replacement and coronary artery bypass grafting (CABG). Patients with triple vessel or left main CAD demonstrated a much lower survival than those with single or double vessel CAD ($p < 0.05$).

LVEF—The effect of LVEF on survival for the entire patient cohort is shown in *Figure 24.4*. Patients with a moderately depressed (35–55%) and severely depressed (< 35%) LVEF demonstrate significantly lower survival than those with a normal LVEF (> 55%). When examining only those patients with MVR + CABG, similar survival curves for the three groups of LVEF were obtained.

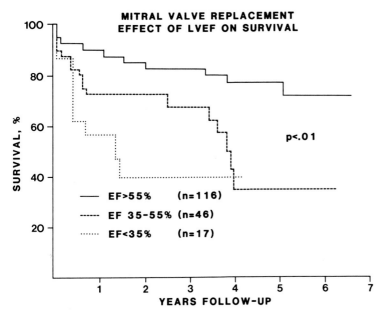

Figure 24.4 Effect of preoperative ejection fraction (EF) on survival following mitral valve replacement.

IABP—An IABP was placed in 24 patients; 22 had coronary artery disease. The probability of survival after 4 years was significantly less in the patients who required placement of an IABP pre- or intraoperatively compared with those who did not require an IABP (p < 0.001) (*see Figure 24.5*).

Age—Age demonstrated a significant effect both in the patients with MVR alone and in the patients with MVR + CABG (*see Figure 24.6*). Age ≥ 60 conferred a significantly lower survival in both groups. Patients with MVR alone and younger than 60 years had a 6-year survival of better than 90%, whereas patients with MVR + CABG over age 60 had a 6-year survival of 40%. Interestingly, the younger patients with MVR + CABG behaved similarly to the older patients with MVR alone (*see Figure 24.6*).

NYHA class—The preoperative NYHA class demonstrated an important effect on survival in the overall group (*see Figure 24.7*) as well as in the patients with and without CABG (*see Figure 24.8*). Patients in NYHA class IV had a lower survival than those in class III; and furthermore within each NYHA class, those with coronary artery disease did worse at 6 years than those without coronary artery disease.

Valve lesion—The valve lesion (mitral regurgitation, mitral stenosis, or mixed) affected survival in the overall group (*see Figure 24.9*) as well as in the patients with MVR + CABG (*see Figure 24.10*). Those with mitral regurgitation demonstrated a

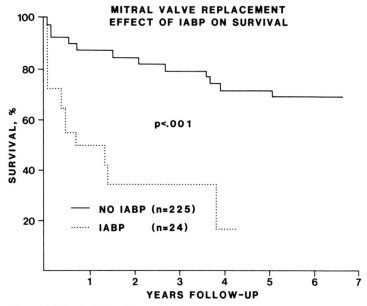

Figure 24.5 Survival following mitral valve replacement, stratified by use of the intra-aortic balloon pump (IABP) preoperatively or intra-operatively.

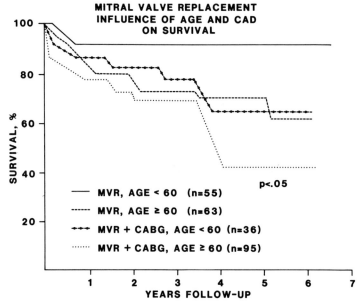

Figure 24.6 Effect of age on survival following mitral valve replacement (MVR) alone, and following MVR and coronary artery bypass grafting (CABG).

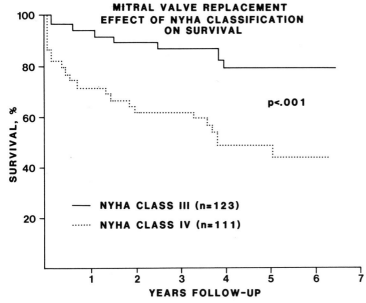

Figure 24.7 Survival following mitral valve replacement, stratified by preoperative New York Heart Association (NYHA) class.

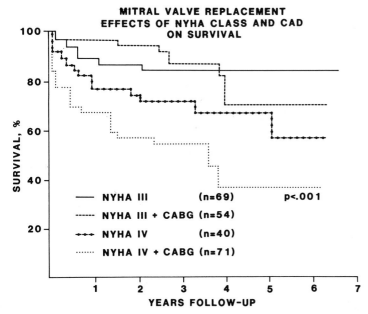

Figure 24.8 Survival following mitral valve replacement, stratified by NYHA class and by the absence or presence of concomitant coronary artery bypass grafting (CABG). CAD = Coronary artery disease.

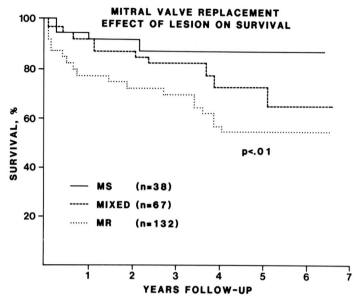

Figure 24.9 Survival following mitral valve replacement, stratified by valve lesion. MR = Mitral regurgitation; MS = mitral stenosis.

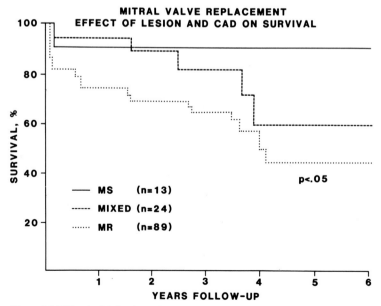

Figure 24.10 Survival following mitral valve replacement and coronary artery bypass grafting, stratified by valve lesion. CAD = Coronary artery disease; MR = mitral regurgitation; MS = mitral stenosis.

significantly lower survival than those with mitral stenosis or mixed lesions. Patients with mitral stenosis or mixed lesions + CABG all had rheumatic heart disease and incidental CABG, whereas 68 of the 89 patients with MVR + CABG had mitral regurgitation etiologically related to their coronary artery disease.

Etiology—The etiology of the mitral valvular disease influenced survival (*see Figure 24.11*). Those with ischemic mitral valve disease had significantly lower survival than those with rheumatic or other etiologies.

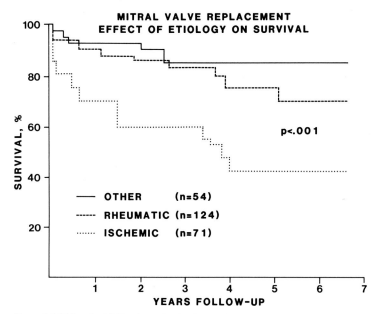

Figure 24.11 Survival following mitral valve replacement, stratified by etiology of the mitral valve lesion.

Valve substitute—The type of valve substitute was similarly distributed between the MVR and MVR + CABG groups. No significant difference in survival as a function of the type of mitral prosthesis was seen after 4 years of follow-up.

Postoperative NYHA class—The distribution of postoperative NYHA class in survivors is shown in *Figure 24.12*. Patients with MVR + CABG experienced a very similar distribution of NYHA class compared with those with MVR alone, although the two groups began very differently preoperatively (*see Table 24.1*). Compared with the preoperative NYHA class, 87% of patients improved their NYHA class postoperatively, 3% remained the same, and 10% worsened.

Discussion

Patients undergoing mitral valve replacement and coronary artery bypass were very different from those undergoing isolated mitral valve replacement. The combined procedure (MVR + CABG) was performed in patients who were older and predominantly male. There was a somewhat lower incidence of heart failure overall in this group (84% *vs.* 97%) but a higher incidence of angina alone or in combination with heart failure, a higher proportion of class IV patients, and a

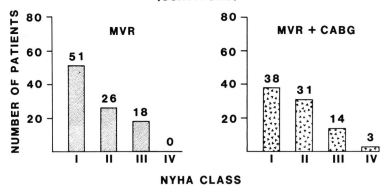

Figure 24.12 Postoperative NYHA class in survivors following mitral valve replacement (MVR) alone and following MVR and coronary artery bypass grafting (CABG).

greater utilization of the IABP. Patients undergoing MVR + CABG had a higher incidence of isolated mitral regurgitation and a lower incidence of isolated mitral stenosis or mixed lesions. There was a greater incidence of ischemic mitral valve disease (i.e. papillary muscle infarction, rupture of the chordae or papillary muscle head, or annular dilation due to left ventricular dilation), and a lower incidence of rheumatic and other etiologies of mitral valve disease.

The preoperative LVEF was lower in the patients with the combined procedure, lower in patients with an ischemic etiology of their mitral valve disease, and lower in the patients with mitral regurgitation. The last result may seem surprising, since in mitral regurgitation the ejection fraction should remain unchanged or increase as the ventricle unloads into the left atrium[11–13]. However, 69% of the patients with mitral regurgitation had coronary artery disease. A depressed LVEF may occur in coronary artery disease with resting ischemia or prior myocardial infarction[14, 15], but may also occur in the absence of coronary disease with chronic or severe degrees of mitral regurgitation[16, 17]. Thus, the compositive LVEF is one which reflects predominantly the depressed EF of ischemic mitral regurgitation and chronic, severe mitral regurgitation in the absence of coronary disease.

The most powerful determinants of outcome were related to preoperative left ventricular function, namely the LVEF and the use of the IABP. Patients with an LVEF < 35% had the lowest survival. The 10% of the patient population of 249 which required IABP augmentation had a very poor prognosis (*see Figures 24.4 and 24.5*). Many studies have shown the LVEF to be an important determinant of outcome, both in patients with coronary artery disease treated medically or by myocardial revascularization[7–9] and in patients undergoing mitral valve replacement without associated coronary artery disease[17–20]. Patients with an intermediate depression of preoperative LV function (35–55%) experienced a survival curve early after surgery similar to patients with normal preoperative LV function, but demonstrated rapid attrition after 3.5 years; thereafter they were similar to those with the most severely depressed LV function. This effect was demonstrated in the overall group (*see Figure 24.4*) which in turn reflected predominantly the patients with MVR + CABG. The addition of CABG apparently delays, but does not eliminate, the eventual deterioration in LV function. One can speculate that progression of coronary artery disease may add to or be causally related to later deterioration in LV function, which in turn adversely affects survival. If so, this is an earlier effect than would be anticipated in patients with coronary artery disease and no mitral involvement.

Advanced age adversely affected outcome, both in the group with MVR alone and in the group with MVR + CABG. Thus, age was an important determinant of outcome, independent of LV function and the presence or absence of coronary artery disease. Several studies have confirmed the important effect of age on survival after MVR[17, 21] and after myocardial revascularization[7–9].

The effect of preoperative NYHA class on postoperative survival after MVR has been controversial. Some studies have shown an effect, especially those in which coronary patients are included[22], while others have shown no effect, usually those in which coronary disease was excluded[17]. Thus, our demonstration of NYHA class as an important determinant of outcome may reflect the inclusion of patients with coronary disease in the study population.

Any statistical analysis of data should always be weighed against the biological importance of each variable. Thus, while the extent of coronary disease, the valve lesion (specifically, mitral regurgitation), and the ischemic etiology of mitral disease dropped out of the prediction analysis, this was only because these variables correlated so highly with depressed LV function. Thus, mitral regurgitation (*see Figure 24.9*), ischemic etiology (*see Figure 24.11*), and extent of CAD (*see Figure 24.3*) are important biological determinants of outcome, even though statistically they are not represented as important variables in the prediction of outcome.

Mortality and causes of death

From the above analysis, it has become apparent that the results of surgical therapy for mitral valve disease reflect the preoperative status of the patient and the underlying disease etiology. The importance of these factors outweighed intraoperative considerations such as the choice of valve substitute and the use of cardioplegia, at least up to the intermediate period of follow-up for this study (maximum 81 months, mean 29 months).

Analysis of the operative and early mortalities (*see Table 24.2*) demonstrated higher mortality ($p < 0.01$) in the combined MVR + CABG group compared with the patients with MVR alone. This reflects the lower LVEF, more advanced age, greater proportion of NYHA class IV patients, coexistent coronary disease, more frequent mitral regurgitation, and greater frequency of ischemic etiology of the mitral valve disease in the patients with combined MVR + CABG. Reported operative mortalities for the combined procedure vary widely, ranging from 0 to 22%[3, 23–29]. The early mortalities in the current series are not discordant with these published reports. With regard to the late mortalities, if one begins with the original patient cohort (*see Table 24.2*), there does not appear to be a statistically significant difference between the two groups once the early period (30 days) is passed. However, when one examines mortality in surviving cohorts by the life table method, there were significant differences between the two groups (*see Figure 24.2*).

Examination of the causes of death (*see Table 24.3*) reveals that 65% (41 out of 63) of all deaths were due to cardiac non-valve-related causes—primarily pump failure early, and congestive heart failure late. This was especially true in the 81%

of deaths in the MVR + CABG group. The other causes of death were insignificant in the MVR + CABG group. A higher proportion of patients with MVR alone died of cardiac valve-related causes (18% *vs.* 5%).

Finally, this experience presents an eloquent argument for earlier surgical therapy in patients with mitral regurgitation, particularly when this is related to and etiologically caused by coronary artery disease. The single most powerful determinant of outcome proved to be the status of LV function preoperatively. Once deterioration in LV function has occurred, there seems to be little that any therapy can accomplish in terms of improvement in long-term survival.

Summary

The following conclusions may be reached based upon the data presented in this study.

1. Mortality after mitral valve replacement is strongly influenced by the preoperative status of the patient.
2. Survival after mitral valve replacement is worse for patients with coronary artery disease than for patients without coronary disease.
3. The presence of triple vessel or left main coronary artery disease adversely affects outcome, and demonstrates a much lower survival than for patients with single or double vessel coronary disease.
4. The single most important preoperative determinant of outcome is left ventricular function, represented by the LVEF.
5. The dominant cause of death can be classified as cardiac non-valve-related; that is, due to pump failure early and congestive heart failure late. This is especially true for patients undergoing concomitant mitral valve replacement and coronary artery bypass grafting, in whom cardiac non-valve related deaths constituted 81% of all cases.

Acknowledgements

The authors thank Marjorie Raymond, Carolyn Conklin and Michele DeRobertis for their valued assistance in the compilation of data for this study. Special thanks go to Morgan Stuart of the Scientific Data Center for statistical analysis of the data.

References

1. SALOMON, N.W., STINSON, E.B., GRIEPP, R.B., *et al.* (1977). Patient-related risk factors as predictors of results following isolated mitral valve replacement. *Ann. Thorac. Surg.*, **24**, 519
2. GANN, D., COLIN, C., HILDNER, F.J., *et al.* (1977). Mitral valve replacement in medically unresponsive congestive heart failure due to papillary muscle dysfunction. *Circulation*, **56** (Suppl II), 101
3. MILLER, D.C., STINSON, E.B., ROSSITER, S.J.. *et al.* (1978). Impact of simultaneous myocardial revascularization on operative risk, functional result, and survival following mitral valve replacement. *Surgery*, **84**, 848–56
4. BRUCSCKE, A.V.T., PROUDFIT, W.L. and SONES, F.M., JR. (1973). Progress study of 590 consecutive nonsurgical cases of coronary disease followed 5–9 years. I. Arteriographic correlations. *Circulation*, **47**, 1147
5. PROUDFIT, W.L., BRUSCHKE, A.V.T. and SONES, F.M., JR. (1978). Natural history of obstructive coronary artery disease: 10 year study of 601 non-surgical cases. *Prog. Cardiovasc. Dis.*, **21**, 53
6. OBERMAN, A., JONES, W.B., RILEY, C.P., *et al.* (1972). Natural history of coronary artery disease. *Bull N.Y. Acad. Med.*, **48**, 1109

7. RAHIMTOOLA, S.H. (1982). Coronary bypass surgery for chronic angina–1981. *Circulation*, **65**, 225–38

8. CUTTER, G.R., OBERMAN, A., KOUCHOUKOS, N., *et al.* (1982). Epidemiologic study of candidates for coronary artery bypass surgery. *Circulation*, **66** (Suppl III), III–6–15

9. KENNEDY, J.W., KILLIP, T., FISHER, L.D., *et al.* (1982). The clinical spectrum of coronary artery disease and its surgical and medical management, 1974–1979. The coronary artery surgery study. *Circulation*, **66** (Suppl III), III–16-23

10. DIXON, W.J. (ed.) (1981). *BMDP Statistical Software*. Berkley: University of California Press

11. KENNEDY, J.W., YARNALL, S.R., MURRAY, S.J., *et al.* (1970). Quantitative angio-cardiography. IV. Relationships of left atrial and ventricular pressure and volume in mitral valve disease. *Circulation*, **41**, 817–24

12. MILLER, G.A.H., KIRKLIN, J.W. and SWAN, H.J.C. (1965). Myocardial function and left ventricular volumes in acquired valvular insufficiency. *Circulation*, **31**, 374–84

13. BOLEN, J.L. and ALDERMAN, E.L. (1977). Ventriculographic and hemodynamic features of mitral regurgitation of cardiomyopathic, rheumatic and non-rheumatic etiology. *Am. J. Cardiol.*, **39**, 177–83

14. EHSANI, A., RAHIMTOOLA, S.H., SINNO, M.Z., *et al.* (1975). Left ventricular performance after acute myocardial infarction: Spectrum of functional abnormalities and significance of wall motion disturbances. *Arch. Intern. Med.*, **135**, 1539

15. MASSIE, B., BOTVINICK, E.H., BRUNDAGE, B.H., *et al.* (1978). Relationship of regional myocardial perfusion to segmental wall motion. Physiological basis for understanding the presence and the reversibility of asynergy. *Circulation*, **58**, 1154

16. SCHULER, G., PETERSON, K.L., JOHNSON, A., *et al.* (1979). Temporal response of left ventricular performance to mitral valve surgery. *Circulation*, **59**, 1218

17. PHILLIPS, H.R., LEVINE, F.H., CARTER, J.E., *et al.* (1981). Mitral valve replacement for isolated mitral regurgitations. Analysis of clinical course and late postoperative left ventricular ejection fraction. *Am. J. Cardiol.*, **48**, 647

18. CHAFFIN, J.S. and DAGGETT, W.M. (1979). Mitral valve replacement: A nine-year follow-up of risks and survivals. *Ann. Thorac. Surg.*, **27**, 312–9

19. KENNEDY, J.W., DOCES, J.G. and STEWART, D.K. (1979). Left ventricular function before and following surgical treatment of mitral valve disease. *Am. Heart. J.*, **97**, 592–8

20. SCHULER, G., PETERSON, K.L., JOHNSON, A., *et al.* (1979). Temporal response of left ventricular performance to mitral valve surgery. *Circulation*, **59**, 1218–31

21. HAMMERMEISTER, K.E., FISCHER, L., KENNEDY, J.W., *et al.* (1978). Prediction of late survival in patients with mitral valve disease from clinical, hemodynamic, and quantitative angiographic variables. *Circulation*, **57**, 341–9

22. SALOMON, H.W., STINSON,M E.B., GRIEP, R.B., *et al.* (1976). Surgical treatment of degenerative mitral regurgitation. *Am. J. Cardiol.*, **38**, 463–8

23. BERGER, T.J., KARP, R.B. and KOUCHOUKOS, N.T. (1975). Valve replacement and myocardial revascularization. *Circulation*, **51**, 52 (Suppl I), 126–32

24. CIARAVELLA, J.M., JR., OCHSNER, J.L. and MILLS, M.L. (1977). Combined procedure of coronary artery bypass grafting and valve repair. *Ann. Thorac. Surg.*, **23**, 20–5

25. FLEMMA, R.J., JOHNSON, W.D., LEPLEY, D., JR., *et al.* (1971). Simultaneous valve replacement and aorto-coronary saphenous vein bypass. *Ann. Thorac. Surg.*, **12**, 163–70

26. GANN, D., COLIN, C., HILDNER, F.J., *et al.* (1977). Mitral valve replacement in medically unresponsive congestive heart failure due to papillary muscle dysfunction. *Circulation*, **56** (Suppl II), 101–4

27. GLANCY, D.L., STINSON, E.B., SHEPHERD, R.L., *et al.* (1973). Results of valve replacement for severe mitral regurgitation due to papillary muscle rupture or fibrosis. *Am. J. Cardiol*, **32**, 313–21

28. KAY, J.H., ZUBIATE, P., MENDEZ, A.M., *et al.* (1976). Myocardial revascularization and mitral repair or replacement for mitral insufficiency due to coronary artery disease. *Circulation*, **54** (Suppl III), 94–6

29. LOOP, F.D., FAVALORA, R.G., SHIREY, E.K., *et al.* (1972). Surgery for combined valvular and coronary heart disease. *J. Am. Med. Assoc.*, **220**, 372–6

25

IHSS, the mitral valve and its treatment

Robert Leachman

Obstructive cardiomyopathy or idiopathic hypertrophic subaortic stenosis (IHSS) was characterized with regard to anatomic, physiologic, and clinical features in the comprehensive report by Braunwald[1] and associates at the National Institutes of Health. This report was a detailed study of 64 patients and a review of the literature to that time. They defined the dynamic nature of the obstruction and its variation in response to position, exercise, blood volume changes, valsalva maneuver, and with a variety of administered drugs. They concluded that during systole the hypertrophied muscle in the outflow tract narrowed sufficiently to produce the obstruction. This dynamic obstruction was thought to be similar to that occurring in the infundibulum of the right ventricle in some patients operated on for pulmonary valve stenosis. The idea of functional obstruction to left ventricular outlet had first been proposed by Sir Russell Brock[2]. He recorded blood pressures at the time of surgery that confirmed the presence of subaortic stenosis from a patient operated on with a diagnosis of aortic valve stenosis. The aortic valve was found to be normal and the left ventricular muscle severely hypertrophied. He concluded that this hypertrophy caused the obstruction and might be secondary to systemic arterial hypertension.

Donald Teare[3] in 1957 reported eight cases of asymmetrical hypertrophy of 'muscular hamartoma' of the heart. Sudden death occurred in seven of the eight cases. He believed the lesions were not glycogen tumors, but was impressed by their tumor-like appearance. He also noted the proximity of the hypertrophied area to the mitral valve.

This presentation is to review the subsequent developments in the understanding of the anatomy, the natural course of the disease and modification of the course by medical or surgical treatment.

Any discussion of diseases of the mitral valve must include obstructive cardiomyopathy, since the anterior leaflet is the obstructing element in its relation to the ventricular septum. The mitral valve was implicated in the left ventricular outlet obstruction by Bjork[4] in 1960 and Moberg[5] in 1963. In one of Bjork's patients, the anterior leaflet was thought to be a sub-aortic membrane because of its anomalous position and was excised. There were other reports of an abnormal mitral valve as a cause of sub-aortic obstruction. Jue and Edwards[6] emphasized the actual and/or potential sub-aortic stenosis in atrioventricular canal defect. Freedom, Dische, and Rowe[7] described complicated malformations associated with accessory endocardial cushion tissue. There were also anatomic descriptions of abnormal attachment of the mitral chordae tendineae with the ventricular septum,[8, 9] similar to Bjork's patient with the leaflet bound to the septum under the right aortic cusp. They emphasized that the anterior leaflet of the mitral valve is an integral part of the left ventricular outflow tract. The presence of accessory tissue of the mitral valve has also been found to cause sub-aortic stenosis.[10, 11]

The concept of a dynamic infundibulum in the left ventricle continued to have wide acceptance and certainly was consistent with the changing obstruction encountered. The outlet of the left ventricle, however, is composed of the upper part of the interventricular septum and a portion of the anterior and posterior walls, but the posterolateral limit is the anterior leaflet of the mitral valve. Any obstruction to the outlet therefore requires an abnormal relation of the anterior leaflet to the upper part of the septum. The changing functional obstruction occurs as a consequence of left ventricular end-systolic volume and the factors that influence it.

The important role of the mitral valve was emphasized in 1969 with the description of the abnormal anterior systolic motion of the anterior leaflet. Pridie[12] presented echocardiographic findings to the British Cardiac Society in 1968, and Shah, Gramiak, and Kramer[13] published echocardiographic features of IHSS in 1969. They published an abstract in 1968 after presenting an exhibit on ultrasound study of IHSS[14]. Not only was the abnormal anterior movement noted, but the anterior leaflet was unusually close to the septum in diastole. In 1974, Henry et al.[15] stated that the outflow obstruction was due to the abnormal forward motion of the valve and that degrees of obstruction are correlated with the anterior position of the leaflet at the beginning of systole. An alternative was that an abnormal position of the papillary muscles resulted in the abnormal motion. Henry et al.[15] concluded that the papillary muscles did not pull the mitral leaflets forward. There is still some disagreement as to whether the systolic anterior motion seen by echo is entirely leaflet or whether the chordae tendineae and papillary muscles contribute to it.

The finding of early systolic closure of the aortic valve has correlated well with the hemodynamic findings. In a group of our patients with this finding, early systolic closure occurred only with a resting outflow tract gradient.[16]

In spite of these findings, the possibility that a congenital abnormality of the mitral valve is the cause of obstructive cardiomyopathy has been more or less rejected. That the anterior leaflet is the obstructing element seems clear. Whether the anterior leaflet and the mitral valve is anomalous in its relation to the ventricular septum, a congenital malformation, or distorted in its relation to the outflow tract by asymmetric hypertrophy is problematical. Perhaps both phenomena are true.

In 1970 we had the opportunity to see a 57-year-old lady with the unique combination of mitral stenosis and hypertrophic sub-aortic stenosis. The calcific mitral valve was replaced with a low-profile disc valve and post-operative catheterization study confirmed that the left ventricular outlet obstruction had been eliminated.[17] We subsequently learned that Schumacher and King[18] had also replaced the mitral valve in a patient in whom he also practiced a simultaneous myomectomy. This case and 27 others subsequently reported[19] in which only the mitral valve was replaced provided convincing evidence that the obstruction is a consequence of the anterior leaflet of the mitral valve.

The frequently fatal outcome of IHSS was recognized even prior to the hemodynamic characterization of the disease. Spodick and Littman[20] presented eight cases and reviewed 66 other published case reports of idiopathic hypertrophy and in this autopsy study noted that 86% of patients were less than 50 years of age at death, and that 65% had died within 2 years of the onset of the disease. It should be emphasized that this was a retrospective autopsy study and there was no information as to the onset of disease, only the onset of symptoms.

It is generally agreed that the course of IHSS is variable and unpredictable; however, from the reports of Frank and Braunwald[21] the mortality rate during approximately 3 years of follow-up was 1 out of 42 (2.3%) patients in NYHA Class I, and 5 out of 40 (12.5%) in Class II, and 4 out of 16 (25%) in patients in Class IV. Maron, Lipson and Roberts[22] also identified eight families with an unusually high mortality from IHSS. Seventy-five per cent of 41 relatives of these index patients had died of their heart disease. Adelman, Wigle, and Ranganathan[23] also noted that 75% of their untreated patients deteriorated or died during the observation period. Within 10 years of detection of a murmur, 93% became symptomatic and 66% deteriorated to NYHA Class III or IV within 5 years of onset of symptoms. McKenna and associates[24] noted that a diagnosis in childhood, blackouts and a family history of the disease were indicators of a poor prognosis. Those diagnosed in childhood had an annual mortality of 5.9% while those over 15 years at diagnosis died at a frequency of 2.5% per year. They did not find prognostic significance in electrocardiographic or hemodynamic information.

Hadarson et al.[25] observed 119 patients for an average of 4.6 years and concluded that embolism, atrial fibrillation, arterial hypertension, and infective endocarditis were the most common complications, other than death which was estimated to occur in 35% at 10 years and 15% at 5 years. These mortality statistics are similar to other reports. Maron and Epstein[26] noted an annual mortality of about 4% per year in patients first diagnosed in childhood.

It seems most likely that the symptoms of dyspnea, fatigue and chest pain are mostly related to hemodynamic alterations. Syncope and vertigo may be hemodynamic in origin, but may also be related to ventricular arrhythmia commonly noted in patients with IHSS.[27, 28] It also seems likely that sudden death may be related to ventricular arrhythmia. The occurrence of atrial fibrillation during cardiac catheterization provides an opportunity to see how dramatically these patients deteriorate with atrial arrhythmia, to the point of collapse and syncope. The apparent beneficial effect of beta-blocking drugs may be mostly in the prevention of these supraventricular arrhythmias, which were noted by McKenna to occur in 46% (14 of 30) of patients monitored.

Most patients with IHSS are now treated with propranolol or similar drugs. In some patients there may be demonstrable hemodynamic improvement in outflow gradient and symptomatic improvement as well. The major effect of beta blockade seems to be in blocking the effect of increased sympathetic activity, such as during exercise or with stimulation with isoproterenol. There is little effect on resting gradient, nor on left ventricular end-diastolic pressure. Resting cardiac output was reported to decrease both with intravenous and oral propranolol administration.[29] The acute administration of intravenous propranolol to three of our patients with IHSS resulted in a decrease in outflow gradient during exercise, but there was also a failure to increase cardiac output during exercise to the pre-drug level. We believe that the pharmacologic effect to prevent the increase in heart rate and an increase in cardiac output explains why some of these patients feel worse with beta blocking drugs. It would seem that an increase in cardiac output is more rate dependent in the non-compliant hypertrophied ventricle. Further, it is likely that the pre-systolic volume is smaller at rapid rates, increasing the dynamic obstruction.

The long-term effect of propranolol on patients with IHSS was presented by Frank and associates.[30] They treated 22 patients with doses of propranolol averaging 462 mg per day. These very large doses produced what they considered 'complete' beta receptor blockade. In a mean follow-up period of 5 years, there were no deaths and symptoms improved. These good results were in contrast to those in ten patients treated with observation or digitalis, diuretics, and anti-arrhythmics, among whom there were four deaths during a mean observation period of 5 years. There were no long-term hemodynamic data, but the authors speculated that improved diastolic compliance was the cause of patient improvement. They speculated that these very large doses of propranolol may have decreased ventricular arrhythmias. In our experience many patients have refused to take propranolol, especially in large doses because they do not feel well with the drug. Particularly, they say they have no energy and tire more rapidly than without the drug.

The introduction of calcium channel blocking drugs with their potential effect on ventricular muscle relaxation was followed by a trial use in IHSS. Kaltenbach[31] and others treated 22 patients with 480 mg daily and noted symptomatic improvement in breathlessness and chest pain. Hemodynamic data were obtained in ten treated patients with findings of a reduced outflow gradient in five, an unchanged or larger gradient in three, no resting gradient in one and no measurement in the other. There was no change in end-diastolic pressure or ejection fraction.

In eight patients receiving oral verapamil, hemodynamic studies were done at rest and exercise after intravenous verapamil and there was a reduction in left ventricular systolic and end-diastolic pressure without change in intraventricular gradient. Rosing and others[32] were able to decrease resting outflow gradient with little change in heart rate or cardiac output following verapamil infusion with IHSS. Eight of the 27 patients had an increase in exercise tolerance. The same investigators concluded that verapamil resulted in an 'impressive improvement' in symptoms of patients treated with 120 mg oral verapamil, four times daily for 12 months. It was subsequently emphasized, however, that verapamil may result in serious complications in these patients.[33] Of 120 patients treated there were three deaths and several episodes of pulmonary edema. They suggest that the drug is contraindicated in those patients with high pulmonary capillary wedge pressure and/or a history of paroxysmal noctural dyspnea in the presence of outflow obstruction. It should also be used cautiously in the presence of sick sinus syndrome or A–V junctional blockade. They also noted in one patient a striking increase in outflow gradient with a drop in systemic blood pressure after verapamil infusion.

Similar clinical findings have been reported by Hasin et al.[34] They also described a decrease in septal thickness, as measured by echocardiogramphy, from 1.6 to 1.4 cm during a mean observation period of 15 months. There was no significant change in systolic anterior motion of the anterior mitral leaflet.

A reduction in septal thickness 4–9 months after oral verapamil therapy was noted by Troesch and associates[35] of Zurich.

These early beneficial reports have been followed by the investigation of nifedipene which similarly has been reported to result in symptomatic improvement in some patients. One such patient was reported by Lorell[36] and it was noted that dyspnea and chest pain were relieved while taking an unspecified dose of nifedipine. Hemodynamic data were obtained at rest and twenty minutes following

20 mg sublingual nifedipine: cardiac index increased from 2.0 to 2.6 l/min/m^2, while pulmonary artery pressure declined from 60 peak systolic to 35, left ventricular end-diastolic pressure from 40 to 29 mm Hg and with normalization of the diastolic contour of the left ventricular pressure. Recent abstracts, however, emphasize the adverse reactions to nifedipine in these patients and lead to the conclusions that syncope, pulmonary edema and hypotension may be limiting factors in its use.[37, 38] It is possible, however, that it might be beneficial in some patients unable to take propranolol or verapamil.

At the present time, surgical treatment is indicated for those patients who are symptomatic and who remain symptomatic or deteriorate with medical treatment. Varying surgical treatments have been utilized, including right ventricular septectomy, left ventricular septectomy or septal myotomy, and mitral valve replacement alone or in combination with other procedures.

The early efforts to correct hypertrophic sub-aortic stenosis surgically are somewhat obscure. Sir Russell Brock[2] in 1957 reported the first attempt to surgically treat these patients with bougies and an expandable dilator introduced into the ventricle and passed into the aorta through the outflow tract. He encountered no resistance in either of two patients and did not relieve the obstruction. He concluded that 'functional subvalvar aortic stenosis seems to be an inoperable state.' Cleland[39] in November 1958, resected part of a very hypertrophied ventricular septum through an aortotomy with resultant symptomatic improvement and the associated characteristic left bundle-branch block. Morrow and Braunwald[40] reported two cases operated with the pre-operative diagnosis of discrete sub-aortic membrane in whom no obstruction was encountered. No definitive surgical procedure was performed, but they supported the idea of functional sub-aortic obstruction.

Wigle, Heinbecker and Gunton[41] reported, in September 1962, on two patients operated by left ventricular septal myomectomy, one of whom was operated on 4 years prior to preparation of the manuscript. Both patients died within 2 weeks following surgery. A third patient was reported to be improved after operation by Bigelow utilizing the technique suggested by Cleland. Bjork[4] reported resection of the hypertrophic septum and acknowledged Cleland's successful resection. Morrow and Brockenbrough[42] had reported in 1961 on two patients operated in January and February, 1961. Planned muscle resection was 'unsuccessful in one patient', but a ventriculomyotomy was performed in both. Both were said to be improved although still symptomatic. One had complete left bundle-branch block, the other did not. Cleland and co-workers had postulated that the surgically created left bundle-branch block might improve the hemodynamics by altering late systole. Morrow and Brockenbrough concluded that the conduction delay was not important since one patient with and one patient without the electrical change had relief of the obstruction. They emphasized that the operation relieved the obstruction by 'interference with the sphincter-like contraction ring.' In this same report, it was recorded that the concept of subaortic ventriculomyotomy had been suggested to Mr William Cleland and Mr H. Burkell by Dr Morrow.

The credit for the popularization, if not the development, of left ventricular septal myomectomy has to go to Andrew G. Morrow.[43] The group of patients operated by this group at the National Heart Institute also provides the largest and most complete information with regard to long term follow-up. Maron et al.[44] reported the long-term status of 124 patients operated on between 1969 and 1975 with an average follow-up of 5.2 years. The majority were operated for symptoms refractory to medical therapy. Eight per cent died in relation to surgery. The majority of survivors were symptomatically improved; however, 6% had persistent and another 6% recurrent severe symptoms. An additional 9% died between 7 months and 13 years after operation of causes thought to be releated to IHSS.

Post-operative hemodynamics were obtained in 79 patients within 9 months of surgery and in another 25 between 1 and 15 years after surgery. No resting gradient was present in the post-operative state in 85 of the 102 patients, while 79 had a resting gradient of more than 50 mm Hg pre-operatively and 28 less than 50 mm Hg. There was no clear correlation between the clinical status and the hemodynamic result of surgical treatment. It was noted that end-diastolic pressure was elevated to abnormal levels in 75% of the patients post-operatively and that there was no correlation between this value and late deaths. The annual mortality rate of the surgical survivors was calculated to be 1.8%; if the surgical mortality was included, the mortality was 3.5% per year.

Survival studies after surgical treatment were also reported by Hardarson et al.[25] Twenty-two patients were operated on: seven died post-operatively, 13 were symptomatically improved, and two unchanged. Current surgical mortality is considerably better than that in the early reports. Reis et al[45] reported 14 patients operated on by ventriculoseptomyomectomy with no surgical deaths and with an average follow-up of 11.4 months. All patients were reported improved and the pre-existing resting gradient present in 13 was abolished in all but one. Six patients with pre-operative moderate to severe mitral regurgitation had trivial or no mitral insufficiency post-operatively.

Adelman and associates[23] from Toronto in a review of 60 patients reported surgical results in 25 observed for an average of 3.6 years. Three patients died early post-operatively and there were three deaths 3–5 years after surgery. There was a tendency for those patients clinically improved after surgery to have better post-operative hemodynamics: no outflow gradient and a lower end-diastolic pressure. They concluded that 75% of surgically treated patients had sustained improvement, while only 25% of those with equal disability had sustained improvement with propranolol.

We have previously reported the clinical experience with right ventricular septostomy from our institution.[46] The clinical results were inconsistent although the resting outflow tract gradient was significantly reduced in most patients and the technique has not recently been recommended. Harkin[47] first reported resection of the inter-ventricular septum from the right ventricular side in a comment on the presentation of Dobell and Scott.

There are available for analysis at present, three groups of patients operated at our institution by different techniques: 12 patients had ventriculoseptal myomectomy alone, another 13 had mitral valve replacement alone, and a third group of 11 had a combination of both mitral valve replacement and myomectomy. All patients had pre- and post-operative hemodynamic and angiographic study within 1 month of surgery. Symptomatic improvement was essentially the same in all three groups of patients. There was no deterioration in symptoms during the 5 years of follow-up. There were three late deaths, two in the mitral valve replacement group, and one in the myomectomy and mitral replacement group. Actuarial attrition rates are 1.6% per year when calculated for the entire group, 3.8% per year from mitral replacement alone, and 2% per year for the combined procedure. The three patients who died were females, all had mitral valve replacements, one with associated myomectomy. They died between 22 and 38 months post-operatively. None had a post-operative outflow tract gradient, one had an elevated left ventricular end-diastolic pressure. All were Class IV pre-operatively and all had atrial fibrillation and persistent pulmonary arterial hypertension after the operation.

The hemodynamic results of the three groups were different, however. Resting outflow tract gradient was entirely eliminated only in the groups of patients with mitral valve replacement. It was improved, if not abolished, in those patients with myomectomy. In this and a previous study group, it was also noted that end-diastolic pressure was greatly improved in the valve replacement group. In a previous group of patients who had only mitral valve replacement, it was noted the left ventricular end-diastolic pressure was normalized. This did not seem to be related to obstruction to inflow by the prosthesis since single projection ventricular volumes calculated from pre- and post-operative angiograms showed the end-diastolic volume and decrease in end-diastolic pressure was observed within 2 weeks of operation and leads us to speculate that the mitral valve apparatus—the chordae tendineae and papillary muscles—might be part of a mechanism that regulates ventricular compliance. Removal of these structures could eliminate a check-rein effect on ventricular expansion and allow the hypertrophic ventricle to expand farther.

Most investigators have concluded that the basic abnormality in IHSS is in the ventricular myocardium and that the outflow obstruction is secondary to this idiopathic septal hypertrophy. We[48] have studied by echocardiography five patients who had only mitral valve replacement for treatment of IHSS an average of 48 months previously. No muscle was resected. It is of interest that by relieving the obstruction in these patients, the ventricular septum was reduced in thickness from 2.2 cm to 1.6 cm in the outflow tract. This leads us to believe that the outflow obstruction is causally related to the hypertrophy and reversible when the obstruction is relieved. If the fundamental abnormality is an overgrowth of ventricular septum from unknown cause, it would seem unlikely that it would regress with relief of the obstruction by only replacing the mitral valve.

Conclusions

It seems clear that the cause of the dynamic outlet obstruction in obstructive cardiomyopathy is the anterior leaflet of the mitral valve as it opposes the ventricular septum. It is not clear whether a developmental abnormal relation of the mitral valve to the septum is the cause of the disease or whether an abnormal hypertrophy of the septum forces the mitral apparatus into this abnormal position. It is my personal belief that in the majority of these patients there is a congenital anomaly of the mitral valve and its relation to the left ventricular cavity and septum.

The disease presents and progresses in an unpredictable way. There is some relation between chest pain and syncope to early death. Approximately 30% of patients, in our experience, have moderate to severe mitral regurgitation. While the regurgitation may be relieved by septectomy in some patients, it seems to persist in many. Increasing left ventricular end-systolic volume by decreasing mitral regurgitation may also help in eliminating outflow gradient. Symptomatic patients with the familial form of the disease also seem to be at higher risk.

The overall annual mortality rate is about 3.5–5% per year and does not seem to be greatly modified by usual medical therapy although very large dose propranolol treatment may improve the outlook. Control of supraventricular and ventricular arrhythmias detected by long-term monitoring may also reduce the incidence of sudden death. Surgical treatment provides better relief of symptoms and seems to increase survival. In the reported surgical survivors there is an annual attrition rate of about 1.5% per year.

It is our current practice to give relatively low-dose beta-blocking drugs to asymptomatic patients and to observe their progress. Symptomatic patients are treated with larger doses of beta blockers or calcium channel blockers as tolerated. If symptoms persist in spite of drug therapy, surgical treatment is indicated with myomectomy alone, particularly in the younger patient without mitral regurgitation. Mitral valve replacement alone or with myomectomy is recommended particularly in those patients with severe mitral regurgitation and in those who have persistent outflow tract gradient or regurgitation following ventricular septal myomectomy.

References

1. MORROW, A.G., LAMBREW, C.T. and BRAUNWALD, E. (1964). Idiopathic hypertrophic subaortic stenosis: II. Operative treatment and the results of pre- and postoperative hemodynamic evaluations. *Circulation*, Suppl. **IV, 120**

2. BROCK, R. (1957). Functional obstruction of the left ventricle (acquired aortic subvalvar stenosis). *Guy's Hospital Report*, 221

3. TEARE, D. (1958). Asymmetrical hypertrophy of the heart in young adults. *Brit. Heart J.*, **20,** 1

4. BJORK, V.O., HULTQUIST, G. and LODIN, H. (1961). Subaortic stenosis produced by an abnormally placed anterior mitral leaflet. *J. Thorac. Cardiovasc. Surg.*, **41,** 5

5. MOBERG, P.F. and SODERBERG, H. (1963). On the pathogenesis of idiopathic hypertrophic subaortic stenosis. *J. Cardiovasc. Surg.*, **4,** 602

6. JUE, K.L. and EDWARDS, J.E. (1967). Anomalous attachment of mitral valve causing subaortic atresia. Observations in a case with other cardiac anomalies and multiple spleens. *Circulation*, **35,** 928

7. FREEDOM, R.M., DISCHE, M.R. and ROWE, R.D. (1977). Pathologic anatomy of subaortic stenosis and atresia in the first year of life. *Am. J. Cardiol.*, **39,** 1035

8. EDWARDS, J.E. (1965). Pathology of left ventricular outflow tract obstruction. *Circulation*, **31,** 586

9. SELLERS, R.D., LILLEHEI, C.W. and EDWARD, J.E. (1964). Subaortic stenosis caused by anomalies of the atrioventricular valves. *J. Thorac. Cardiovasc. Surg.*, **48,** 2, 289–302

10. KURIBAYASHI, R., IMAI, T., YAGI, Y. and GOMI, H. (1979). Subaortic stenosis caused by an accessory tissue of the mitral valve. *J. Cardiovasc. Surg.*, **20,** 591–6

11. HATEM, J., SADE, R.M., TAYLOR, A., USHER, B.W. and UPSHUR, J.K. (1981). Supernumerary mitral valve producing subaortic stenosis. *Chest*, **79,** 483–6

12. PRIDIE, R.B. and OAKLEY, CELIA. (1969). Mitral valve in hypertrophic obstructive cardiomyopathy. Proceedings of the British Cardiac Society. *Brit. Heart J.*, **31,** 390

13. SHAH, P.M., GRAMIAK, R. and KRAMER, D.H. (1969). Ultrasound localization of left ventricular outflow obstruction in hypertrophic obstructive cardiomyopathy. *Circulation*, **40,** 3–11

14. SHAH, P.M., GRAMIAK, M.D. and KRAMER, D.H. (1969). Ultrasound localization of obstruction in hypertrophic obstructive cardiomyopathy. *Am. J. Cardiol.*, **23,** 138

15. HENRY, W.L., CLARK, C.E., GRIFFIFTH, J.M. and EPSTEIN, S.E. (1975). Mechanism of left ventricular outflow obstruction in patients with obstructive asymmetric septal hypertrophy (Idiopathic subaortic stenosis). *Am. J. Cardiol.*, **35,** 337–45

16. KRAJCER, Z., ORZAN, F., PECHACEK, L.W., GARCIA, E. and LEACHMAN, R.D. (1978). Early systolic closure of the aortic valve in patients with hypertrophic subaortic stenosis and discrete subaortic stensosis: Correlation with preoperative and postoperative hemodynamics. *Am. J. Cardiol.*, **41,** 823

17. ELLIS, J.G., TERNENY, O.J., WINTERS, W.L. and LEACHMAN, R.D. (1971). Critical role of the mitral valve leaflet in hypertrophic subaortic stenosis and amelioration of the disease by mitral valve replacement. *Chest*, **59,** 4, 378–82

18. SCHUMACKER, H.B. and KING, H. (1965). New operative approach in the management of hypertrophic subaortic stenosis. *J. Thorac. Cardiovasc. Surg.*, **49,** 3, 497–503

19. COOLEY, D.A., GRACE, R.R., WUKASCH, D.C. and LEACHMAN, R.D. (1976). Replacement and/or repair of

the mitral valve as treatment of idiopathic hypertrophic subaortic stenosis. *Cardiovasc. Disease*, **3**, 4, 382–93

20. SPODICK, D.H. and LITTMANN, D. (1958). Idiopathic myocardial hypertrophy. *Am. J. Cardiol.*, **1**, 610–23

21. FRANK, S. and BRAUNWALD, E. (1968). Idiopathic hypertrophic stenosis. Clinical analysis of 126 patients with emphasis on the natural history. *Circulation*, **37**, 759–88

22. MARON, B.J., LIPSON, L.C. and ROBERTS, W.D (1978). 'Malignant' hypertrophic cardiomyopathy: Identifications of a subgroup of families with unusually frequent premature deaths. *Am. J. Cardiol.*, **41**, 1133

23. ADELMAN, A.G., WIGLE, E.D., RANGANATHAN, N., et al. (1972). The clinical course in muscular subaortic stenosis: A retrospective and prospective study of 60 hemodynamically proved cases. *Ann. Int. Med.*, **77**, 515–25

24. MCKENNA, W., DEANFIELD, J., FARUQUI, A., ENGLAND, DIANE, OAKLEY, C. and GOODWIN, J. (1981). Prognosis in hypertrophic cardiomyopathy: Role of age and clinical, electrocardiographic and hemodynamic features. *Am. J. Cardiol.*, **47**, 532–8

25. HARDARSON, T., CURIEL, R., DE LA CALZADA, C.S. and GOODWIN, J.F. (1973). Prognosis and mortality of hypertrophic obstructive cardiomyopathy. *Lancet*, **ii**, 1462–7

26. MARON, B.J. and EPSTEIN, S.E. Clinical course of patients with hypertrophic cardiomyopathy. In *Congenital Heart Disease in Adults* (ed. W.C. Roberts), pp. 253–64

27. MCKENNA, W.J., CHETTY, S., OAKLEY, CELIA M. and GOODWIN, J.F. (1980). Arrhythmia in hypertrophic cardiomyopathy: Exercise and 48 hour ambulatory electrocardiographic assessment with and without beta adrenergic blocking therapy. *Am. J. Cardiol.*, **45**, 1, 1–5

28. SAVAGE, D.D., SEIDES, S.F., MARON, B.J., MYERS, DEBRA and EPSTEIN, S.E. (1979). Prevalance of arrhythmias during 24-hour electrocardiographic monitoring and exercise testing in patients with obstructive and non-obstructive hypertrophic cardiomyopathy. *Circulation*, **59**, 5, 866–75

29. STENSON, R.E., FLAMM, M.D., HARRISON, D.C. and HANCOCK, E.W. (1973). Hypertrophic subaortic stenosis. Clinical and hemodynamic effects of long-term propranolol therapy. *Am. J. Cardiol.*, **31**, 763–73

30. FRANK, M.J., ABDULLA, A.M., CANDEO, M.I. and SAYLORS, R.D. (1978). Long-term medical management of hypertrophic obstructive cardiomyopathy. *Am. J. Cardiol.*, **42**, 993–1001

31. KALTENBACH, M., HOPF, R., KOBER, G., BUSSMANN, W.D., KELLER, M. and PETERSEN, Y. (1979). Treatment for hypertrophic obstructive cardiomyopathy with verapamil. *Brit. Heart J.*, **42**, 35–42

32. ROSING, D.R., KENT, K.M., BORER, J.S., SEIDES, S.F., MARON, B.J. and EPSTEIN, S.E. (1979). Verapamil therapy: A new approach to the pharmacologic treatment of hypertrophic cardiomyopathy. I. Hemodynamic effects. *Circulation*, **60**, 6, 1201–13

33. EPSTEIN, S.E. and ROSING, D.R. (1981). Verapamil: Its potential for causing serious complications in patients with hypertrophic cardiomyopathy. *Circulation*, **64**, 3, 437–41

34. HASIN, Y., LEWIS, B.S., LEWIS, N., WEISS, A.T. and GOTSMAN, M.S. (1982). Long-term effect of verapamil in hypertrophic cardiomyopathy. *Int. J. Cardiol.*, **1**, 243–51

35. TROESCH, M., HIRZEL, H.O., JENNI, R. and KRAYENBUHL, H.P. (1982). Reduction of septal thickness following verapamil in patients with asymmetric septal hypertrophy. Abstract, 52nd Science Session. *Circulation*, **66**, Suppl II, 155

36. LORELL, B., PAULUS, W.J., GROSSMAN, W., et al. (1980). Improved diastolic function and systolic performance in hypertrophic cardiomyopathy after nifedipine. *New Eng. J. Med.*, **303**, 801–3

37. RUDDY, T.D., KOILPILLAI, C., LIU, P.P., et al. (1982). Evaluation of chronic nifedipine therapy in nonobstructive hypertrophic cadiomyopathy. *Abs. Circulation*, **66**, Suppl II, 24

38. ROSING, D.R., CANNON, R.O., WATSON, R.M., KENT, K.M., LAKATOS, E. and EPSTEIN, S.E. (1982). Comparison of verapamil and nifedipine effects on symptoms and exercise capacity in patients with hypertrophic cardiomyopathy. *Circulation*, **66**, Suppl II, 24

39. GOODWIN, J.F., HOLLMAN, A., CLELAND, W.P. and TEARE, D. (1960). Obstructive cardiomyopathy simulating aortic stenosis. *Brit. Heart J.*, **22**, 403–14

40. MORROW, A.G. and BRAUNWALD, E. (1959). Functional aortic stenosis. A malformation characterized by resistance to left ventricular out-flow without anatomic obstruction. *Circulation*, **20**, 181–9

41. WIGLE, E.D., HEIMBECKER, R.O. and GUNTON, R.W. (1962). Idiopathic ventricular septal hypertrophy causing muscular subaortic stenosis. *Circulation*, **26**, 325–40

42. MORROW, A.G. and BROCKENBROUGH, E.C. (1961). Surgical treatment of idiopathic hypertrophic subaortic stenosis: Technic and hemodynamic results of subaortic ventriculomyotomy. *Ann. Surg.*, **154**, 2, 181–9

43. MORROW, A.G., ROBERTS, W.D., ROSS, J. JR., et al. (1968). Obstruction to left ventricular outflow. Current concepts of management and operative treatment. *Ann. Int. Med.*, **60**, 6, 1255–80

44. MARON, B.J., MERRILL, W.H., FREIER, P.A., KENT, K.M., EPSTEIN, S.E. and MORROW, A.G. (1978).

Long-term clinical course and symptomatic status of patients after operation for hypertrophic subaortic stenosis. *Circulation*, **57**, 6, 1205–13

45. REIS, R.L., BOLTON, M.R., KING, J.F., PUGH, D.M., DUNN, M.I. and MASON, D.T. (1974). Anterior-superior displacement of papillary muscles producing obstruction and mitral regurgitation in idiopathic hypertrophic sub-aortic stenosis. *Circulation*, **49** and **50**, Suppl. II, 181–8

46. COOLEY, D.A., BLOODWELL, R.D., HALLAM, G.L., LASORTE, A.F., LEACHMAN, R.D. and CHAPMAN, D.W. (1967). Surgical treatment of muscular subaortic stenosis. Results from septectomy in twenty-six patients. *Circulation*, **35** and **36**, Suppl. I, 124–32

47. HARKIN, D.E., DOBELL, A.R.C. and SCOTT, H.F. (1964). Hypertrophic subaortic stenosis. *J. Thorac. Cardiovasc. Surg.*, **47**, 26

48. LEACHMAN, R.D. and KRAJCER, Z. (1981). Significant reduction of asymmetrical septal hypertrophy following mitral valve replacement in patients with idiopathic hypertrophic subaortic stenosis. *Abs. Circulation*, **64**, Suppl IV, 314

26

Thromboembolism after mitral valve replacement

Lawrence H. Cohn

Thromboembolism (TE) is a well-recognized complication of mitral valvular heart disease following insertion of a prosthetic or bioprosthetic cardiac valve. Because of chronic supraventricular dysrrhythmias, dilatation of the left atrium behind the stenotic or regurgitant valve and chronic low output state in some patients with mitral regurgitation and left ventricular dysfunction, patients are predisposed to stasis in the left atrial appendage producing atrial thrombus and systemic clinical TE. In addition, the valve devices implanted have a variety of irregular surfaces and contours with varying degress of obstruction and stasis depending on valve design.

This chapter will focus on some of the etiologic features and risk factors for TE in the post-mitral valve replacement state, presentation of comparative data outlining the risk of TE after replacement with various types of prosthetic and bioprosthetic mitral valves, data on prevention of TE and identification of subsets of patients that are at particularly high risk of TE. Analysis of these data should provide the clinician with a reasonable expectation of the risk of TE after replacement with various devices in a variety of clinical subsets of patients and recommendations for prevention and treatment.

Diagnosis and reporting of thromboembolism

The diagnosis of TE in patients with prosthetic or bioprosthetic valves may be difficult. Certainly a cerebrovascular accident, femoral embolus, or other major clinical phenomenon related to an embolus are easy to detect. Difficult to diagnose are transient ischemic attacks, evidence of myocardial ischemia and myocardial infarction, and minor changes in cerebration or vision that may be fleeting, sudden unexplained death, which is often attributed to arrhythmia but which could conceivably be due to TE. As Edmunds[1] has pointed out, even if post-mortem examinations are performed, a small coronary or cerebral embolus may be missed. Thus, most observers believe that thromboemboli are under-reported because of the difficulty in assessing clinical thromboemboli. Edmunds also points out convincingly that the under-reporting of emboli may be related to the fact that thrombi are simply embolized to various 'silent' parts of the body. The brain receives 14% of the cardiac output but it accounts for approximately 80% of recognized emboli in patients with prosthetic heart valves[2-6]. According to Edmunds[1], if one assumes valve-related emboli are actually distributed to the body in proportion of blood flow, one must multiply the incidence of detected emboli by a factor of 5.7 (0.8 × 100 ÷ 14) to estimate the actual incidence of emboli produced by prosthetic heart valves.

Incidence of thromboembolism after mitral valve replacement

Table 26.1 is a tabulation of the thromboembolic complications of currently used mitral valve mechanical prostheses. These data reflect current data on the standard prosthetic mitral valves: Starr–Edwards, Bjork–Shiley and St. Jude. This table summarizes emboli/100 patient-years and probability of freedom from TE at specific time periods, varying from 5 to 10 years. The less hemodynamically efficient Starr–Edwards ball valve has the highest incidence, the pivoting disc valves a lesser incidence. In the mechanical valve series, all patients are anticoagulated.

TABLE 26.1 Thromboembolic complications of current prosthetic mitral valve replacement devices*

Valve	Reference	Maximum follow-up (year)	Emboli/ 100 patient-years	% (No.) free from TE
Starr–Edwards	7	10	6.4	70 (10)
	8	10	6.1	51 (10)
Bjork–Shiley	9	10	4.2	81 (5)
	10	10	2.1	
St Jude	11	3	3.6	95 (3)
	12	4	2.8	90 (4)

*Maximum number of patients = 50.
TE = Thromboembolism.

In *Table 26.2* is a compilation of representative series of porcine and pericardial valves and the incidence of TE after MVR. Most of the patients in these series are not anticoagulated but the differences and reasons for this will be discussed. The rates of TE after tissue valve MVR are slightly lower than any of the prosthetic valves.

TABLE 26.2 Thromboembolic complications of current bioprosthetic mitral valve replacement devices*

Valve	Reference	Maximum follow-up (year)	Emboli/100 patient-years	% (No.) free of TE
Porcine: Hancock and	13	10	2.1	90 (9)
Carpentier–Edwards	14	10	2.1	92 (6)
	15	11	2.2	81 (11)
	16	8	2.4	92 (6)
Bovine pericardium	17	10	0.6	96 (10)
	18	4	2.1	71 (4)

*At least 50 patients.
TE = Thromboembolism.

Incidence of valve thrombosis

Thrombosis of prosthetic or bioprosthetic valves has occasionally been reported in low output cardiac failure since the inception of valve surgery in 1960. Of· note, however, is the total thrombosis rate in patients with the pivoting disc valves such as the Bjork–Shiley[19]. The other currently used pivoting disc valves have a lesser incidence of thrombosis experience compared with the Bjork–Shiley but their clinical usage is considerably shorter. The incidence of total thrombosis of the mitral Bjork–Shiley valve has been reported to be 2–7%, (mean, 4.3%) with warfarin (see Table 26.3). Most patients developing thrombosis have had changes in or inadequate anticoagulation. Other factors implicated have been the design of the valve disc causing change to convexoconcave disc with the Bjork–Shiley valve, although thrombosis of the 'C–C' valve has been reported[19], or possibly technique of implantation[20]. For patients having other non-cardiac operations with this valve in place we taper the coumadin for 2 days prior to surgery, then begin intravenous clinical Dextran the night of operation at a rate of 500 ml/24 hours and continue each day until oral anticoagulation is therapeutic. Meticulous anticoagulation and management of changes in anticoagulation for other health conditions are critical with this valve.

TABLE 26.3 Incidence of thrombosis of mitral Bjork–Shiley valve

Reference	Patients	Thrombosis (%)
20	127	3 (2.4)
21	85	6 (7.1)
9	302	17 (5.6)
22	224	14 (6.3)
23	167	3 (1.8)

Factors affecting the incidence of thrombeomboli after MVR

Factors that affect thromboemboli after MVR include anticoagulation, presence of chronic atrial fibrillation, the presence or absence of intra-atrial thrombus, type of valve lesion (mitral stenosis vs. mitral regurgitation), and size of the left atrium.

Long-term anticoagulation

Long-term anticoagulation is the most important factor affecting the incidence of TE in patients with prosthetic mitral valves and in certain subsets of patients with bioprosthetic valves. Adequacy of anticoagulation correlates with the incidence of thromboembolic complications and inadequate anticoagulation predisposes to thromboemboli and as noted, thrombosis in some valves. In a recent review of the 20-year experience with the Starr–Edwards valve from Starr's group[24], data prior to 1973 demonstrated an incidence of emboli in the Starr–Edwards bare strut valve at 6.6/100 patient-years but after 1973, the incidence of emboli decreases significantly to 4.8/100 patient-years. Simultaneously, the incidence of anticoagulation-related complications, i.e. bleeding, increased significantly as the incidence of thromboemboli also decreased. Similarly, in the Bjork–Shiley valve[9], non-anticoagulation results in a vastly higher incidence of TE than when anticoagulated.

Thus, all patients with mechanical valves should receive long-term anticoagulation. When anticoagulants are omitted in patients, the incidence of TE increases markedly in both the cloth-covered Starr–Edwards valve and the Bjork–Shiley valve. When coumadin derivatives are stopped after a few months in patients with cloth-covered prostheses, the incidence of thromboembolic complications increases significantly. Likewise temporary interruption of anticoagulation increases the risk of TE, particularly in the tilting disc or pivoting disc type of valve. As noted above, the incidence of thrombosis of the Bjork–Shiley valve increased markedly whenever patients had temporary interruption of warfarin. In most cases a period of about 10 months seems to be required for organized thrombus to build up on the valve to cause acute thrombosis.

In patients with prosthetic heart valves, bleeding complications most frequently involve the central nervous, genitourinary, or gastrointestinal systems[5, 25]. In general, fatal hemorrhages involve the central nervous system[2, 10], and less frequently the gastrointestinal tract or retroperitoneal area. Patients with prosthetic heart valves seem to have a higher incidence of central nervous system hemorrhages[2, 6, 25, 26, 27] than anticoagulated patients without prosthetic valves which may be due to bleeding complicating small embolic infarcts within the nervous system[27, 28].

Several factors affect the incidence of bleeding complications in anticoagulated patients[29]: the degree of suppression of prothrombin time is the most important factor, drug interaction and age over 60 years[28]; however, the increase is small. Hypertension and heart failure do not appear to increase bleeding complications[28] but trauma does, and is the inciting cause in approximately 25% of patients[6]. In the very best of hands, anticoagulation has serious complications. In the study by Forfar from Scotland[30] in a very well-controlled local clinical group of over 500 patients on long-term anticoagulation, this author found that the incidence of coumadin-related hemorrhagic complications increased with time so that the probability of an anticoagulation hemorrhage at 7 years was 22%. In some series, difficulty with anticoagulation or repeated thromboembolic complications despite good anticoagulation in patients with prosthetic valves have necessitated valve change to bioprosthetic valve[31]. Overall, the morbidity of coumadin anticoagulation is about 5–15%/year while the mortality is estimated to be 1%/year.

Acetylsalicylic acid (aspirin) inhibits the function of circulating platelets and has been advocated for use in place of coumadin in some patients in both bioprosthetic[32, 33] and prosthetic valves[34, 35]. No long-term study is available on the efficacy of aspirin alone but in many patients with bioprosthetic valves this therapy is reasonable. With prosthetic valves aspirin without coumadin does not provide adequate protection against thromboembolic complications[1].

Aspirin and dipyrimidol have been used in addition to coumadin for thromboembolic prophylaxis in patients with mechanical valves. Several studies have shown that coumadin and 500–1000 mg aspirin with dypyrimidol, 400 mg/day, reduce incidence of thromboemboli[36–38]. However, this combination increases the incidence of bleeding complications[35–38]. In a personal survey, several years ago[33], of 19 major cardivascular centers more than 50% of surgeons use aspirin and dipyrimidole for prophylaxis in patients with bioprosthetic mitral valves.

In many centers heparin anticoagulation is started immediately postoperatively as soon as the chest tubes are out to reduce early thromboembolic phenomena[39]. Though logical, there is no hard data to support widespread use. Since thrombosis of any type of valve can occur in an early low output state, heparin in this situation may be of real aid. Many authors have observed the incidence of thromboemboli is higher during the first 3–12 months after bioprosthetic or bare strut ball valves[13–17, 40–42] but less so in pivoting disc valves where a more constant rate occurs[23, 25]. Our data from the Brigham and Women's Hospital and many others have documented that 80% of events occur in the first 10–12 weeks postoperatively [13–17, 43]. Hence, in almost all centres in all patients who will have bioprosthetic valves regardless of cardiac rhythm, anticoagulation for 10–12 weeks is carried out to protect the patients in this vulnerable period. For example, in a report by Hetzer[42], emboli/100 patient-years in the first 3 months was 13.3 and 0.4 thereafter.

Cardiac rhythm

Though not as pertinent in the discussion of thromboemboli following mechanical valve replacement since all patients with these devices must take anticoagulation, the presence or absence of chronic atrial fibrillation does seem to play an important role in the incidence of thromboemboli following bioprosthetic valve replacement. The incidence of thromboemboli is lower in patients in sinus rhythm than in patients in chronic atrial fibrillation after bioprosthetic mitral valve replacement[40, 43–46]. Atrial fibrillation, commonly thought to be a relatively benign rhythm, has been shown, in large numbers of patients, to affect long-term mortality negatively[47, 48].

In data published by the insurance industry with some 3000 patients in atrial fibrillation, it is apparent that chronic atrial fibrillation has a negative influence on long-term survival because of thromboemboli[47] (*see Figure 26.1*).

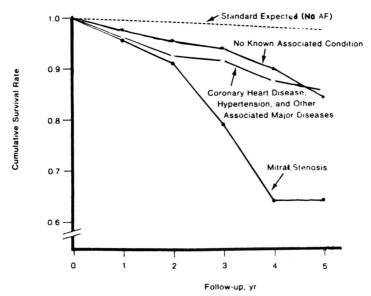

Figure 26.1 Cumulative survival rate observed in insured men and women with chronic atrial fibrillation (AF) associated with mitral stenosis, other major conditions, or none. Expected survival was derived from the 1965–1979 Select Basic Tables. (Reproduced from reference 47, by kind permission of authors and publishers.)

Analysis of our own data at the Brigham and Women's Hospital has shown that atrial fibrillation contributes significantly to long-term emboli in patients with mitral valve bioprostheses[13, 33, 44]. This has been noted by other large centers using both Hancock and Carpentier–Edwards bioprosthetic valves. Most cardiologists and cardiac surgeons now recommend long-term anticoagulation in a patient with a bioprosthetic valve if the predominant rhythm is chronic atrial fibrillation but some can show no difference with or without anticoagulation[46] in patients with this rhythm. Thus, the choice of bioprosthetic versus mechanical valve in a patient with atrial fibrillation is less clear. Some have actually recommended that the bioprosthetic valves in chronic atrial fibrillation should not be used[1]. Early data from our institution documenting the difference in thromboemboli in patients with atrial fibrillation using either bioprosthetic or mechanical valves, did show a difference favoring bioprosthetic valves even in this setting[49]. Other clinical considerations that might suggest a bioprosthetic valve despite chronic atrial fibrillation are pregnancy or other medical conditions or operations where anticoagulation would be hazardous, or inability to take anticoagulation.

Hetzer[43] noted in a recent analysis of 254 patients with mitral bioprostheses that all thromboemboli occurred in patients with atrial fibrillation. Interestingly, in their patient group with chronic atrial fibrillation, the hemorrhagic rate from anticoagulation was more than five times higher than the embolic incidence (5.4 vs. 0.7/100 patient-years). Patients in chronic atrial fibrillation and no long-term anticoagulation did not suffer either emboli or bleeding. They likewise showed that 6 out of 10 emboli occurred during the first postoperative month and eight within the first 3 postoperative months. All emboli in the 10 patients that suffered the emboli out of the 254 occurred within the first year. In addition, Williams et al.[50] showed the same TE rate in all patients with mitral porcine valves without anticoagulation.

Since it is well known that atrial fibrillation adversely effects cardiac output and increases the risk of TE restoration of sinus rhythm appears to be the best protection against the hazard of atrial fibrillation. Since the presence of chronic atrial fibrillation is a determinant in many institutions of the type of valve replacement device that will be used, it is probably important to determine at what time limit of chronic mitral fibrillation is reversible. Betriu and co-workers[51] from the Montreal Heart Institute studied a large number of patients undergoing mitral valve replacement and attempted to estimate the degree of time after which cardioversion is not successful. In their institution the probability of return to sinus rhythm was more that 90% for patients presenting with atrial fibrillation of less than 1 year's duration and only 8% for patients in whom atrial fibrillation was longer than 1 year. In a report by Szekeley[52] of patients with rheumatic heart disease who had had no cardiac operation emboli/100 patient-years in patients in sinus rhythm was 0.67 compared with a rate of 5.26 if in atrial fibrillation. Thus, it would appear that this factor may be an important determinant of long-term morbidity and mortality following mitral valve replacement.

In the future, with improvements in mitral valve replacement devices and cardiac surgical procedures, it may well be that the appearance of atrial fibrillation in a patient with mild to moderate mitral valve disease might be an early indication for mitral valve reconstruction. If not reconstruction, mitral valve replacement might prevent the development of chronic atrial fibrillation which appears to adversely effect long-term morbidity and mortality to a significant degree.

Atrial factors

The presence of a very large left atrium following mitral valve replacement or the presence of intra-atrial thrombus at the time of operation in patients with mitral valve disease have been considered controversial in terms of their role in promoting long-term morbidity and mortality from TE after mitral valve replacement. Most surgeons believe that the presence of any of these factors is, in fact, an indication for chronic anticoagulation regardless of the type of valve[40, 53, 54]. Since most of these factors occur in conjunction with atrial fibrillation, it is very difficult to sort out individually their effect on long-term thromboembolic rates. Some reports suggest that these factors increase the incidence of TE but others fail to confirm this correlation. Nevertheless, as indicated, most recommend coumadin anticoagulation if one or more of these factors, or if atrial fibrillation is present in patients with bioprosthetic valves.

Hetzer et al. in a recent review[43] showed that the presence of one of these findings, that is, increased atrial size, left atrial thrombus or previous TE, in conjunction with atrial fibrillation increases the probability of a postoperative embolus in a patient with bioprosthetic valve significantly. If any patient in their series had all four findings, the probability was one in three that they would sustain a postoperative thromboembolic event. Interesting data from Spampinato[55], however, in 202 patients with chronic atrial fibrillation, giant left atrium and atrial thrombi showed that their incidence of TE without anticoagulation did not seem to be any different from those that received postoperative anticoagulation. Similarly, Ionescu[17], in his excellent series of Ionescu–Shiley valves, does not anticoagulate any patient regardless of the size of the left atrium and has documented a very low thromboembolic rate.

Ventricular factors

A final factor in determining the probability of a TE is the patient's valve lesion and the state of ventricular function leading to overall cardiac performance. The probability of TE in a patient with mitral regurgitation is higher than that in mitral stenosis[13, 40]. This generally reflects a somewhat chronically lower cardiac index in these patients, dilated left ventricle and left atrium and decreased cardiac performance as measured by systolic pump indices. Also patients with complete heart block in whom atrio-ventricular coordination is lost seem to be at a higher risk for thromboemboli.

Conclusions

The reporting of TE is imprecise since the definition of TE varies from institution to institution, though improving reports of incidence of TE are identical from valve to valve.

All patients with mechanical mitral valves require anticoagulation. Without anticoagulation, the incidence of TE increases 3–5 times[1]. Aspirin and dipyrimidole may decrease TE further but the cost, inconvenience and potential for increased bleeding have not made this combination popular. Anticoagulation has major morbidity and mortality; cessation exposes the patient to risk of TE and in tilting disc valves, the possibility of total thrombosis.

For the currently available mechanical valves, TE per 100 patient-years varies from 4 to 6%/patient-year and about 2%/patient-year for mitral bioprostheses. In the latter, chronic atrial fibrillation affects the incidence of TE. All patients with bioprosthetic valves are anticoagulated for 2–3 months and then individualized according to heart rhythm or atrial risk factors, though many believe anticoagulation makes no difference in patients with atrial fibrillation, increased left atrial size or intra-atrial clot.

Atrial fibrillation is not a benign rhythm and sinus rhythm should be maintained whenever possible even if it means earlier operations in less symptomatic individuals.

TE will be decreasing in the future, particularly with new bioprosthetic mitral valves. Better hemodynamics due to better valve design will allow better emptying of the left atrium and less stasis. Earlier operations to prevent development of chronic atrial fibrillation will also be indicated, particularly as mitral valve reconstruction becomes more popular.

References

1. EDMUNDS, L.H. (1982). Thromboembolic complications of current cardiac valvular prostheses. *Ann. Thorac. Surg.*, **34**, 96
2. CLELAND, J. and MOLLOY, P.J. (1973). Thromboembolic complications of the cloth-covered Starr–Edwards prosthesis No. 2300 aortic and No. 6300 mitral. *Thorax*, **28**, 41
3. DALE, J. (1976). Arterial thromboembolic complications in patients with Starr–Edwards aortic ball valve prostheses. *Am. Heart J.*, **91**, 653
4. OXMAN, H.A. CONNOLLY, D.C. and ELLIS, F.M., JR. (1975). Mitral valve replacement with the Smeloff–Cutter prosthesis. *J. Thorac. Cardiovasc. Surg.*, **69**, 247
5. SHEAN, F.C., AUSTEN, W.G., BUCKLEY, M.J., *et al.* (1977). Survival after Starr–Edwards aortic valve replacement. *Circulation*, **44**, 1
6. FRIEDLI, B., AERICHIDE, A., GRONDIN, P. and CAMPEAU, L. (1971). Thromboembolic complications of heart valve prostheses. *Am. Heart J.*, **81**, 702
7. FUSTER, V., PUMPHREY, C.W., MCGOON, M.D., CHESEBRO, J.H., PLUTH, J.R. and MCGOON, D.C. (1982). Systemic thromboembolism in mitral and aortic Starr–Edwards prostheses: a 10–19 year follow-up. *Circulation*, **66**, I–161
8. STARR, A., GRUNKEMEIER, G., LAMBERT, L., OKIES, J.E. and THOMAS, D. (1976). Mitral valve replacement: a 10-year follow-up of non-cloth-covered *vs.* cloth-covered caged-ball prostheses. *Circulation*, **54**, III–47
9. BJORK, V.O. and HENZE, A. (1979). Ten years' experience with the Bjork–Shiley tilting disc valve. *J. Thorac. Cardiovasc. Surg.*, **78**, 331
10. KLEINMAN, L.H., FLEMMA, R.J., MULLEN, D.C., WEIRAUCH, E., ANDERSON, A.J. and LEPLEY, D. (1982). Mitral valve replacement with the Bjork–Shiley prosthesis: a 10-year evaluation. *Circulation*, **66**, II–274
11. NICOLOFF, D.M., EMERY, R., AROM, K.V., *et al.* (1981). Clinical and hemodynamic results with the St. Jude Medical cardiac valve prosthesis: a three-year experience. *J. Thorac. Cardiovasc. Surg.*, **82**, 674
12. CHAUX, A., GRAY, R. and MATLOFF, J. (1982). Incidence of thromboembolism after St. Jude prosthetic cardiac valve replacement. *Circulation*, **66**, II–311
13. DISESA, V., COLLINS, J.J., JR. and COHN, L.H. (1984). Mitral valve replacement with the porcine bioprosthesis. In *Mitral Valve Disease: Diagnosis and Treatment* (eds M. Ionescu and L.H. Cohn). London: Butterworths. (In press)
14. OYER, P.E., STINSON, B., MILLER, D.C., *et al.* (1982). Clinical analysis of the Hancock porcine bioprosthesis. In *Bioprosthetic Heart Valves* (eds L.H. Cohn and V. Gallucci), p. 539. New York: Yorke Medical Books
15. GALLUCCI, V., VALFRE, C., MAZZUCCO, A., *et al.* (1982). Heart valve replacement with the Hancock bioprosthesis: a 5–11 year follow-up. In *Bioprosthetic Heart Valves* (eds L.H. Cohn and V. Gallucci), p. 9. New York: Yorke Medical Books
16. DELOCHE, A., PERIER, P., BOUREZAK, S., *et al.* (1982). A 14-year experience with valvular bioprostheses: valve survival and patient survival. In *Bioprosthetic Heart Valves* (eds L.H. Cohn and V. Gallucci), p. 25. New York: Yorke Medical Books
17. IONESCU, M.I., SMITH, D.R., HASAN, S.S., CHIDAMBARAM, M. and TANDON, A.P. (1982). Clinical durability of the pericardial xenograft valve: ten years' experience with mitral replacement. *Ann. Thorac. Surg.*, **34**, 265

18. BECKER, R.M., SANDOR, L., TINDEL, M. and FRATER, R.W.M. (1981). Medium-term follow-up of the Ionescu–Shiley heterograft valve. *Ann. Thorac. Surg.*, **32**, 120
19. WRIGHT, J.O., HIRATZKA, L.F., BRANDT, B., III and DOTY, D.B. (1982). Thrombosis of the Bjork–Shiley prosthesis. *J. Thorac. Cardiovasc. Surg.*, **84**, 138
20. MESSMER, B.J., OKIES, J.E., HALLMAN, G.L. and COOLEY, D.A. (1971). Mitral valve replacement with the Bjork–Shiley tilting disc prosthesis. *J. Thorac. Cardiovasc. Surg.*, **62**, 938
21. MORENO–CABRAL, R.J., MCNAMARA, J.J., MAMIYA, R.T., BRAINARD, S.C. and CHUNG, G.K. (1978). Acute thrombotic obstruction with Bjork–Shiley valves. *J. Thorac Cardiovasc. Surg.*, **75**, 321
22. COPANS, H., LAKIER, J.B., KINSLEY, R.H., COLSEN, R.R., FRITZ, V.U. and BARLOW, J.B. (1980). Thrombosed Bjork–Shiley mitral prostheses. *Circulation*, **61**, 169
23. KARP, R.B., CYRUS, R.J., BLACKSTONE, E.H., KIRKLIN, J.W., KOUCHOUKOS, N.T. and PACIFICO, A.D. (1981). The Bjork–Shiley valve: intermediate-term follow-up. *J. Thorac. Cardiovasc. Surg.*, **81**, 602
24. TEPLEY, J.F., GRUNKEMEIER, G.L., SUTHERLAND, D.H., LAMBERT, L.E., JOHNSON, V.A. and STARR, A. (1981). The ultimate prognosis after valve replacement: an assessment of 20 years. *Ann. Thorac. Surg.*, **32**, 111
25. DALE, J. (1977). Arterial thromboembolic complications in patients with Bjork–Shiley and Lillehei–Kaster tilting disc valve prostheses. *Am. Heart J.*, **93**, 715
26. AKABARIAN, M., AUSTEN, W.G., YURCHAK, P.M. and SCANNELL, J.G. (1978). Thromboembolic complications of prosthetic cardiac valves. *Circulation*, **37**, 826
27. LIEBERMAN, A., HOSS, W.K., PINTO, R., *et al.* (1978). Intracranial hemorrhage and infarction in anticoagulated patients with prosthetic heart valves. *Stroke*, **9**, 18
28. COON, W.W. and WILLIS, P.W. (1974). Hemorrhagic complications of anticoagulant therapy. *Arch. Int. Med.*, **133**, 386
29. DEYKIN, D. (1970). Warfarin therapy. *N. Engl. J. Med.*, **283**, 801
30. FORFAR, J.C. (1979). A 7-year analysis of hemorrhage in patients on long-term anticoagulant treatment. *Br. Heart J.*, **42**, 128
31. REITZ, B.A., STINSON, E.B., GRIEPP, R.B. and SHUMWAY, N.E. (1980). Tissue valve replacement of prosthetic heart valves for thromboembolism. *Am. J. Cardiol*, **41**, 512
32. HETZER, R., GERBODE, F., KEITH, W.J., *et al.* (1979). Thrombotic complications after valve replacement with porcine hetergrafts. *World J. Surg.*, **3**, 505
33. COHN, L.H. (1979). Bioprosthetic valves: anticoagulation or not? In *Bioprosthetic Cardiac Valves* (ed. F. Sebening). Munchen: Deutsche Herzzentrum
34. MOGGIO, R.A., HAMMOND, G.L., STANSEL, H.C., JR, and GLENN, W.W.L. (1978). Incidence of emboli with cloth-covered Starr–Edwards valve without anticoagulation and with varying forms of anticoagulation. *J. Thorac. Cardiovasc. Surg.*, **75**, 296
35. WEINSTEIN, G.S. and MAVROUDIS, C. and EBERT, P.A. (1982). Preliminary experience with aspirin for anticoagulation in children with prosthetic cardiac valves. *Ann. Thorac. Surg.*, **33**, 549
36. SULLIVAN, J.M., HARKEN, D.E. and GORLIN, R. (1971). Pharmacologic control of thrombotic complications of cardiac valve replacement. *N. Engl. J. Med.*, **284**, 1391
37. ALTMAN, R., BOULLON, F., ROUVIER, J., *et al.* (1976). Aspirin and prophylaxis of thromboembolic complications in patients with substitute heart valves. *J. Thorac. Cardiovasc. Surg.*, **72**, 127
38. CHESEBRO, J.H., FUSTER, V., PUMPHREY, C.W., *et al.* (1981). Combined warfarin-platelet inhibitor anti-thrombotic therapy in prosthetic heart valve replacement. *Circulation*, **64**, IV–76
39. CHEUNG, D., FLEMMA, R.J., MULLEN, D.C., *et al.* (1981). Ten-year follow-up in aortic valve replacement using the Bjork–Shiley prosthesis. *Ann. Thorac. Surg.*, **32**, 138
40. BARNHORST, D.A., OXMAN, H.A., CONNOLLY, D.C., *et al.* (1975). Long-term follow-up of isolated replacement of the aortic or mitral valve with the Starr–Edwards prosthesis. *Am. J. Cardiol.*, **35**, 728
41. MACMANUS, Q., GRUNKEMEIER, G., THOMAS, D., *et al.* (1977). The Starr–Edwards Model 6000 valve. *Circulation*, **56**, 623
42. BLOODWELL, R.D., OKIES, J.E., HALLMAN, G.L. and COOLEY, D.A. (1979). Aortic valve replacement. *J. Thorac. Cardiovasc. Surg.*, **58**, 457
43. HERTZER, R., TOPALIDIS, T. and BORST, H.G. (1982). Thromboembolism and anticoagulation after isolated mitral valve replacement with porcine heterografts. In *Bioprosthetic Heart Valves* (eds L.H. Cohn and V. Gallucci), p. 172. New York: Yorke Medical Books
44. COHN, L.H., MUDGE, G.H., PRATTER, F. and COLLINS, J.J., JR. (1981). Five to eight-year follow-up of patients undergoing porcine heart valve replacement. *N. Engl. J. Med.*, **304**, 258
45. GEHA, A.S., HAMMOND, G.L., LAKS, H., STANSEL, H.C. and GLENN, W.W.L. (1982). Factors affecting performance and thromboembolism after procine xenograft cardiac valve replacement. *J. Thorac. Cardiovasc. Surg.*, **83**, 377
46. HILL, J.D., LAFOLLETTE, J. SZARNICKI, R.J., *et al.* (1982). Risk-benefit analysis of warfarin therapy in Hancock mitral valve replacement. *J. Thorac. Cardiovasc. Surg.*, **83**, 718

47. GAJEWSKI, J. and SINGER, R.B. (1981). Mortality in an insured population with atrial fibrillation. *J. Am. Med. Assoc.*, **245**, 1540

48. KANNEL, W.B., ABBOTT, R.D., SAVAGE, D.D. and MCNAMARA, P.M. (1982). Epidemiologic features of chronic atrial fibrillation. *N. Engl. J. Med.*, **306**, 1018

49. COHN, L.H., SANDERS, J.H. and COLLINS, J.J., JR. (1976). Actuarial comparison of Hancock porcine and prosthetic disc valves for isolated mitral valve replacement. *Circulation*, **54** (III), III–60

50. WILLIAMS, J.B., KARP, R.B., KIRKLIN, J.W., *et al.* (1980). Considerations in selection and management of patients undergoing mitral valve replacement with glutaraldehyde-fixed porcine bioprostheses. *Ann. Thorac. Surg.*, **30**, 247

51. BETRIU, A., CHAITMAN, B.R., ALMAZAN, A., GUITERAS, VAL, P. and PELLITIER, C. (1982). Preoperative determinants of return to sinus rhythm after valve replacement. In *Bioprosthetic Heart Valves* (eds L.H. Cohn and V. Gallucci), p. 184. New York: Yorke Medical Books

52. SZEKELY, P. (1964). Systemic embolism and anticoagulant prophylaxis in rheumatic heart disease. *Br. Med. J.*, **ii**, 1209–13

53. HANNAH, H. and REIS, R.L. (1976). Current status of porcine hetergraft prostheses. *Circulation*, **54**, 27

54. EDMINSTON, W.A., HARRISON, E.C., DUICK, G.F., *et al.* (1978). Thromboembolism in mitral porcine recipients. *Am. J. Cardiol.*, **41**, 508

55. SPAMPINATO, N., STASSANO, P., GAGLIARDI, C., TECCHIA, L.B. and PANTALEO, D. (1982). Mitral bioprostheses in 202 patients with chronic atrial fibrillation, giant left atrium, and atrial thrombi: Long-term results with no anticoagulation. In *Bioprosthetic Heart Valves* (eds L.H. Cohn and V. Gallucci), p. 169. New York: Yorke Medical Books

27

Antithrombotic therapy following mitral valve replacement

Laurence A. Harker

Introduction

Thromboembolism has been a major complication in patients receiving older ball and cage or tilting disc type of mitral heart valves, and patients with such prostheses have required long-term anticoagulation[1–5]. While the risks of thromboembolism have been substantially reduced due to advances in the engineering design of prosthetic valves[4, 5], actuarial analysis shows that even in this decade thromboembolism is a continuing time-dependent risk for patients with mitral valve replacement[1–7]. The frequency of clinically detectable thromboembolism from mechanical prosthetic heart valves continues to be a significant problem. For example, at the Mayo Clinic, where patients with heart valves are routinely anticoagulated, the frequency of thromboembolism during the first postoperative year is about 5% for a recent aortic and 10% for the mitral Starr–Edwards prosthesis, respectively[1]. Thereafter, the annual frequency is about 1% and 2%, respectively[8]. Interestingly, the thromboembolic frequency is higher in patients on inadequate oral anticoagulation and highest in those unable to take oral anticoagulants[1, 2, 8]. Left atrial enlargement, atrial fibrillation and the presence of left atrial thrombus at surgery are all risk factors with respect to thromboembolism in prosthetic mitral valve patients[1, 2].

The mechanism of thrombus formation in association with mitral valve prosthesis

Whereas normal endothelium is non-reactive with circulating blood, non-endothelialized surfaces activate platelets and coagulation factors to initiate thrombus formation. Three major variables determine the state and extent of thrombus: (1) mechanical effects in which blood flow is predominant; (2) alterations in the constituents of the blood; and (3) abnormal surfaces exposed to flowing blood.

The structure and localization of thrombi are profoundly influenced by blood flow. Venous thrombi form under stagnant low shear conditions and the composition of the thrombus is similar to that seen in shed blood that has been allowed to clot in the test tube ('red thrombus'). These conditions of relatively slow-flow probably retard the removal of activated coagulation factors. In contrast, the high-shear rheological conditions in arterial flow favors the diffusion of platelets towards the vessel wall and the composition of a thrombus forming in arteries is platelet-enriched ('white thrombus'). Indeed, red cells increase platelet diffusion at high shear rates thereby enhancing platelet deposition on non-endothelialized surfaces. Moreover, the localization of thrombi within the arterial circulation is influenced by hemodynamic factors. For example, platelet deposition is localized at sites of bifurcation and around orifices of right angle branches thus favoring the growth of thrombus at these locations. Noteworthy is the fact that aortic endothelium also shows an increased turnover rate at these same sites of shear stress.

The distinctions between arterial and venous thrombogenesis are illustrated by kinetic studies using labeled platelets and fibrinogen. In patients with ongoing arterial thromboembolism, the principal role of platelets in the thrombotic process is reflected as isolated platelet consumption, i.e. shortened platelet survival and increased turnover without detectable consumption of circulating fibrinogen. Circulating fibrinogen is not consumed in this setting presumably because procoagulant material is swept away from the thrombogenic focus by the rapid arterial flow before coagulation becomes fully activated. Ongoing venous thrombosis is manifested kinetically as the equivalent consumption of both platelets and fibrinogen; this process reflects fibrin extension under static or low shear flow conditions. The composition of the thrombus has important therapeutic implications; fibrin formation and venous thrombosis are most effectively inhibited by anticoagulants such as heparin or warfarin, whereas arterial thrombi appear to be prevented by agents that modify platelet behavior.

In association with mitral valve prostheses there is formation of both fibrin thrombus and platelet ('white') thrombus. Fibrin thrombi form secondary to stasis, as a consequence of atrial dilatation, atrial fibrillation and the interrupted flow characteristic of the heart. Platelet thrombi form on the non-endothelialized prosthetic surface under high-shear conditions. Platelet deposition has been observed intraoperatively on the sewing ring of the prosthesis as well as on the parivascular damaged cardiac surfaces using the technique of indium-111 labeled autologous platelets and gamma-camera imaging. moreover, the thrombotic material forming on prosthetic surfaces not only potentially interferes with valve function but undergoes embolization[9]. Indium-111 platelet-labeled thrombi have been demonstrated to embolize to renal cortex, brain, cardiac and skeletal muscle[10]. Most of the emboli are small and therefore not clinically detected. Thus the reported frequency of thromboembolism in patients is undoubtedly an underestimate of the true frequency of events.

Platelet survival measurements in patients with prosthetic heart valves have been shown to be of value in identifying patients at risk and in predicting the effects of therapy[11, 13]. With respect to mechanical prosthetic heart valves, this thromboembolic risk is related at least in part to the surface area of the valve. Thus, as the prosthetic surface area increases, the thromboembolic risk rises in parallel and the platelet survival time shortens proportionately. In patients with homograft valves, no detectable shortening of platelet survival has been found and a marked reduction in the frequency of thromboembolic events is observed[11, 13]. Platelet survival time has also been useful in evaluating the effects of various pharmacologic agents. When dipyridamole is administered in doses of 100 mg four times a day to patients with mitral prosthetic heart valves the platelet survival time is normalized, implying an interruption of the thrombotic process[11]. Sulfinpyrazone has also been reported to normalize platelet survival at doses of 200 mg four times daily[12]. By contrast, aspirin alone has usually been reported to be ineffective in modifying platelet survival[11, 14], although aspirin was found to increase platelet survival in one study[15]. A similar effect has been reported for suloctidil[16].

Trials of antithrombotic therapy

In the experience of the majority of clinicians, inadequate anticoagulant control has been the principal factor predisposing to clinically significant thrombosis of most prosthetic heart valves[1–8, 17–19]. Patients on anticoagulant therapy plus a platelet inhibitor drug have the lowest frequency of thromboembolism (see Table 27.1)[20–25]

TABLE 27.1 Antithrombotic therapy in patients with mechanical prosthetic heart valves

| | | | Treatment | | | Thrombo- |
| | | Follow-up | | | No. of | embolism |
Reference	Methods	(years)	Drug	(mg/day)	Patients	(%)
20	Prospective, randomized, blind	1	A/C + placebo		84	14
			A/C + D	400	79	1
21	Prospective, randomized	1–3	A/C		39	21
			A/C + D	400	40	5
22	Prospective, randomized, blind	1	A/C		154	5
			A/C + D	375	136	3
23	Prospective randomized	1-2	A/C		87	13
			A/C + D	300	78	4
24	Prospective, randomized, blind	1	A/C + placebo		38	9
			A/C + ASA	1,000	39	2
			ASA	1,000	77	15
21	Prospective, randomized	2	A/C		65	20
			A/C + ASA	500	57	5

A/C = Anticoagulant; D = dipyridamole; ASA = aspirin.

Dipyridamole at 400 mg/day (100 mg four times daily) supplementing the anticoagulant therapy has been shown to be effective in reducing thromboembolism[20–23]. One gram of aspirin per day together with oral anticoagulation has also been reported to reduce the frequency of thromboembolism[24], although the frequency of gastrointestinal bleeding is significant in the group receiving aspirin together with oral anticoagulation. A later trial using 500 mg of aspirin per day in combination with oral anticoagulants[25] reported a reduction in the frequency of thromboembolism without significant increase in the frequency of bleeding. However, in a subsequent recent trial of 500 mg aspirin per day with anticoagulants, gastronintestinal bleeding was found to be excessive in the warfarin aspirin group and no reduction in thromboembolism was found compared with warfarin therapy alone[26].

    While thromboembolism in patients with porcine hetergraft valves is uncommon (see Table 27.2)[6, 7, 27–32], a substantial risk of thromboembolism is seen when risk factors are combined (advanced disease, atrial fibrillation, left atrial enlargement,

TABLE 27.2 Antithrombotic therapy in porcine heterograft mitral valves

Reference	Follow-up (years)	Treatment	No. of Patients	Thromboembolism (%)
6	3	None	214	12, 75% early*
27	2	A/C 6 weeks	56	5, 10% if LAE or AF
28	5	None	104	12
29	4	None	47	2
30	3	A/C 3 months	335	3, 67% early*
31	1	A/C 3 months	107	4
7	3	A/C	22	23
32	5–7 1/2	A/C if LAE or AF	118	10, 33% < 1 month

A/C = anticoagulant; LAE = left atrial enlargement; AF = atrial fibrillation.
* ≤ 3 months.

previous thromboembolic events and inadequate anticoagulant therapy[7]. Several studies report that the majority of thromboembolic events are observed in the initial 3 months following valve placement[6, 24, 33]. Those patients with very large left atria, atrial fibrillation or previous thromboembolism have the highest frequency of thromboembolic events.

Management recommendations

On the basis of the available information patients with mechanical prosthetic heart valves should receive oral anticoagulation together with dipyridamole at a dose of 400 mg per day (100 mg four times daily). This regimen is preferred over the combination of oral anticoagulants and low-dose aspirin because of the uncertain efficacy and the increased frequency of gastrointestinal bleeding associated with the latter regimen[26]. An alternative therapy for those unable to tolerate the dipryidamole–anticoagulant regimen may be anticoagulation together with sulfinpyrazone (200 mg four times daily)[12], although no prospective randomized clinical trials with this combination have been reported to date. However, it should be noted that sulfinpyrazone decreases the warfarin requirement to about one-half that required without sulfinpyrazone. There is no good evidence that antiplatelet regimens can substitute for anticoagulation.

Patients with porcine heterograft valves are probably benefited by routine anticoagulation for the initial 3 months postopertively, although no clinical trial confirmation has been reported. Moreover, patients with heterograft values and a previous history of thromboembolism or patients who have very large left atria or atrial fibrillation may be candidates for indefinite oral anticoagulant therapy.

Summary

Following the placement of mitral valve prosthesis, systemic embolization originates from the valve or the left atrium. The frequency of clinically manifested thromboembolism from mechanical prosthetic heart valves in anticoagulated patients during the first post-operative year is about 5% for the aortic and about 10% for the mitral prosthesis; thereafter the frequency is 1% and 2–3% per year, respectively. The presence of left atrial enlargement or atrial fibrillation increases the frequency of thromboembolism, and therapy with a combination of anticoagulant therapy plus a platelet inhibitor minimizes the clinical frequency of these events. Thromboembolism in patients with procine hetergraft valves is uncommon, although thrombeombolism may develop in those patients with very large left atria, atrial fibrillation or histories of previous thromboembolism.

On the basis of the available data, the following therapy is recommended:

(1)   Patients with mechanical prosthetic heart valves are anticoagulated with an oral agent such as warfarin and also given dipyridamole (100 mg four times daily) irrespective of the previous history of thromboembolic disease. Patients unable to tolerate the dipryidamole may be placed on oral anticoagulants and sulfinpyrazone (200 mg four times daily) or oral anticoagulants plus aspirin, although serious excessive bleeding may be seen with aspirin and oral anticoagulants together.

(2)   Patients with porcine heterograft valves should probably receive oral anticoagulation for 3 months following valve placement, and patients with previous thromboembolism, very large left atria or atrial fibrillation are candidates for longer anticoagulant therapy.

(3)   Patients with heart valve prostheses who experience recurrent thromboembolism despite adequate anti-thrombotic therapy require re-operation.

References

1. BARNHORST, D.A., OXMAN, H.A., CONNOLLY, D.C., et al. (1975). Long-term follow-up of isolated replacement of the aortic and mitral valve with the Starr–Edwards prosthesis. Am. J. Cardiol., 35, 228

2. BARNHORST, D.A., OXMAN, H.A., CONNOLLY, D.C., et al. (1976). Isolated replacement of the mitral valve with the Starr–Edwards prosthesis. J. Thorac. Cardiovasc. Surg., 71, 230

3. DALE, J. (1976). Arterial thromboembolic complications in patients with Starr–Edwards aortic ball valve prostheses. Am. Heart J., 91, 653

4. BJORK, V.O. and HERZE, A. (1979). Ten years experience with the Bjork–Shiley tilting disc valve. J. Thorac. Cardiovasc. Surg., 78, 331

5. SCHOEVAERDTS, J.C., JAUMEN, P., PONLOT, R., CHALANT, C.H. and GRUNKEMEIER, G.L. (1979). Twelve years results with a caged-ball mitral prosthesis. Thorac. Cardiovasc. Surgeon, 27, 45

6. SALOMON, N.W., STINSON, E.B., GRIEPP, R.B. and SHUMUDY, N.E. (1977). Mitral valve replacement: Long-term evaluation of prosthesis-related mortality and morbidity. Circulation, 56 (Suppl II), 94

7. EDMISTON, W.A., HARRISON, E.C., DUICK, G.F., PARNASSUS, W. and LAU, F.Y.K. (1978). Thromboembolism in mitral porcine-valve recipients. Am. J. Cardiol., 41, 508

8. FUSTER, V., McGOON, M.D., CHESEBRO, J.H., PUMPHREY, C.W., PLUTH, J.R. and McGOON, D.C. (1981). Systemic thromboembolism in mitral and aortic Starr–Edwards prosthesis: A long term follow-up (10–21 years). Circulation, 64, (Suppl IV), 257

9. ROBERTS, W.C. and HAMMER, W.J. (1976). Cardiac pathology for valve replacement with a tilting disc prosthesis (Bjork–Shiley type): A study of 46 necropsy patients and 49 Bjork–Shiley prostheses. Am. J. Cardiol., 37, 1024

10. DEWANJEE, M.K., KAYE, M.P. and FUSTER, V. (1980). Noninvasive radiosotope technique for detection of platelet deposition in mitral valve prosthesis and quantitation of cerebral, renal and pulmonary microembolism in dogs. Circulation, 62, (Suppl III), 8

11. HARKER, L.A. and SLICHTER, S.J. (1970). Studies of platelet and fibrinogen kinetics in patients with prosthetic heart valves. N. Eng. J. Med., 283, 1302

12. STEELE, P., RAINWATER, J. and VOGEL, R. (1979). Platelet suppressant therapy in patients with

prosthetic cardiac valves. Relationship of clinical effectiveness to alteration of platelet survival time. *Circulation*, **60**, 910

13. RAJAH, S.M. (1976). Platelet survival in patients with homograft and prosthetic heart valves: Correlation with incidence of thromboembolism. *Br. J. Haematol.*, **33**, 148

14. STEELE, P., RAINWATER, J., VOGEL, R. and GENTON, E. (1978). Platelet-suppressant therapy in patients with coronary artery disease. *J. Am. Med. Assoc.*, **240**, 228

15. DALE, J. MYHRE, E. and ROOTWELT, K. (1975). Effects of dipyramidole and acetylsalicylic acid on platelet function in patients with aortic ball-valve prostheses. *Am. Heart J.*, **89**, 613.

16. BEYS, C., FERRANT, A. and MORIAU, M. (1981). Effects of suloctidil on platelet survival time following cardiac valve replacement. *Thromb. Res.*, **46**, 550

17. BEN-ZVI, J., HILDNER, F.J., CHANDRARATMA, P.A. and SANET, P. (1974). Thrombosis on Bjork–Shiley aortic valve prosthesis: Clinical, arteriographic, echocardiographic, and therapeutic observations in seven cases. *Am. J. Cardiol.*, **34**, 538

18. COPANS, H., LAKIER, J.B., KINSLEY, R.H., COLSEN, P.R., FRITZ, V.U. and BARLOW, J.B. (1980). Thrombosed Bjork–Shiley mitral prostheses. *Circulation*, **61**, 169

19. MOREMO–CABIAL, R.J., McNAMARA, J.J., MAMIYD, R.T., BRAINARD, S.C. and CHUNG, S.K.T. (1978). Acute thrombotic obstruction with Bjork–Shiley valves. Diagnostic and surgical considerations. *J. Thorac. Cardiovasc. Surg.*, **75**, 321

20. SULLIVAN, J.M., HARKEN, D.E. and GORLIN, R. (1971). Pharmacologic control of thromboembolic complications of cardiac valve replacement. *N. Engl. J. Med.*, **284**, 1391

21. KASHARA, T. (1977). Clinical effect of dipyridamole ingestion after prosthetic heart valve replacement. *J. Jap. Assoc. Thorac. Surg.*, **25**, 1007

22. GROUPE DE RECHERCHE P.A.C.T.E. (1978). Prevention des accidents thromboemboliques systemiques chez les porteurs de prostheses valvulaires artificielles. *Coeur*, **9**, 915

23. RAJAH, S.M. In *Proceedings of the Prostaglandins and the Cardiovascular System Symposium. Wilrijk, Belgium,* December, Vol. **6**, p. 54

24. DALE, J., MYHRE, E., STORSTEIN, O., STORMORKEN, H. and EFSKIND, L. (1977). Prevention of arterial thromboembolism with acetylsalicylic acid. A controlled clinical study in patients with aortic ball valves. *Am. Heart J.*, **94**, 101

25. ALTMAN, R., BOULLON, F., ROUVIER, J., RACA, R., DE LA FUENTE, L. and FAVALORO, R. (1976). Aspirin and prophylaxis of thromboembolic complications in patients with substitute heart valves. *J. Thorac. Cardiovasc. Surg.*, **72**, 127

26. CHESEBRO, J.H., FUSTER, V., PUMPHREY, C.W., McGOON, D.C, PLUTH, J.R., PUGA, F.J., ORZULAK, T.A., PIEHLER, J.M., SCHAFF, H.V. and DANIELSON, G.K. (1981). Combined warfarin-platelet inhibitor antithrombotic therapy in prosthetic heart valve replacement. *Circulation*, **64** (Suppl IV), 76

27. COHN, L.H., SANDER, J.H. and COLLINS, J.J. (1976). Actuarial comparison of Hancock porcine and prosthetic disc valves for isolated mitral valve replacement. *Circulation*, **54** (Suppl III), 60

28. HANNAH, H. and REIS, R.L. (1976). Current status of porcine heterograft prostheses. *Circulation*, **54** (Suppl III), 27

29. McINTOSH, C.L., MICHAELIS, L.L., MORROW, A.G., ITSCOITZ, S.B., REDWOOD, E.R. and EPSTINE, S.E. (1975). Atrioventricular valve replacement with the Hancock porcine xenograft: A five year clinical experience. *Surgery*, **78**, 768

30. CEVESE, P.G., GALLUCCI, V., MOREA, M., VOLTA, S.D., FASOLI, G. and CASAROTTO, D. (1976). Heart valve replacement with the Hancock bioprosthesis, analysis of long-term results. *Circulation*, **54** (Suppl II), 111

31. JONES, E.L., CRAVER, J.M., HATCHER, C.R. and MORGAN, E.A. (1976). Clinical experience with the Hancock porcine xenograft valve. *Am. J. Cardiol.*, **39**, 303

32. LAKIER, J.B., KHAJA, F., MAGILLIGAN, D.J. and GOLDSTEIN, S. (1980). Porcine xenograft valves. Long-term (60–89 months) follow-up. *Circulation*, **62**, 313

33. PIPKIN, R.D., BUCH, W.S. and FOGARTY, T.J. (1976). Evaluation of aortic valve replacement with a porcine xenograft without long-term anticoagulation. *J. Thorac. Cardiovasc. Surg.*, **71**, 180

The diagnosis and treatment of congenital mitral valve disease

28

The pathology of congenital mitral valve disease

Maurice Lev and Saroja Bharati

Isolated congenital mitral valve anomalies are rare. On the other hand, congenital abnormalities of the mitral valve associated with minor and major cardiac abnormalities are frequently seen in various types of congenital heart disease. This may complicate the surgical outcome in these lesions. We will therefore discuss first isolated mitral valve disease and then deal with those seen with major cardiac lesions. There will be some overlap with lesions seen in the isolated type and that seen associated with other cardiac abnormalities.

The types of isolated lesions of the mitral valve are as follows:

1. Congenital mitral stenosis:
   (a) annular;
   (b) at the level of the leaflets.
2. Parachute mitral valve.
3. Arcade mitral valve.
4. Floppy mitral valve—without Marfan's syndrome.
5. Accessory mitral valve:
   (a) in anterior leaflet;
   (b) in posterior leaflet.
6. Supravalvular mitral stenosis.
7. Straddling mitral valve (complete, basilar or peripheral):
   (a) anterior leaflet;
   (b) posterior leaflet.
8. Displaced mitral valve.
9. Congenital mitral insufficiency:
   (a) annular;
   (b) quadricuspid or pentacuspid;
   (c) cleft in the anterior leaflet.
10. Ebstein's anomaly of the mitral valve.
11. Mitral atresia.

Congenital mitral stenosis (see Figure 28.1)[1-3] may rarely occur as a result of annular narrowing alone. Usually the valvular apparatus, though normally formed, is also small. In a second variety there is a ridge of thickening which is seen at the leaflet midway between the annulus and the edge. Here again although the entire valve can be divided into anterior and posterior leaflets, the circumferential ridge of

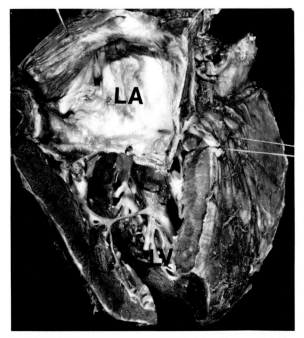

Figure 28.1 Isolated congenital mitral stenosis. LA = Left atrium; LV = Left ventricle.

thickening makes the valvular structure small. In other cases, the body of the valve is irregularly thickened and the line of closure and the edge are thickened and nodose. The chordae are thick and shortened. The papillary muscles are often hypertrophied. The stenosis in these cases may be not only at the annulus, but at the body and line of closure. Congenital mitral stenosis may also be produced by a parachute or arcade mitral valve.

Parachute mitral valve—Usually the anterior papillary muscle is absent and the entire leaflet is peripherally connected to a single or a group of posterior papillary muscles. Rarely, the posterior papillary muscle may be absent or very poorly formed. Thus, the entire leaflet may be connected to a single or group of anterior papillary muscles. In a parachute mitral valve usually the annulus and the leaflets are smaller than normal.

Arcade mitral valve[4]—Classically, in this lesion, the anterior and posterior group of papillary muscles join together in an arcade fashion as they fuse with the entire edge of the leaflet structure without the presence of the chordae. Rarely the arcade may be formed with very few or moderately well-formed chordae interposed in the arcade formed by the anterior and posterior papillary muscles and the edge of leaflet structure. In a rare heart either the anterior or the posterior group of papillary muscles join the leaflet directly without the chordal intervention. In other words, only one papillary muscle participates in the arcade while the other papillary muscle and the chordal connections are normal. In a still rarer specimen, one may find a combination of a parachute with an arcade formation. Arcade mitral valve may produce mitral stenosis or insufficiency.

Floppy mitral valve (see Figure 28.2)[5]—Classically the posterior leaflet is redundant, nodose, thickened and the excess of valvular tissue balloons into the left

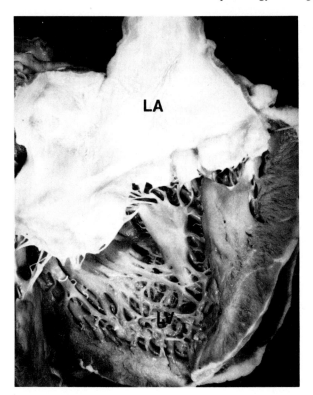

Figure 28.2 Floppy mitral valve. LA = Left atrium; LV = Left ventricle.

atrial cavity. In our experience, we have found this with valvular *elongation* and annular widening. This is frequently associated with some calcification of the annulus of the posterior leaflet. Histologically we have shown that the architecture of the valve is altered in addition to the elongated valvular structure. There is more of spongiosa than fibrosa element present in the leaflet and there may be a mixture of the two. Uncommonly, both the anterior and the posterior leaflets may be floppy in nature. Rarely the anterior leaflet alone may be floppy. In floppy mitral valve usually the chordae may be elongated and profuse in their connection.

Accessory mitral valve—Isolated accessory mitral openings may not be hemodynamically significant if they are small in nature. However, a moderately sized or a large opening may result in mitral insufficiency. Classically the opening is seen in the posterior leaflet with separate chordal and papillary muscle connections. Accessory mitral orifice may also be seen in the anterior leaflet as well. In some cases, the annulas may be small, with mitral stenosis and insufficiency.

Supravalvular mitral stenosis—Here there is a ridge of endocardial thickening or rarely a membrane present just above the annulus in a circumferential manner, this ridge being below the level of the left atrial appendage. This may be seen in combination with a parachute and/or an arcade mitral valve. It is not uncommon to find isolated bands or strands extending into the atrium or to the mitral valve forming an incomplete supravalvular ridge above the annulus of the mitral valve. The hemodynamic significance of these is not known today. It is possible that they may facilitate in the development of thromboembolic phenomena.

Straddling mitral valve[6]—This rare anomaly may be seen with a large common atrioventricular canal type of a ventricular septal defect where the defect extends more towards the anterior part of the ventricular septum. In a complete form of straddler the anterior leaflet of the mitral valve passes through the defect to the right ventricle and is connected by way of an accessory anterolateral papillary muscle in the right ventricle. Thus a part of the annulus with the leaflet structure and part of the peripheral connections are present in the right ventricle. More rarely only some of the peripheral connections alone may be seen in the right ventricle. This is called the peripheral type of straddling mitral valve. In the basilar type, one may sometimes find only part of the annulus (base) of the leaflet in the right ventricular cavity. Although the anterior mitral valve is usually involved in straddling, occasionally the posterior leaflet of the mitral valve may straddle. The annulus may be small or large and usually the anterior papillary muscle of the left ventricle is absent or poorly formed.

Displaced mitral valve[7]—This is extremely rare. Here the mitral valve is completely connected with the morphologically right ventricle and hence the term displaced is used. That is the annulus, the leaflet with its entire peripheral connections, are present in the right ventricle. Usually this is accompanied by straddling of the tricuspid valve to the opposite chamber. The displaced mitral orifice is small and stenotic.

Congenital mitral insufficiency (see Figure 28.3)[8–10]–This is rare. In one type, the annulus alone is widened without any other abnormality in the valvular apparatus. A second, more common, variety is one in which the valve consists of four or even five leaflet structures. A quadricuspid mitral valve has been considered normal by

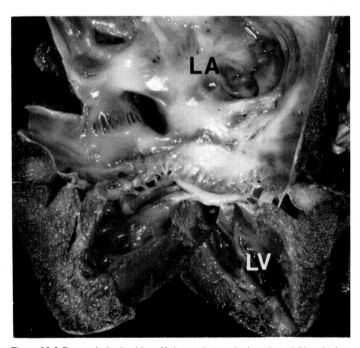

Figure 28.3 Congenital mitral insufficiency. LA = Left atrium; LV = Left ventricle.

some. This is because normally the mitral valve does not have true commissures. Instead, there are two intercalated leaflet structures between the anterior and posterior leaflets. In some cases, these intercalated leaflet structures may be very well developed, giving rise to quadricuspid mitral valve. In addition, the posterior leaflet may be divided into two or three components. Thus, one may find a well-developed pentacuspid or multileaflet structure of the mitral valve. These we have seen in older individuals with evidence of mitral insufficiency being present. It thus appears that although this is a congenitally abnormally formed mitral valve, as the individual ages, with time, mitral insufficiency may develop. A third type of congenital mitral insufficiency may develop as a result of an isolated cleft in the anterior leaflet of the mitral valve. The cleft may be present in the anterior or posterior or may be in the middle of the leaflet, with the apex of the cleft extending towards the annulus of the mitral valve.

Ebstein's malformation of the mitral valve[11]—The only one of its kind was reported by us some years ago. This was seen with atrioventricular concordance and normally related great arteries. Here the posterior leaflet is displaced downwards into the posteroinferior wall of the left ventricular cavity, although the annulus is in its normal location. The chordae and the papillary muscles may be very small.

Mitral atresia[12]—When this lesion is seen without hypoplasia of the aortic tract complex, there is a good sized ventricular septal defect. Here the left ventricle, although smaller than normal, is usually well developed as in the aortic orifice and valve.

Congenital mitral valve disease seen in other cardiac malformations

The congenital cardiac malformations which may be accompanied by lesions of the mitral valve are as follows:

1. Coarctation of the aorta, paraductal.
2. Coarctation, fetal.
3. Supravalvular aortic stenosis.
4. Aortic stenosis, valvular.
5. Subaortic stenosis:
   (a) membranous;
   (b) ridge, discrete;
   (c) muscular;
   (d) excess of endocardial tissue.
6. Floppy mitral valve with Marfan's syndrome.
7. Acessory structures related to mitral valve:
   (a) anomalous chordae and strands;
   (b) anomalous muscle bundles.
8. ASD—fossa ovalis type.
9. Origin of coronary from pulmonary artery.
10. Double outlet right ventricle.
11. Complete transposition.
12. Congenital polyvalvular disease.

Coarctation of the aorta[2, 13]—In the paraductal type the previously described parachute or arcade mitral valve with stenosis and/or insufficiency may be present.

Fetal coarctation—In addition to arcade and parachute type of deformities, the annulus alone may be small, with a shrunken leaflet structure resulting in mitral stenosis.

Supravalvular aortic stenosis—Rarely this may be associated with a small mitral annulus and leaflet structure resulting in mitral stenosis.

Aortic stenosis (valvular)[2]—This may be associated with isolated or parachute or arcade type of mitral valve.

Subaortic stenosis:

1. *Membranous.* Since the membrane involves the base of the anterior mitral leaflet, one should expect any type of abnormality to occur such as parachute or arcade mitral valve.
2. *Discrete ridge.* What has been described for the mebranous type may be seen with this defect.
3. *Excess of endocardial tissue* attached to the anterior mitral valve may obstruct the outflow tract into the aorta on the one hand or produce an abnormal anterior movement of the mitral valve on the other. This may also be seen in cases of aortic stenosis and supravalvular aortic stenosis.
4. *Muscular subaortic stenosis.* In our experience, in general, the mitral valve is normally formed. Occasionally the chordae may be elongated and thickened. We believe that the myocardial disarray pattern seen histologically also extends to the anterio-lateral papillary muscle, thus resulting in abnormal anterior movement of the mitral valve.

Floppy mitral valve in Marfan's syndrome[14]—Here the other manifestations of Marfan's syndrome both clinically and in the heart are present. In the heart, dissecting aneurysm of the ascending aorta, aneurysm of sinuses of the aortic valve with insufficiency may be accompanied by a floppy mitral valve. The mitral annulus is wide with redundancy of the posterior leaflet and chordal connections may be elongated, producing mitral insufficiency.

Accessory structures related to mitral valve—Abnormal muscle bundles or papillary muscles may go to the base of the anterior or posterior or both leaflet structures. This may result in insufficiency or stenosis of the mitral valve. Sometimes these muscle bundles and strands or chordae may extend towards the outflow tract of the left ventricle, thus resulting in left ventricular outflow obstruction. Accessory mitral valves may also be seen (*see Figure 28.4*).

Atrial septal defect of fossa ovalis type—There may be a congenital type of mitral stenosis. This is rare. More frequently, a floppy mitral valve is present in large atrial septal defect of any type. We have seen this resulting in mitral stenosis or insufficiency.

Origin of coronary from pulmonary artery—Infarction of the anterior papillary muscle may result in mitral insufficiency or the associated fibroelastosis of the left ventricle may involve the chordae and papillary muscles resulting in insufficiency.

In fibroelastosis of the dilated or contracted type, all types of mitral valve abnormalities may be seen (*see Figure 28.5*). In the simplest form the fibroelastosis may involve the chordae of the mitral valve to produce mitral insufficiency.

Double outlet right ventricle—Any type of mitral valve abnormality may be seen with any type of double outlet right ventricle. For example, in subaortic or non-committed type of DORV one may encounter a parachute or arcade, or supravalvular mitral lesion. On the other hand we have noted the frequent

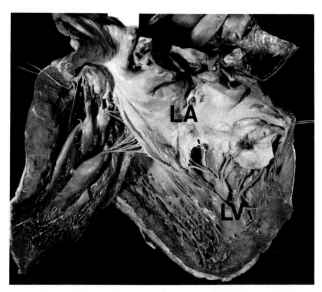

Figure 28.4 Marfan's syndrome with mitral regurgitation and accessory mitral valve. LA = Left atrium; LV = left ventricle.

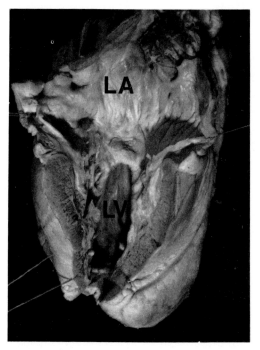

Figure 28.5 Contracted type of fibroelastosis with arcade mitral valve. LA = Left atrium; LV = left ventricle.

occurrence of straddling mitral valve in the Taussig–Bing group of hearts (*see Figure 28.6*).[15]

Complete transposition—Although uncommon, any type of previously described mitral valve abnormality may be seen in this anomaly.

Congenital polyvalvular disease[16]—In our material, we have seen a dysplastic type of valvular structure in all the four valves. This is frequently present in trisomy 13–15 and 18. The mitral valve and the other valves are irregularly thickened and

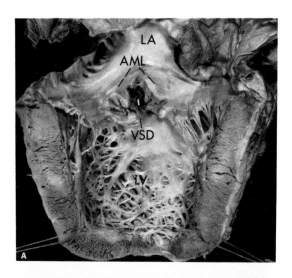

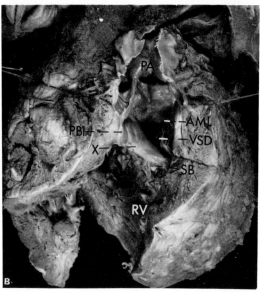

Figure 28.6 Taussig–Bing complex with straddling mitral valve. (A) Left ventricular view. (B) Right ventricular view. LA = Left atrium; AML = anterior mitral leaflet; VSD = ventricular septal defect; PBI = first parietal band; x = abnormal muscle passing from the first parietal band to septal band; PA = pulmonary artery. (Reproduced from reference 6, by kind permission of authors and publishers.)

nodose, resulting in stenosis or insufficiency. Histologically the valve structure is greatly altered.

Displaced mitral valve—This is usually seen with regular or inverted transposition with or without straddling of the tricuspid valve.

The discussion of the mitral valve lesions seen in association with other cardiac lesions is by no means complete. Tetralogy of Fallot, cor triatriatum sinister, premature narrowing of the foramen ovale, single ventricle without transposition, single ventricle with regular transposition, and many more lesions may be associated with congenital mitral valve abnormalities. All of these are important for the surgeon to know beforehand, since the type of surgery to be performed may be different.

Acknowledgement

Aided by Grant HL 30558–01 from the Heart, Lung and Blood Institute of the National Institutes of Health.

References

1. EMERY, J.L. and ILLINGWORTH, R.S. (1951). Congenital mitral stenosis. *Arch. Dis. Child.*, **26**, 304
2. FERENCZ, C., JOHHNSON, A.L. and WIGLESWORTH, F.W. (1984). Congenital mitral stenosis. *Circulation*, **9**, 161
3. VAN DER HORST, R.L. and HASTREITER, A.R. (1967). Congenital mitral stenosis. *Am. J. Cardiology*, **20**, 773
4. LAYMAN, T.E. and EDWARDS, J.E. (1967). Anomalous mitral arcade; a type of congenital mitral insufficiency. *Circulation*, **35**, 389
5. BHARATI, S., GRANSTON, A.S., LIEBSON, P.R., LOEB, H.S., ROSEN, K.M. and LEV, M. (1981). The conduction system in mitral valve prolapse syndrome with sudden death. *Am. Heart J.*, **101**, 667
6. BHARATI, S., MCALLISTER, H.A., JR. and LEV, M. (1979). Straddling and displaced atrioventricular orifice and valves. *Circulation*, **60**, 673
7. LIBERTHSON, R.R., PAUL, M.H., MUSTER, A.J., ARCILLA, R.A., ECKNER, F.A.O. and LEV, M. (1971). Straddling and displaced atrioventricular orifices and valves with primitive ventricles. *Circulation*, **43**, 213
8. TALNER, N.S., STEIN, A.M. and SLOAN, H.E., JR. (1961). Congenital mitral insufficiency. *Circulation*, **23**, 339
9. KEITH, J.D. (1962). Congenital mitral insufficiency. *Prog. Cardiovas. Dis.*, **5**, 264
10. FLEGE, J.B., JR., VLAD, P. and EHRENHAFT, F.T. (1967). Congenital mitral incompetence. *J. Thorac., Cardiovasc. Surg.*, **53**, 138
11. RUSCHAUPT, D.G., BHARATI, S. and LEV, M. (1976). Ebstein's type malformation of the mitral valve in the absence of corrected transposition: A hitherto underscribed anomaly. *Am. J. Cardiol.*, **38**, 109
12. LEV, M. (1966). Some newer concepts of the pathology of congenital heart disease. *Med. Clin. North America*, **50**, 3
13. KHOURY, G., HAWES, C.R. and GROW, S.B. (1969). Coarctation of the aorta with obstructive anomalies of the mitral valve and left ventricle. *J. Pediatrics*, **75**, 652
14. RAGHIB, G., JUE, K.L., ANDERSON, R.C. and EDWARDS, J.E. (1965). Marfan's sydrome with mitral insufficiency. *Am. J. Cardiol.*, **16**, 127
15. MUSTER, A.J., BHARATI, S., PAUL, M.H., *et al.* (1979). Taussig–Bing anomaly with straddling mitral valve. *J. Thorac. Cardiovasc. Surg.*, **77**, 832
16. BHARATI, S. and LEV, M. (1973). Congenital polyvalvular disease. *Circulation*, **47**, 575

29

The pathology of complete atrioventricular orifice

Saroja Bharati and Maurice Lev

Introduction

In this chapter, we will deal only with the pathology of the common atrioventricular orifice (CAVO) or canal of the complete type. We will:

(1) Define what we mean by CAVO.
(2) Detail the anatomic variations seen in the valvular apparatus.
(3) Discuss the sizes of the ventricular chambers.
(4) Deal with the sizes of the atrial and ventricular components of CAVO.
(5) Discuss the major associated cardiac abnormalities.
(6) Detail the extracardiac abnormalities frequently seen in CAVO.

We believe that the above factors singly or in any combination may alter the surgical outcome immediately or many years later.

Definition

By common atrioventricular orifice (CAVO) of the complete type we mean that condition in which the central fibrous body is absent, and hence, in which there is a defect in the distal part of the atrial septum combined with a defect in the upper part of the ventricular septum resulting in an opening between both atria and both ventricles. This opening is guarded by a single or a common atrioventricular valve with a bare or nude area devoid of valvular tissue on the summit of the ventricular septum (*see Figure 29.1*)[1].

The valvular apparatus

The valvular apparatus of the CAVO consists of the following leaflets in the classic complete form (*see Figure 29.1*). There is an anterior bridging leaflet, a posterior bridging leaflet and two small lateral leaflets, one for each ventricle. The periphery of the anterior bridging leaflet in the majority of cases is anchored on to the ventricular septum at the level of the non-coronary and the left aortic cusps. These connections may be by way of chordae tendineae, or the valve may be directly

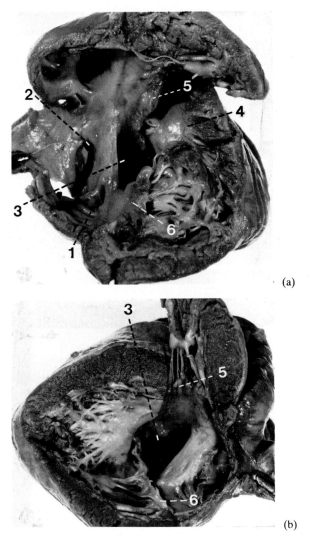

Figure 29.1 Complete atrioventricular orifice. (*a*) Right atrial and ventricular view. (*b*) Left ventricular view. 1 = Entry of coronary sinus; 2 = patent foramen ovale; 3 = common atrioventricular orifice with patent foramen primum and foramen interventriculare; 4 = septal band of crista supraventricularis; 5 = anterior bridging leaflet; 6 = Posterior bridging leaflet. (Reproduced from reference 4, by kind permission of the publishers.)

anchored on to the septum to a varying length beneath the aortic valve. Thus, one may call this a non-free-floating leaflet. The posterior bridging leaflet is almost always anchored on to the posterior wall of the septum by way of chordae. The lateral leaflets are usually small structures connecting the anterior and posterior bridging leaflets one on the right ventricular and the other on the left ventricular side.[1] One may therefore consider that in CAVO there is an anterior, posterior and lateral component for the leaflet structure in the right (tricuspid) and left (mitral) side. This may be interpreted as trileaflet structures of the tricuspid and mitral valves.[2]

In the complete form of CAVO, in many cases the anterior bridging leaflet may not be anchored on to the septum at all but by way of papillary muscles. This may be called a free-floating leaflet.

The peripheral connections to the above two types of the leaflets in addition to the chordal connections are by way of anterior and posterior groups of papillary muscles in each ventricular chamber. Although the first type (non-free-floating) is seen usually in cases of Down's syndrome, without any other major cardiovascular anomalies, it may be seen in other major cardiac lesions. The second type which is the free-floating leaflet is almost always seen when there is a major associated cardiac abnormality. These include patent ductus arteriosus, coarctation, tetralogy of Fallot, double outlet right ventricle, complete transposition, common atrium and other lesions.[1, 3] However, a free-floating anterior bridging leaflet may be seen without any other associated cardiac lesions.

The variations seen in CAVO

Although the classic description of CAVO is given above, it should be noted that very frequently the leaflet connections are quite variable. This is important for the surgeon to be aware of, so that he can tailor the creation of the mitral valve appropriately. For example, the anterior bridging leaflet may be divided or not divided as it bridges over the ventricular septum. This may or may not require special surgical methods for shaping a new mitral valve. As for the connections beneath the aortic valve, the anterior bridging leaflet (ABL) may only in part be attached and in part may be a free-floater. It may be connected only by way of chordae in some and in others it may be directly attached to the septum without the chordae. These connections beneath the aortic valve may extend along the curve of the ventricular septum to a considerable extent or the leaflet may be connected only to the summit alone. Likewise, the posterior bridging leaflet (PBL) may be divided or may be a single leaflet and occasionally may be anchored only minimally. The PBL is usually smaller than the anterior bridging leaflet.

The papillary muscle connections also may vary quite frequently. The antero-lateral papillary muscle of the right ventricle may be absent or small. Hence, the connections and the valvular apparatus may be directed towards the left ventricle almost completely. Likewise, the anterior papillary muscle of the left ventricle may be absent or very small and the entire leaflet may be prolapsed towards the right ventricular cavity. If a mitral valve is created, we now will be dealing with a 'parachute type of mitral valve'. The same type of situation may be seen for the posterior papillary muscle in both ventricles. Uncommonly the papillary muscles either in the right or left ventricles may proceed to the base of the valve directly rather than by way of chordal connections.

Accessory orifices and accessory muscle bundles

Accessory orifices although uncommon, are important especially while creating a new mitral valve. These may be small, large or medium sized and may be present in ABL or PBL either on the right or left ventricular side.

Accessory muscle bundles may be seen in the right ventricular sinus part thus reducing the cavity size or may be seen in the outflow tract of the right ventricle.

Likewise, accessory muscle bundles may be seen in the left ventricular outflow tract resulting in sub-aortic obstruction.

Nature of the leaflet structure

It is quite common to find the CAVO leaflets to be thickened, irregular and nodose resembling a dysplastic valve. This, particularly when seen in the left side, may pose a problem for the surgeon. This type of a dysplastic valve is commonly seen in Down's syndrome. Histologically, the architecture of the valve is distinctly altered with more of the element of spongiosa seen throughout. This may result in mitral insufficiency in some cases post-operatively. This may occur in the immediate or late post-operative period due to tear of the sutures or the dysplastic valve *per se* may not function as a normal mitral valve.

Sizes of ventricular chambers

We now have to take into account the sizes of the chambers in CAVO. Broadly speaking, CAVO may be classified into a balanced form, a dominant right or a dominant left form[1]. By *balanced* form (*see Figure 29.1*) we mean that there is hypertrophy of both ventricles and the chamber sizes are adequate for the given age, height and weight of the individual. By *dominant right* type (*see Figure 29.2*)

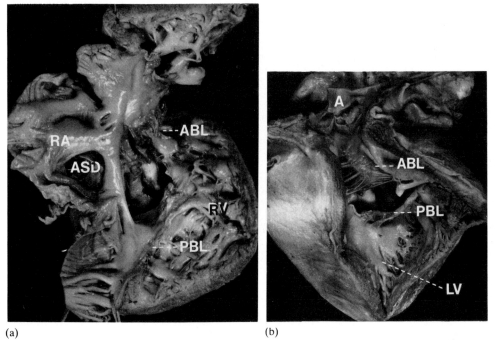

(a)   (b)

Figure 29.2 Dominant right type of common atrioventricular orifice, complete form. (*a*) Right atrial and right ventricular view. (*b*) Left ventricular view. RA = Right atrium; ASD = atrial septal defect, foramen ovale type; ABL = anterior bridging leaflet; PBL = posterior bridging leaflet; RV = right ventricle; LV = left ventricle; A = aorta. Note the small left ventricle with deficiency of valvular structure for the mitral component.

we mean the right ventricle is not only hypertrophied and enlarged but the left ventricle is smaller than normal for the given age, height and weight of the patient. In the *dominant left* type (*see Figure 29.3*) the left ventricle is hypertrophied and enlarged, while the right ventricle is *smaller* than normal for the age, height and weight of the individual.

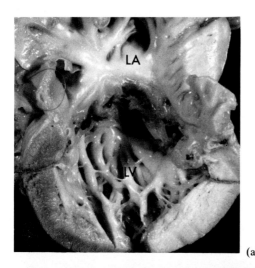

(a)

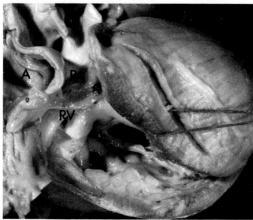

(b)

Figure 29.3 Dominant left form of common atrioventricular orifice, complete type. (*a*) Left atrial and left ventricular view. (*b*) Right ventricular view. LA = Left atrium; LV = left ventricle; A = aorta; RV = right ventricle; PA = pulmonary trunk. (Reproduced from reference 1, by kind permission of publishers.)

In general, in the balanced form, the valvular tissue is adequate for the creation of the tricuspid and mitral valves (*see Figure 29.1*). On the other hand, the valvular tissue is deficient on the left side (mitral component) (*see Figure 29.2 (b)*) in the dominant right side, and in the dominant left side the tricuspid component of the CAVO leaflet is deficient (*see Figure 29.3 (b)*). Therefore, it is clear that is a ventricular chamber is smaller than normal, we may end up post-operatively with tricuspid or mitral stenosis in some cases. The smallness of a chamber is variable. This may be diminutive, or markedly smaller than normal. Obviously, a total correction may not be applicable in these cases. On the other hand, if the smallness of the chamber is moderate or border line, total surgical correction may give good results.

Size of the CAVO

The combined defect in the atrial and the ventricular septum may be small, moderate or large. It is not uncommon to find the atrial component larger than the ventricular component. In some, the reverse may be true, or both may be small. Occasionally both may be large, resulting in cor biloculare. This largeness of one component of the defect may alter the physiology. In addition, with a large ventricular component in CAVO, the ABL may anchor more anteriorly than usual beneath the left ventricular out-flow tract and may result in subaortic obstruction postoperatively.

Associated cardiac abnormalities[1, 3]

CAVO is seen with almost any type of major cardiac abnormality. As a matter of fact, in our material CAVO with an associated cardiac abnormality is seen more frequently than when it occurs alone. The associated cardiac abnormalities are: patent ductus arteriosus, coarctation, paraductal and fetal coarctation, aortic stenosis, tetralogy of Fallot (*see Figure 29.4*), double outlet right ventricle, complete transposition, single ventricle, corrected transposition, pulmonary stenosis and common atrium.

Subaortic area in CAVO

Although the subaortic area is smaller than normal in CAVO, usually there is no hemodynamically significant left ventricular obstruction in many cases. The subaortic obstruction may be due to several factors. Subaortic stenosis may be seen due to a fibroelastic discrete ridge, a membraneous shelf or a shelf of endocardial tissue beneath the aortic valve. It also may be due to anomalous chordal or valvular insertion, more anteriorly than usual. These may result in significant left ventricular obstruction postoperatively.

We have previously pointed out the inverse relationship of Down's syndrome and splenic abnormalities in CAVO. Sixty per cent of CAVOS are associated with Down's syndrome with normal spleen. On the other hand, when CAVO is seen with common atrium, DORV, complete transposition and total or partial anomalous pulmonary venous drainage there is usually a splenic abnormality such as polysplenia or asplenia. These are seen in isolated levocardia, dextrocardia or mesocardia, *without* Down's syndrome.

Conduction system in CAVO (*see Figure 29.5*)[4]

The sinoatrial node is in normal position. The AV node originates in the myocardium of the distal (downstream) wall of the right atrium and the adjacent

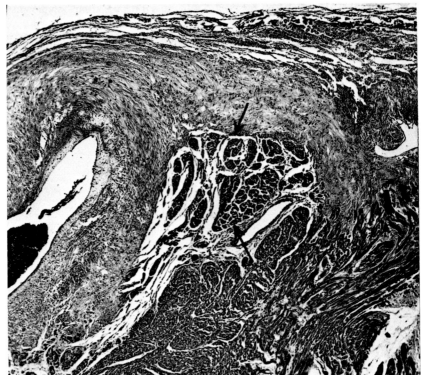

(a)

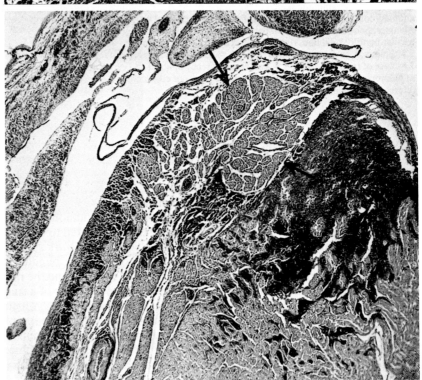

(b)

Acknowledgement

Aided by Grant HL 30558–01 from the National Heart, Lung and Blood Institute, National Institutes of Health, Bethesda, Md.

References

1. BHARATI, S. and LEV, M. (1973). The spectrum of common atrioventricular orifice. *Am. Heart J.*, **80**, 553
2. CARPENTIER, A. (1977). Surgical anatomy and management of mitral component of atrioventricular defects. In *Pediatric Cardiology* (eds R.H. Anderson and E.A. Shinebourne), pp. 477–87. Edinburgh: Churchill–Livingstone
3. BHARATI, S., KIRKLIN, J.W., MCALLISTER, H.A., JR. and LEV, M. (1980). The surgical anatomy of common atrioventricular orifice associated with tetralogy of Fallot, double outlet right ventricle, and complete regular transposition. *Circulation*, **61**, 1142
4. LEV, M. (1958). The architecture of the conduction system in congenital heart disease 1. Common atrioventricular orifice. *Arch. Path.*, **65**, 174

Figure 29.6 (*a*) Atrioventricular bundle at the level of the common atrioventricular orifice. Arrows point to bundle. (Hematoxylin and eosin. Original magnification ×40; reduced to one-half in reproduction.) (*b*) Atrioventricular bundle at level of interventricular foramen. Arrows point to bundle. (Weigert and Van Gieson Stain. Original magnification ×60; reduced to one-half in reproduction.) (Reproduced from reference 4, by kind permission of publishers.)

30

Diagnosis, evaluation and treatment of congenital abnormalities of the mitral valve

Rene A. Arcilla

Summary

Abnormal development of any of the basic structures of the mitral valve apparatus can result in mitral regurgitation, stenosis, atresia or A–V valve malposition with straddling mitral valve. In about 90% of cases, varying cardiac anomalies are also present. These coexisting lesions make clinical recognition of the mitral valve disease difficult. As a rule, two-dimensional echocardiography and cardiac catheterization with angiocardiography are needed for diagnosis and evaluation of valve dysfunction as well as ventricular performance. Precise identification of the anatomic abnormality, including that of the valvular and subvalvar structures, is essential to the surgical management. Unfortunately, these are not always obtainable by current laboratory techniques and surgical exploration may then be the only source for such details.

Mitral regurgitation is often successfully corrected or palliated by annuloplasty with or without valvuloplasty. The surgical management of congenital mitral stenosis is difficult. Recent trends suggest that reconstructive surgery is possible in many but valve replacement may still be necessary in some children. In certain types of mitral atresia complex, and in straddling/overriding mitral valve, right-heart bypass surgery offers the best physiologic palliation, provided that the pulmonary vascular disease is not yet present. In babies or young children with pulmonary hypertension, pulmonary artery banding may be initially necessary prior to eventual right-heart bypass.

Introduction

The mitral valve apparatus has four major components: mitral annulus, two leaflets, two papillary muscles and multiple chordae tendineae extending from both leaflets to both papillary muscle groups. Abnormal development of any may result in regurgitation, stenosis, atresia or A–V valve malposition with straddling of the mitral valve.

Clinical recognition of mitral valve disease is usually easy in the absence of associated intracardiac defects which mask the clinical presentation. Unfortunately, its occurrence as an isolated defect is only about 10%. In the rest, varying cardiac anomalies are also present. Awareness of the cardiac complexes where mitral valve anomalies tend to coexist is helpful to the diagnostic process.

As a general rule, echocardiography and cardiac catheterization are needed to establish the diagnosis. Each compliments the other. Two-dimensional echocardiography provides anatomic details of the mitral valve which may not be as well identified in angiocardiograms such as leaflet thickening and mobility, commissural fusion and relative orifice size, and location as well as size of papillary muscles. Cardiac catheterization confirms the diagnosis, and provides physiologic data that help assess valvular as well as ventricular function.

This presentation is a review of the diagnosis, assessment and management of congenital mitral valve anomalies. Evaluation of severity takes into consideration two related aspects: severity of valve dysfunction and extent of ventricular function.

Congenital mitral regurgitation

This may be due to abnormal development of the leaflets such as cleft anterior (aortic) leaflet, leaflet agenesis or underdevelopment, wide separation of commissures, and double-mitral orifice. It may also be due to abnormal sub-leaflet structures such as chordae elongation, agenesis/hypoplasia of chordae or of papillary muscles, or abnormal position of papillary muscles resulting in relative elongation of chordae. It is not clear whether annulus dilatation alone may cause incompetence although this was the only indentifiable finding at surgery in some children[1].

Excluding endocardial cushion defects where mitral incompetence is always present, other intracardiac defects are observed in about 70%. The most common are secundum atrial septal defect, ventricular septal defect, and patent ductus arteriosus. Coarctation of the aorta and aortic stenosis are, comparatively speaking, much less frequent in this condition than in congenital mitral stenosis.

Isolated congenital mitral regurgitation is difficult to clinically differentiate from rheumatic mitral insufficiency. In both, the typical auscultatory finding is an apical pansystolic murmur that is well transmitted to the left axilla. Additional information which favour a congenital etiology are early-age onset (if known), absent rheumatic history, mid-systolic click suggesting mitral valve prolapse, and evidence for chromosomal abnormality or other skeletal anomalies.

There are no diagnostic echocardiographic findings. The mitral valve echoes are often unremarkable. However, the left ventricle appears enlarged, and the estimated left ventricular output is abnormally high. Leaflet prolapse may be recognized but the nature of the chordal anomaly responsible for the prolapse may not be identified even by two-dimensional echocardiography. Quantitation of the regurgitation by this non-invasive technique is not possible although the left ventricular enlargement and the high left ventricular output reflect the severity of the disease.

The valvular incompetence is identified by combined Doppler–echocardiography, and is confirmed by retrograde left ventricular angiography which shows contrast opacification of the left atrium during ventricular systole. The underlying anatomic abnormality responsible for the regurgitation may sometimes be identified such as cleft anterior leaflet or mitral valve prolapse. If the regurgitation is pronounced, these structural abnormalities may be masked by the contrast-filled regurgitant stream. It is not uncommon then that the precise anatomic defect may be recognized only at the time of surgery. Simultaneously obtained pulmonary capillary wedge and left ventricular diastolic pressures fail to demonstrate significant pressure gradients. In children, both may be in the normal range or only mildly elevated in the presence of regurgitant fractions of less than 50%, suggesting increased ventricular distensibility (*see Figure 30.1*). The pulmonary arterial pressures also vary from normal to systemic levels; those with pulmonary hypertension often reveal high regurgitant fractions of 50% or greater.

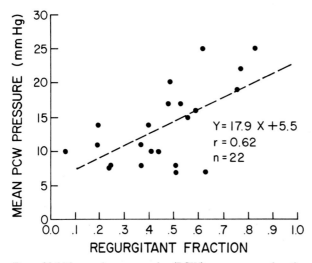

Figure 30.1 Mean pulmonary wedge (PCW) pressures as a function of regurgitant fraction in children with isolated mitral regurgitation.

The regurgitation may be quantified by determining the total left ventricular stroke output (LVO) and the forward or systemic stroke output. In the absence of tricuspid insufficiency, systemic output is equivalent to right ventricular stroke output (RVO). The difference between the two ventricular outputs represents regurgitant volume or flow. The degree of regurgitation is expressed by *regurgitant fraction* which expresses the ratio of regurgitant flow to total left ventricular output:

$$\text{regurgitant fraction} = \frac{\text{LVO} - \text{RVO}}{\text{LVO}}$$

Several methods are available for determining regurgitant fraction. One involves angiographic determination of left ventricular and right ventricular volumes in end-diastole and end-systole to estimate their respective outputs[2]. Systemic output, calculated by the Fick method, may also be used instead of the angio-derived right ventricular output[2, 3]. In recent years, non-invasive assessment of valvar regurgitation utilizing the same principle has been carried out using gated equilibrium radionuclide angiography[4–6]. The relative proportions of left ventricular and right ventricular stroke outputs are derived from ventricular time–activity curves without actual volume measurements. The method is safe, and the estimated regurgitant fraction is reproducible and is comparable with that by the angiographic method[5, 6]. As in any laboratory method, inherent difficulties exist such as in the count analysis of the right ventricle due to background activity or scatter, atrial overlap, variable size and geometry and edge delineation. Echocardiographic quantitation of mitral regurgitation has been proposed, utilizing the aortic forward stroke volume and the mitral stroke volume as derived from M-mode aortic valve and mitral valve echograms, respectively[7]. Although theoretically feasible, the flow derivation is not too reliable, especially since the valve echograms are influnced by the spatial movement of the heart during systole and diastole.

Ejection fraction

This is a popular index for ventricular pump performance. It is the ratio of ventricular stroke volume to ventricular end-diastolic volume, and may be derived from angiocardiograms as well as radionuclide angiograms. However, its interpretation is difficult in the presence of mitral regurgitation since the ventricular output is sensitive not only to changes in contractility but also to changes in preload and afterload. Left ventricular preload is increased due to the additional regurgitant volume, and afterload is reduced due to the unloading mechanism afforded by the incompetent valve. Left ventricular ejection fraction should, therefore, be at least in the high normal range in isolated mitral regurgitation, and should proportionately increase with the severity of the regurgitation unless some compromise of pump performance is already present. Interestingly, the ejection fraction remains relatively flat at wide ranges of regurgitant fraction in children (*see Figure 30.2*). An ejection fraction that is still within the normal range does not negate ventricular dysfunction in this condition; on the other hand, a low ejection fraction always indicates poor ventricular function.

The end-systolic wall stress/end-systolic volume ratio (ESWS/ESVI) has been advocated as a better index of left ventricular function since end-systolic volume is relatively independent of preload and varies linearly with afterload[8]. The analysis,

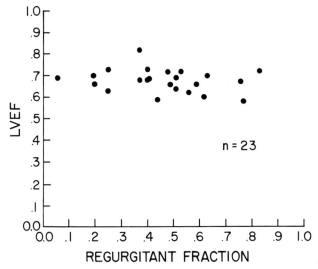

Figure 30.2 Left ventricular ejection fraction (LVEF) plotted against regurgitant fraction in children with isolated mitral regurgitation. Note flat distribution of data points over the wide range of regurgitant fraction.

however, is cumbersome and ideally requires simultaneous recordings of high fidelity pressures and biplane angiocardiograms. In children with isolated mitral regurgitation, where advanced left ventricular dysfunction is uncommon, estimation of the ESWS/ESVI ratio may not be necessary to help identify the ideal candidates for surgery. Abnormal left ventricular regional wall motion has been observed in adults with chronic mitral or aortic regurgitation[9]. We have also observed this in some children with severe mitral regurgitation.

Treatment for moderate or severe mitral regurgitation is surgical. In our experience, mitral annuloplasty with or without valvuloplasty, is superior to valve replacement in children. Our criteria for surgical intervention are as follows:

1. Hemodynamic (major criteria).
   (a) Reduced ejection fraction.
   (b) Regurgitant fraction $\geqslant 50\%$
   (c) Elevated pulmonary artery or pulmonary capillary wedge pressures.
   (d) Left ventricular end-diastolic volume $> 200\%$ of PN.
2. Clinical (minor criteria):
   (a) NYHA functional class II or more.
   (b) Cardiothoracic ratio $> 50\%$ in chest X-rays.
   (c) Left ventricular hypertrophy moderate or severe in EKG.

Surgery is indicated in the presence of : three or more major criteria, or two major plus two or more minor criteria. In more than half of our cases, annuloplasty resulted in normal valve function; in the rest, residual mild or trivial incompetence with essentially normal left ventricular size and function was observed.

When mitral regurgitation coexists with other defects, its presence may still be suspected if the typical apical systolic murmur is observed. However, it may also be missed even during cardiac catheterization unless specifically sought for through selective left ventriculography. Because of the associated shunting defects, assessment by regurgitant fraction estimation is no longer feasible. The relative severity of the valvar incompetence can then be only roughly estimated based on how faintly or totally $(+ \text{ to } ++++)$ the left atrium gets opacified during systolic emptying by the contrast-filled left ventricle (*see Figure 30.3*). This grading method is subjective and is invalidated by arrhythmia during the contrast injection.

The left ventricular size is sometimes helpful in the assessment of the valvar disease in these complicated cases. Since the left ventricle tends to be small in children with atrial septal defect[10], enlargement of this chamber in patients with combined atrial septal defect and mitral incompetence indicates that the regurgitation is not mild. If ventricular septal defect or patent ductus arteriosus coexists with mitral insufficiency, gross left ventricular enlargement despite angiographic demonstration of only a small septal defect or ductus arteriosus also suggests that the mitral regurgitation is of a significant degree.

Surgical repair of the incompetent mitral valve in these complex cases depends on the overall hemodynamics, associated anomalies and assessment of the mitral disease. Closure of an atrial septal defect without correction of significant mitral incompetence may compromise left heart function. On the other hand, closure of large shunting defects without simultaneous repair of an incompetent mitral valve can be effective for palliating severely symptomatic infants or young children. If still needed, and after hemodynamic reassessment, mitral valve surgery may be carried out later.

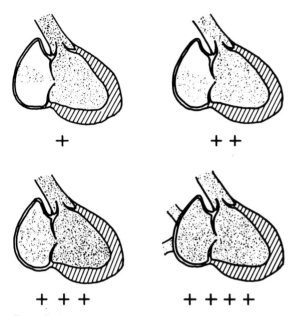

$+$

$++$

$+++$

$++++$

Figure 30.3 Schematic diagram illustrating relative grades of regurgitation. $+$ = Small regurgitant stream that opacifies only small part of left atrium (LA) and disappears during diastole. $++$ = More contrast filling of LA but not of entire chamber. $+++$ = Opacification of entire LA including atrial appendage. $++++$ = Same as $(+++)$, with opacification of some pulmonary veins.

Congenital mitral stenosis

The developmental abnormality involves most, if not all, valve components. The annulus is small, the leaflets are thick and fused, the chordae are short and stubby, and the papillary muscles are grossly abnormal. Depending on the site where the inflow obstruction appears to be greatest, the stenosis may be designated as primarily supravalvar, annular, valvular, or subvalvular. However, such a categorization is often difficult to ascertain by current laboratory methods, and may be possible only during surgical exploration or autopsy.

Excluding hypoplastic left heart syndrome with aortic atresia where mitral stenosis or atresia is always present, associated cardiac defects occur in at least 90%[11]. The most common is coarctation of the aorta. Others include aortic stenosis, patent ductus arteriosus and ventricular septal defect. Occasionally, mitral stenosis may accompany tetralogy of Fallot or other complex lesions with reduced pulmonary flow.

The diagnosis may be clinically suspected in the rare case where the valvular anomaly is isolated or where the associated defect is simple, so that the characteristic apical diastolic murmur is still recognizable. Despite absence of the typical murmur, the stenosis should be considered to be potentially present in symptomatic babies or children with complex lesions that include coarctation, aortic stenosis or others referred to earlier. In most instances, the first suggestion of mitral stenosis is provided by the M-mode echocardiogram which characteristically shows multiple echoes of the mitral valve with decreased opening amplitude (D to E excursion), greatly reduced E to F slope, and absent or miniaturized 'A' wave excursion of the anterior mitral leaflet. The posterior leaflet moves paradoxically anteriorly during diastole, instead of posteriorly, although this is not observed in all patients (*see Figure 30.4*).

The two-dimensional echocardiogram provides more anatomic information. Irrespective of the valvar or subvalvar anatomy, the mitral leaflets appear

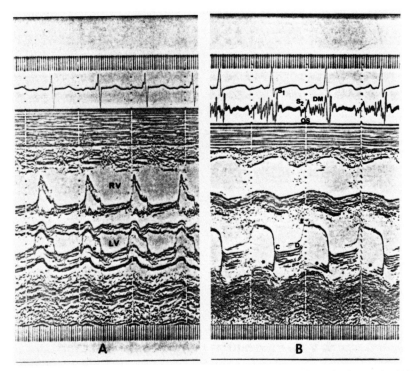

Figure 30.4 M-mode echocardiograms of two children with congenital mitral stenosis. (A) Infant with severe mitral stenosis, double-outlet right ventricle and other complex lesions. Note flat E-to-F slope of anterior mitral leaflet and anterior (paradoxical) motion of posterior leaflet identified by asterisk. (B) Child with similar findings to (A) except that posterior leaflet motion is normal. Note opening snap (OS) in phonocardiogram which coincides with E point of anterior mitral leaflet.

thickened in all planes of examination, and reveal reduced mobility especially at the tips which seem to be anchored (*see Figure 30.5*). The thick papillary muscles are identifiable in several views but are best evaluated in the long axis and short axis views. In 'parachute mitral valve deformity', only a single and prominent papillary muscle (posteromedial muscle) is identifiable. A similar picture is obtained if both papillary muscles are fused or are apposed to each other, giving a semblance of a single hypertrophied muscle. An abnormal echo band stretching obliquely across the left atrial cavity above the mitral valve, seen in the long-axis and apical views, suggests supravalvar mitral ring.

The diagnosis is confirmed by cardiac catheterization which demonstrates reproducible diastolic pressure gradients between simultaneously obtained pulmonary capillary wedge (or left atrial) and left ventricular pressures. At comparable degrees of mitral narrowing, the pressure gradient is higher in patients with large mitral valve flow as in left-to-right shunting defects than in those without

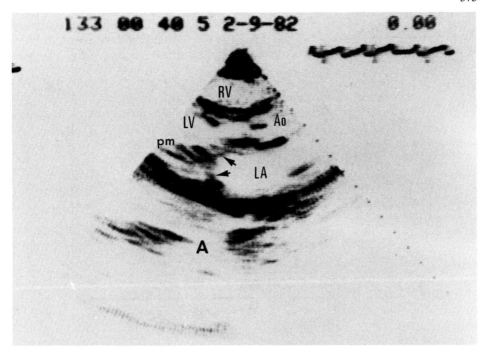

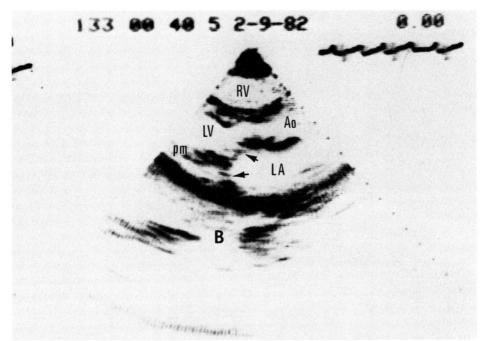

Figure 30.5 Two-dimensional echocardiogram, long axis view, of 65-year-old male with mitral valve area of 1 cm²/m² body surface area. (A) During ventricular diastole. (B) During ventricular systole. Note thick leaflets (shown by arrows), prominent papillary muscle (pm), and limited leaflet excursion. RV = right ventricle; LV = left ventricle; Ao = aorta; LA = left atrium.

such defects. Conversely, patients with severe pulmonary stenosis—hence with reduced pulmonary venous return—may have only small gradients.

Angiocardiography also provides anatomic/functional details such as leaflet thickening, restricted movement of anterior leaflet during diastole as well as systole, and left ventricular size (*see Figure 30.6*). Left ventricular size reflects the volume load of this chamber. It may be normal or slightly reduced in the absence of shunting defects or may be increased in those with associated ventricular septal defect or patent ductus arteriosus. It can be quite small if pulmonary venous return is partly diverted into the right heart chambers by an accompanying atrial septal defect or partial anomalous pulmonary veins. The anatomy of the papillary muscle is not as readily apparent as in the two-dimensional echocardiograms. Nevertheless, abnormal papillary muscles may be observed. In 'parachute mitral valve deformity' the left ventricular angiogram in the lateral or oblique projection often reveals an 'egg-timer' filling defect during diastole. The posterosuperior portion of this filling defect is accounted for by the coned mitral leaflets and chordae, and the anteroinferior portion by the single but large posteromedial papillary muscle[12]. A similar filling defect may be noted when both papillary muscles are apposed or are fused, or when the papillary muscles insert almost directly into the cone-shaped thick mitral valve.

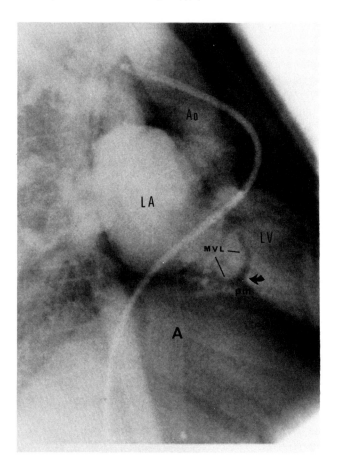

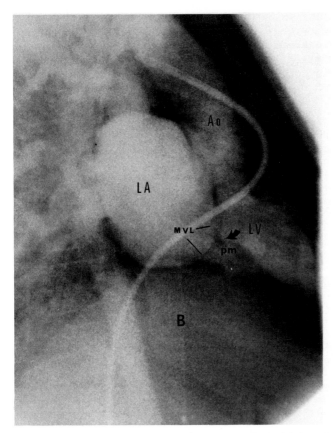

Figure 30.6 Selective angiocardiogram (pulmonary injection) in lateral projection of same patient as in *Figure 30.5*. (A) At onset of ventricular diastole, showing thick mitral leaflets (MVL) which appear anchored (arrow) to thick papillary muscle (pm). (B) During ventricular systole, showing restricted posterior movement of thick leaflets and the thick papillary muscle. See *Figure 30.5* for abbreviations.

The severity of inflow obstruction is best expressed by the mitral valve orifice area. The latter is traditionally calculated at cardiac catheterization utilizing the Gorlin formula[13, 14] which takes into consideration the mean diastolic pressure gradient across the valve, the stroke volume or flow across the valve, and the diastolic filling period. Its estimation in babies or small children is difficult due to problems related to cardiac output determination by the Fick method. If shunting defects are also present, either pulmonary or systemic blood flow is utilized in the equation depending on the shunt site. In small children, especially in those with shunting defects, it is preferable to derive the left ventricular stroke volume angiographically than by the Fick method. A simplified method for valve area calculation has been proposed[15]. This utilizes cardiac output (CO) and mean pressure gradient (MPG) as the only parameters:

$$\text{MVA} = \frac{\text{CO}}{\sqrt{\text{MPG}}}$$

Valve areas calculated by this method from adults with acquired mitral stenosis were highly comparable with those obtained by the Gorlin formula[15]. Our studies on children with congenital mitral stenosis also showed similar results (*see Figure 30.7*).

Non-invasive methods, primarily involving echocardiography, have also been proposed for assessing the severity of mitral stenosis. By and large, these have been

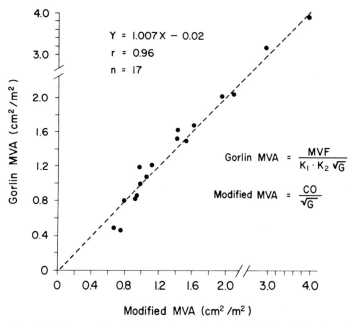

Figure 30.7 Comparison of mitral valve areas calculated by the Gorlin formula (13B) and by a modified equation, in congenital mitral stenosis. The observed values were practically identical.

evaluated using the mitral valve areas of adult patients with acquired mitral stenosis as points of reference. Although useful for diagnosis, the E to F slope of the mitral valve echogram is an unreliable index of the severity of stenosis[16]. The motion pattern of the posterior aortic root has been ascribed to left atrial volume changes during the cardiac cycle, and has been utilized to analyze left atrial emptying in normal subjects as well as in those with mitral stenosis[17]. The left atrial emptying index derived by this approach has been reported useful for predicting the severity of the mitral valve disease[18]. However, this is not a reliable index in children. The 'left atrial emptying index' is rate dependent (*see Figure 30.8*). More importantly, our analysis of posterior aortic root motion has shown that it is related more to right ventricular volume changes than to left atrial events. The peak rate of dimensional change during left ventricular filling (dD/dt) and the filling rate normalized for instantaneous diameter ($dD/dt/D$) have likewise been shown to correlate well with mitral valve area in acquired mitral stenosis[19]. We have not found this to be the case in congenital mitral stenosis, presumably because of the other associated lesions which also influence left ventricular performance in these subjects. Perhaps for the same reason, a recently proposed hydraulic formula for estimating valve area based on echo-derived stroke volume and left ventricular diastolic filling

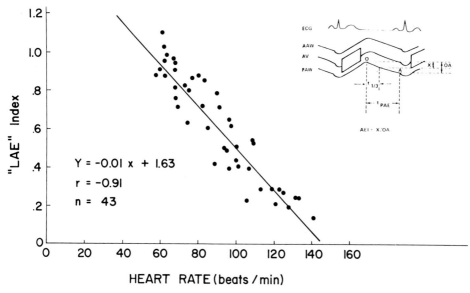

Figure 30.8 Left atrial emptying (LAE) index and heart rate in normal children.

period as the only variables[20] does not appear to be as reliable in small children than in adults with mitral stenosis.

The two-dimensional echocardiogram is better suited for estimating the severity of stenosis than the M-mode echocardiogram. This involves planimetry of the mitral valve orifice at the distal level of the leaflets in the short axis view. Nichol *et al.*[21] has shown excellent correlation between the valve areas obtained by this approach and those by cardiac catheterization. Since the calculation is uninfluenced by the hemodynamics, including presence of associated lesions, it is suited for pediatric patients as well. Nevertheless, there are potential sources for errors related to ultrasonic techniques for cardiac imaging such as inherent resolution, gain control setting or transducer angulation.

The surgical management is difficult due to the unusual anatomy and variability of the valve apparatus, and presence of associated lesions. In hypoplastic left heart syndrome with aortic atresia, surgery is not truly indicated although short-term palliation may be possible. Precise definition of the valve anatomy including that of the tensor apparatus is essential to the surgical planning. Supravalvar mitral ring is corrected by resection; the other types of stenosis are more difficult to repair. Unfortunately, current laboratory methods may not provide full anatomic details and one may have to rely on the findings at the time of surgery. Any surgical attempt carries with it the possibility of valve replacement as an alternative option. For this reason, we have been conservative in managing these children especially those whose mitral valve areas are not less than $1 \, cm^2/m^2$ BSA. We prefer to surgically correct or palliate the coexisting lesions first with the hope that mitral valve surgery can be deferred for as long as possible due to the possibility of valve replacement. On the other hand, Carpentier and co-workers[1] have shown that mitral valve reconstruction is usually possible in most of these patients without need for valve replacement.

Mitral atresia

The mitral valve is thick and has no orifice, and an atrial septal defect serves as the only left atrial outlet. Other intracardiac lesions, usually of a complex nature, are also present. Two general groups may be recognized: where the aorta arises from the left ventricle (group I), or where it originates from the opposite ventricle (group II). A ventricular septal defect (VSD) may or may not be present. In group I without VSD, the left ventricle is virtually non-existent (hypoplastic left heart syndrome with mitroaortic atresia); if a VSD is present, the left ventricle is grossly hypoplastic as is the aorta. In group II, both great vessels arise from a large right ventricle. A ventricular septal defect is usually present, and the left ventricle is also small. Pulmonary stenosis may or may not be present.

The diagnosis is not made clinically but may be suspected in echocardiograms that show thick and distorted mitral echograms with hardly any motion pattern, or without any identifiable mitral valve tracing altogether. The left ventricular cavity is small, tiny or absent. If mitroaortic atresia is present, contrast echocardiography or anigography, with injection into the mid-thoracic aorta via an umbilical arterial line, shows retrograde flow into the blind aortic root.

Cardiac catheterization and angiocardiography are essential for diagnosis, especially in the group II lesions where informtion relative to the anatomy of the great vessels, size of atrial septal defect, and status of the pulmonary vascular bed are essential to the surgical management (*see Figure 30.9*). In the absence of pulmonary stenosis, the pulmonary artery is large and harbors systemic pressures but peripheral vascular resistance may not necessarily be high. Elevated left atrial pressures indicate that the atrial septal defect is small and restrictive. If pulmonary stenosis is present, the pulmonary artery pressure may be normal or elevated and its size smaller than normal.

Surgical 'correction' consisting of a right-heart bypass (modified Fontan) procedure is now possible in the group II lesions and probably represents the only feasible approach. It involves subdividing the right atrium into two compartments—a proximal one carrying caval return directly into the pulmonary circulation, and a distal one draining the pulmonary venous blood from the left atrium via an enlarged atrial septal defect into the right ventricle which serves as the systemic ventricle (*see Figure 30.10*). For this to be possible, pulmonary vascular resistance must ideally be normal and it may be necessary to initially band the pulmonary artery early in infancy while deferring the bypass surgery for sometime later. The preservation of a large atrial defect and or a nearly normal pulmonary vascular bed should be the primary goal of this initial surgical procedure. It is theoretically possible that this type of right-heart bypass procedure may also be feasible in some patients in group I provided that the aorta is not markedly hypoplastic.

Figure 30.9 Selective angiocardiograms in child with mitral atresia, ventricular septal defect, double outlet right ventricle with pulmonary stenosis, and previous Glenn surgery at age 6 years. (**A**) Frontal projection, contrast injection into left atrium (LA) with streaming of contrast into right atrium (RA) and some reflux into pulmonary veins (PV). (**B**) Lateral projection, contrast injection into large right ventricle (RV) with contrast-filling of small left ventricle (LV) and simultaneous opacification of aorta (Ao) as well as pulmonary artery (PA).

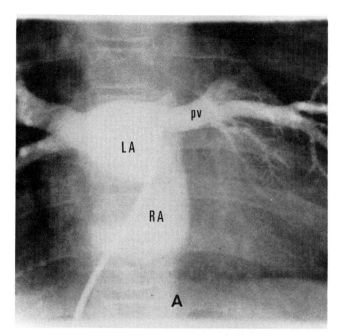

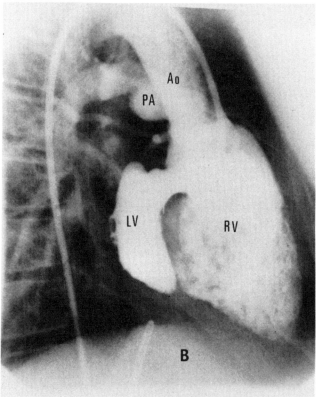

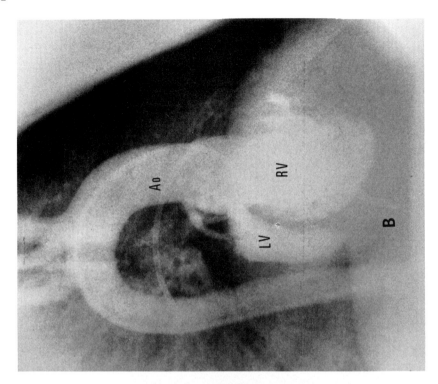

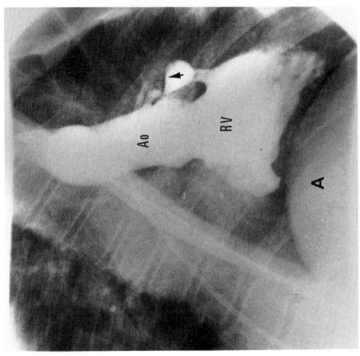

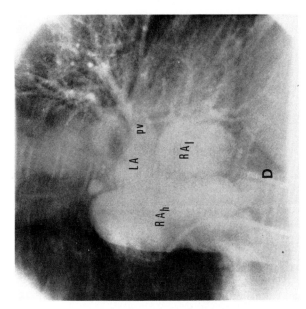

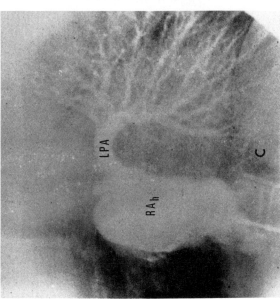

Figure 30.10 Selective angiocardiograms, 1 year after right-heart bypass surgery, on same patient in
Figure 30.9. Right atrium was divided into two compartments with high right atrium (RA_h) leading to
left pulmonary artery (LPA), and lower right atrium (RA_l) communicating with left atrium (LA) via
enlarged atrial septal defect. (A) Right ventricular contrast injection in angled frontal view, showing
opacification of aorta and of stump of previous pulmonary trunk. (B) Same injection, angled oblique
view, demonstrating opacification of both ventricles and aorta. (C) Injection into RA_h, frontal projection, with contrast filling of left pulmonary arteries (LPA). (D) Left pulmonary venous return into left
atrium (LA) and then into lower right atrium (RA_l) prior to ventricular filling.

Straddling mitral valve

This represents a complex positional abnormality of the A–V valve characterized by overriding of the mitral annulus or malattachment of part of the mitral tension apparatus into the right ventricle, resulting in partially double inlet right ventricle and hypoplasia of the ipsilateral left ventricle[2]. A ventricular septal defect is always present. The valve straddles the anterior part only of the ventricular septum which extends up to the crux cordis. The conduction system, i.e. A–V node and His bundle, is usually at its normal position unlike in straddling tricuspid valves[23]. Positional abnormalities of the great vessels and other complex intracardiac anomalies are common.

The clinical findings and hemodynamics vary widely. Combined echocardiography and cardiac catheterization are necessary for diagnosis. The malattachment of the mitral valve into the ventricular septum or contralateral ventricle may be suspected in M-mode or two-dimensional echocardiograms[24]. However, the valve straddling is best established by selective injection of contrast into the left atrium. In the absence of an atrial septal defect, this reveals simultaneous left ventricular as well as right ventricular filling directly from the left atrium via two separate streams (*see Figure 30.11*).

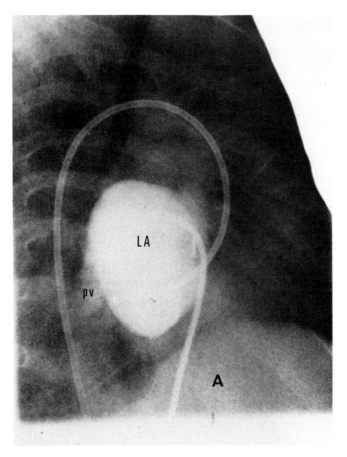

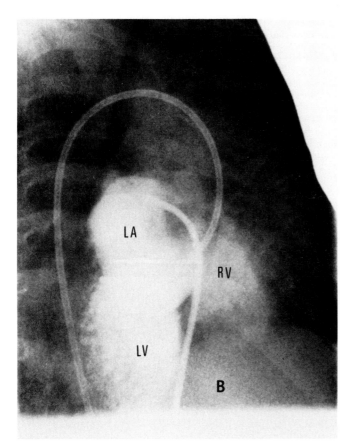

Figure 30.11 Selective angiocardiograms, lateral projection, in infant with complex intracardiac defects which include mitral stenosis, straddling mitral valve, ventricular septal defect and others. (A) Contrast injection into left atrium (LA) through venous catheter advanced via patent foramen ovale, with some opacification of pulmonary vein (PV). (B) Subsequent cineframe during ventricular diastole, showing nearly simultaneous opacification of left ventricle (LV), and right ventricle (RV) without contrast-filling of right atrium.

The surgical repair of this condition is difficult and requires optimal information pertaining to chamber size, A–V valve anatomy, position and size of great vessels, and overall hemodynamics. Of several options available—e.g. total repair with/without valve replacement, Rastelli procedure or modified Fontan procedure—the last appears to be the most feasible provided that the pulmonary vascular bed is still ideal for right heart bypass and A-V valve regurgitation is absent or only trivial.

References

1. CARPENTIER, A., BRANCHINI, B., COUR, J.C., *et al.* (1976). Congenital malformations of the mitral valve in children: Pathology and surgical treatment. *J. Thorac. Cardiovasc. Surg.*, **72**, 854
2. SULAYMAN, R., MATHEW, R., THILENIUS, O.G., REPLOGLE, R. and ARCILLA, R.A. (1975). Hemodynamics and annuloplasty in isolated mitral regurgitation in children. *Circulation*, **52**, 1144
3. SANDLER, H., DODGE, H.T., HAY, R.E. and RACKLEY, C.E. (1963). Quantitation of valvular insufficiency in man by angiocardiography. *Am. Heart J.*, **65**, 501

4. RIGO, P., ALDERSON, P.O., ROBERTSON, R.M., BEAKER, L.C. and WAGNER, H.N., JR. (1979). Measurement of aortic and mitral regurgitation by gated cardiac blood pool scans. *Circulation*, **60**, 306–312

5. THOMPSON, R., ROSS, I. and ELMES, R. (1981). Quantification of valvar regurgitation by cardiac gated pool imaging. *Brit. Heart J.*, **46**, 629–635

6. JANOWITZ, W.R. and FESTER, A. (1982). Quantitation of left ventricular regurgitant fraction by first pass radionuclide angiocardiography. *Amer. J. Cardiol.*, **49**, 85–92

7. CORYA, B.C., RASMUSSEN, S., PHILLIPS, J.F. and BLACK, M.J. (1981). Forward stroke volume calculated from aortic valve echograms in normal subjects and patients with mitral regurgitation secondary to left ventricular dysfunction. *Amer. J. Cardiol.*, **47**, 1215–1222

8. CARBELLO, B.A., NOLAN, S.P. and MCGUIRE, L.B. (1981). Assessment of preoperative left ventricular function in patients with mitral regurgitation: Value of the end-systolic wall stress—end-systolic volume ratio. *Circulation*, **64**, 1212–1217

9. OSBAKKEN, M.D., BOVE, A.A. and SPANN, J.F. (1981). Left ventricular regional wall motion and velocity of shortening in chronic mitral and aortic regurgitation. *Amer. J. Cardiol.*, **47**, 1005–1009

10. MATHEW, R., THILENIUS, O.G. and ARCILLA, R.A. (1976). Comparative response of right and left ventricles to volume overload. *Amer. J. Cardiol.*, **38**, 209–217

11. RUCKMAN, R.N. and VAN PRAAGH, R.V. (1978). Anatomic types of congenital mitral stenosis: Report of 49 autopsy cases with considerations of diagnosis and surgical implications. *Amer. J. Cardiol.*, **42**, 592–601

12. MACARTNEY, F.J., SCOTT, O., IONESCU, M.I. and DEVERALL, P.B. (1974). Diagnosis and management of parachute mitral valve and supravalvar mitral ring. *Brit. Heart J.*, **36**, 641–652

13. GORLIN, R. and GORLIN, S.G. (1951). Hydraulic formula for calculation of the area of the stenotic mitral valve, other cardiac valves, and central circulatory shunts. *Amer. Heart J.*, **41**, 1–45

14. COHEN, M.V. and GORLIN, R. (1972). Modified orifice equation for the calculation of mitral valve area. *Amer. Heart J.*, **84**, 839–840

15. HAKKI, A.H., ISKANDRIAN, A.S., BEMIS, C.E., *et al.* (1981). A simplified valve formula for the calculation of stenotic cardiac valve areas. *Circulation*, **63**, 1050–1055

16. COPE, G.D., KISSLO, J.A., JOHNSON, M.L. and BEHAR, V.S. (1975). A reassessment of the echocardiogram in mitral stenosis. *Circulation*, **52**, 664–670

17. STRUNK, B.L., FITZGERALD, J.W., LIPTON, M., POPP, R.L. and BARRY W.H. (1976). The posterior aortic wall echocardiogram. Its relationship to left atrial volume change. *Circulation*, **54**, 744–750

18. STRUNK, B.L., LONDON, E.J., FITZGERALD, J., POPP, R.L. and BARRY, W.H. (1977). The assessment of mitral stenosis and prosthetic mitral valve obstruction, using the posterior aortic wall echocardiogram. *Circulation*, **55**, 885–891

19. FURUKAWA, K., MATSUURA, T., ENDO, N., *et al.* (1979). Use of digitized left ventricular echocardiograms in assessment of mitral stenosis. *Brit. Heart J.*, **42**, 176–181

20. SEITZ, W.S. and FURUKAWA, K. (1981). Hydraulic orifice formula for echographic measurement of the mitral valve area in stenosis. Application to M-mode echocardiography and correlation with cardiac catheterization. *Brit. Heart J.* **46**, 41–46

21. NICHOL, P.M., GILBERT, B.W. and KISSLO, J.A. (1977). Two-dimensional echocardiographic assessment of mitral stenosis. *Circulation*, **55**, 120–128

22. LIBERTHSON, R.R., PAUL, M.H., MUSTER, A.J., ARCILLA, R.A., ECKNER, F.A.O. and LEV, M. (1971). Straddling and displaced atrioventricular valves in primitive ventricle. *Circulation*, **43**, 213–226

23. MILO, S., HO, S.Y., MACARTNEY, F.J. *et al.* (1979). Straddling and overriding atrioventricular valves: Morphology and classification. *Amer. J. Cardiol.*, **44**, 1122–1134

24. AZIZ, K.U., PAUL, M.H., MUSTER, A.J. and IDRISS, F.S. (1979). Positional abnormalities of atrioventricular valves in transposition of the great arteries including double outlet right ventricle, atrioventricular straddling and malattachment. *Amer. J. Cardiol.*, **44**, 1135–1145

31

Repair of complete atrioventricular canal

Gordon K. Danielson

Successful correction of the complete form of atrioventricular (A–V) canal is now readily achievable. The most challenging technical feature of this anomaly is the associated mitral valvular deformity. From a surgical standpoint, we have found it helpful to classify A–V canal according to Rastelli's original types, based on the anatomy of the common anterior leaflet[1, 2].

Repair is conducted with cardiopulmonary bypass combined with hypothermia at 20°C. Cold blood cardioplegic solution is infused every 30 minutes and topical hypothermia is added to keep the myocardial temperature below 20°C. The repair is performed through a right atriotomy. Ideal exposure is gained by mobilization of the caval cannulae as shown in *Figure 31.1(A)*. After the anatomy of the anterior and posterior common leaflets is determined, the initial step in the repair is the approximation of their mitral components with a few interrupted sutures. If the anterior common leaflet is type A and incompletely divided, or is type C, the leaflet is incised to the annulus at the junction of mitral and tricuspid portions. A similar incision of the posterior common leaflet may be required, as shown by the dotted line, in patients with an interventricular communication beneath this leaflet.

A single prosthetic patch is fashioned in an oval shape and of a size comparable with that of the overall ventricular and atrial septal defect (*see Figure 31.1(b)*). The inferior portion of the patch is sutured with interrupted sutures to the right side of the ventricular septum. All of the sutures are placed prior to lowering the patch into position.

The mitral and tricuspid margins of the naturally divided or incised anterior common leaflet are then sutured to the patch with interrupted horizontal mattress sutures at a level that corresponds to the plane of the normal mitral and tricuspid anuli (*see Figure 31.1(c)*). The incised or naturally divided posterior common leaflet is attached to the patch in a similar manner.

In those cases in which the posterior common leaflet is attached to the interventricular septum by a membrane or fused chordae, the patch shape is altered so it can be sewn directly to the atrial surface of the leaflet (*see Figure 31.1(d)*).

The valve is then tested by injecting saline forcefully into the left ventricle. Additional sutures are added where required. If a central leak is present, the valve annulus is narrowed by a double anuloplasty technique. The final step in the repair is closure of the atrial portion of the septal defect by suturing the most cephalad portion of the patch to the rim of the atrial septum (*see Figure 31.1(e)*). In the

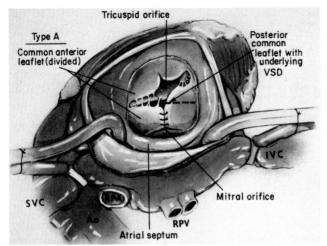

Type A

Common anterior leaflet (divided)

Tricuspid orifice

Posterior common leaflet with underlying VSD

IVC

SVC

RPA

Ao

RPV

Atrial septum

Mitral orifice

(a)

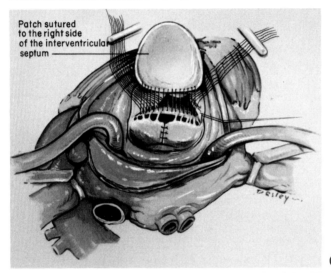

Patch sutured to the right side of the interventricular septum

Desley

(b)

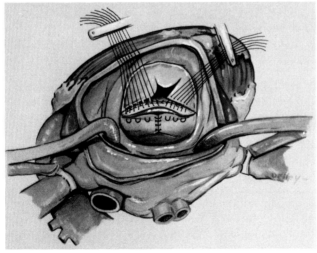

Desley

(c)

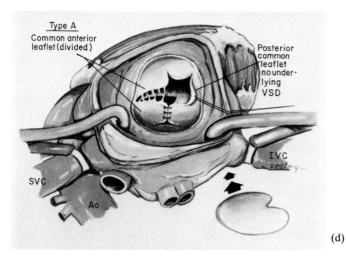

(d)

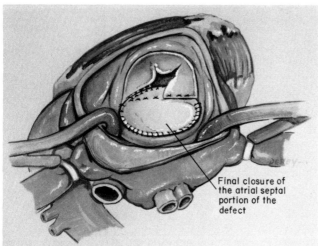

Figure 31.1 Repair of complete atrioventricular canal, type A^2. (*a*) Repair of mitral valve. (*b*) Insertion of oval prosthetic patch the size of the combined atrial and ventricular septal defects. All sutures to the right side of the septum are placed before the patch is lowered into position. (*c*) The patch is sutured to the leaflets at a level that corresponds to that of the normal mitral and tricuspid annuli. (*d*) If the posterior common leaflet is attached to the interventricular septum by a membrane or fused chordae, a patch of different shape is sewn to the atrial surface of the leaflet. (*e*) The final step. The most cephalad portion of the patch is sutured to the rim of the atrial septum. (Reproduced from reference 2, by kind permission of authors and publishers.)

presence of associated pulmonary stenosis, valvotomy and infundibular resection are performed as indicated.

A variation of the repair in which individual patches are used to close the atrial and ventricular septal defects has been employed in some circumstances. This two-patch technique has theoretical advantages for repair in infants, as there is no shortening of leaflet substance which occurs when divided leaflets are attached to a single patch. Another variation, which is designed to decrease the risk of heart block, employs an extension of the atrial portion of the patch which is sutured around the coronary sinus, thus avoiding crossing the plane of the conduction bundle during closure of the atrial septal defect.

We believe that an integral part of the operation for atrioventricular canal is the performance of intraoperative double-sampling indocyanine dye curves. Withdrawal catheters are passed off from the operating table and connected to dual densitometers. The curves are performed by injecting into the left ventricle and sampling simultaneously in the left atrium and ascending aorta. The amount of early-appearing dye in the left atrium quantitates the degree of mitral regurgitation. If severe regurgitation is demonstrated (regurgitant fraction greater than 20–25%), bypass is resumed, the left atrium is entered, and the repair is revised or the valve is replaced with a prosthesis.

Associated mitral valvular deformities can pose special technical problems in the repair both of partial and of complete atrioventricular canal. In our series of 241 patients undergoing operation, 20 (8.3%) had severe deformities of the mitral valve including parachute mitral valve (single papilllary muscle) (2.1%), double orifice mitral valve (4.1%), and miscellaneous defects such as double clefts (2.1%).

Our surgical mortality for complete repair of A–V canal prior to June 1963 was 60%. The standardized operation described earlier was then developed and the mortality dropped to 7% in the next 27 patients. However, all 27 patients were 3 years of age or older. Younger patients were banded, with inconsistent results. Subsequently, we have accepted symptomatic patients of any age for repair[3].

There were 175 patients undergoing repair of complete A–V canal between 1963 and August 1982 (see Table 31.1). The total hospital (30-day) mortality was 14.3%.

TABLE 31.1 Surgical repair of complete atrioventricular canal, 1963 to August 1982

Age	No. of patients	Deaths	
		No.	%
< 12 months	26	7	26.9
1–2 years	56	14	25.0
3–23 years	93	4	4.3
Total	175	25	14.3

The mortality for patients aged 3 years to 23 years was 4.3%. The relatively high mortality in the 1–2 year age group is probably related to the development of pulmonary vascular obstructive disease in many of these patients and to our acceptance of borderline candidates for operation in order not to exclude those patients with pulmonary hypertension who might achieve an excellent long-term result following repair of their defect.

Only one patient required mitral valve replacement at the time of repair.

Ninety-six survivors of reparative operation between 1967 and 1978 were followed up for 2–12 years (mean 5.1 years). There were four late deaths. The New York Heart Association functional classifications of the survivors were: Class I, 70%; Class II, 25%; and Class III 1%.

Postoperative cardiac catheterizations were performed in 23 patients, most of whom were symptomatic. Mitral incompetence was assessed as severe in 1, moderate in 5, mild in 12, and absent in 5. Five patients (5%) required mitral valve replacement during the follow-up interval.

Twenty-three patients had catheterization data before operation and at follow-up 1–8 years later (mean 4.2 years) which allowed calculation of pulmonary arteriolar resistance (*see Table 31.2*). The most favourable group had resistance less than 5 units/m².

TABLE 31.2 Pulmonary arteriolar resistance in patients with complete atrioventricular canal

Preoperative		*At follow-up (1–8 years)*	
Units/m²	*No. of patients*	*Decrease or same*	*Increase*
<5	15	13	2
5–10	6	3	3
>10	2	0	2
Total	23	16	7

There were 208 patients with complete A–V canal who were evaluated at our institution between 1960 and 1978.[4] Forty-six (22%) had pulmonary arteriolar resistance equal to or greater than 5 units/m². Fifteen of the 46 (33%) had Down's syndrome whereas only 17% of the overall group were Down patients. This finding supports the clinical impression that patients with Down's syndrome are more prone to develop pulmonary vascular obstructive disease. The ages of the 46 patients ranged from 5 months to 32 years (mean 6.5 years).

Follow-up ranged from 1 to 21 years, with a mean of 10 years. Of the 33 patients with pulmonary arteriolar resistance 5–13 units/m², 18 were treated medically and 15 surgically. All 13 patients with resistance of 14 units/m² or over were treated medically. The results are shown in *Table 31.3*. The only patients who improved were those treated surgically (54% of the surgical group improved), whereas all of the medically treated patients deteriorated or died.

TABLE 31.3 Repair of complete atrioventricular canal with pulmonary vascular obstructive disease (PVOD)

	Rpa = 5–13 U/m²				*Rpa ≥ 14 U/m²*	
Clinical status	*Surgical*		*Medical*		*Medical*	
at follow-up	*No.*	*(%)*	*No.*	*(%)*	*No.*	*(%)*
Improvement	8	(54)	0	—	0	—
Deterioration	2	(13)	11	(61)	7	(54)
Mortality	5	(33)	7	(39)	6	(46)
Total	15	(100)	18	(100)	13	(100)

Rpa = Pulmonary arteriolar resistance.

In our experience in a follow-up of over 20 years, over 90% of patients with a preoperative pulmonary arteriolar resistance less than 5 units/m² have had a good late result. In contrast to this, only 50–60% of patients with a resistance of 5 units/m² or greater have had a good late result.

A relationship has been found between the pulmonary arterial oxygen saturation and the results in the surgical patients, with pulmonary arteriolar resistance elevated to 5–13 units/m². If the saturation is 85% or greater, the late results are generally good, whereas 80% of patients with a saturation of 84% or less have deteriorated or died at follow-up.

These data have led us to suggest the following criteria of operability:

(1) If the pulmonary arteriolar resistance is less than 5 units, the operative risk is small and the late results are good.

(2) If the pulmonary arteriolar resistance is 5–13 units/m^2 (total pulmonary resistance 7–14 units/m^2), the pulmonary arterial oxygen saturation is determined. If the saturation is 85% or greater, surgical treatment is advised. If the saturation is less than 85%, surgical treatment is not advised except in patients 1–2 years of age (infants are excluded, as there is a greater chance for regression of pulmonary vascular obstructive disease after repair in patients 2 years of age or younger).

(3) If the pulmonary arteriolar resistance is 14 units/m^2 or greater (total pulmonary resistance 15 units/m^2 or greater), surgical treatment is not advised.

Mention should also be made of repair of complete A–V canal associated with additional complex congenital cardiac lesions. Until recently, attempted repairs usually resulted in an unsuccessful outcome. Several recent cases of successful repair of complicated forms of complete A–V canal give encouragement to the present capability to accomplish repair of such complex lesions, even in the infant group. One example is given in the report of a 2-year-old girl who underwent repair of a complete A–V canal associated with isolated dextrocardia, common atrium, total anomalous systemic venous return to a left superior vena cava, and double orifice mitral valve[5].

Complete A–V canal associated with either common ventricle (type IC) or giant ventricular septal defect and insufficiency of both A–V valves requiring valve replacement has also been successfully accomplished[6].

Another example of complete A–V canal associated with other complex cardiac anomalies is given in the report of a 6-year-old girl who had the combination of complete A–V canal, double outlet right ventricle and atrioventricular discordance[7]. In addition, there was dextrocardia, common atrium, bilateral superior venae cavae, and pulmonary stenosis. A previous ascending aorta–left pulmonary artery (Waterston) anastomosis had been performed and subsequently a left Blalock anastomosis was constructed. Repair was accomplished by ligation of the left subclavian artery, take-down of the Waterston anastomosis with pericardial patch enlargement of the left pulmonary artery, repair of the A–V canal in the classical fashion, and insertion of a valved conduit between the pulmonary ventricle and the pulmonary artery. She represents the first successful repair of this anomaly and is doing well 5 years later.

In summary, complete atrioventricular canal can now be repaired satisfactorily at all ages. The most challenging technical feature of this anomaly is the associated mitral valvular deformity. In most circumstances, we prefer primary repair in infancy rather than a two-stage procedure. Many complex forms of complete atrioventricular canal are also now amenable to total correction.

References

1. RASTELLI, G.C., KIRKLIN, J.W. and TITUS, J.L. (1966). Anatomic observations on complete form of persistent common atrioventricular canal with special reference to atrioventricular valves. *Mayo Clin. Proc.*, **41**, 296

2. MCMULLAN, M.H., WALLACE, R.B., WEIDMANN, W.H. and MCGOON, D.C. (1972). Surgical treatment of complete atrioventricular canal. *Surgery*, **72**, 905

3. MCGOON, D.C., MCMULLAN, M.H., MAIR, D.D. and DANIELSON, G.K. (1973). Correction of complete atrioventricular canal in infants. *Mayo Clin. Proc.*, **48,** 769

4. FUSTER, V., FELDT, R.H., RITTER, D.G. and MCGOON, D.C. (1980). Complete atrioventricular canal defect with pulmonary vascular obstructive disease—medical versus surgical management. In *Proceedings of World Congress of Paediatric Cardiology*, Abstract 008. London

5. DANIELSON, G.K., MCMULLAN, M.H., KINSLEY, R.H. and DUSHANE, J.W. (1973). Successful repair of complete atrioventricular canal associated with dextroversion, common atrium, and total anomalous systemic venous return. *J. Thorac. Cardiovasc. Surg.*, **66,** 817

6. DANIELSON, G.K., GIULIANI, E.R. and RITTER, D.G. (1974). Successful repair of common ventricle associated with complete atrioventricular canal. *J. Thorac. Cardiovasc. Surg.*, **67,** 152

7. DANIELSON, G.K., TABRY, I.F., RITTER, D.G. and MALONEY, J.D. (1978). Successful repair of double-outlet right ventricle, complete atrioventricular canal, and atrioventricular discordance associated with dextrocardia and pulmonary stenosis. *J. Thorac. Cardiovasc. Surg.*, **76,** 710

Section 10

Investigational papers

32

In-situ function of the papillary muscles in the intact canine left ventricle

S. Hagl, W. Heimisch, H. Meisner, N. Mendler and F. Sebening

Introduction

The papillary muscles are an essential functional part of the atrioventricular valve apparatus. The knowledge of the contractile behaviour of the papillary muscles is a prerequisite for understanding the tricuspid and mitral valve mechanics. However, most of our present knowledge of papillary muscle dynamics is based on studies of isolated papillary muscle preparations[1, 2] and theoretical considerations[3]. Only a limited number of investigations have made direct measurements of *in-situ* papillary muscle function. The results, obtained by different techniques including cineradiography[4], Walton Brodie strain gauges[5-7], mercury-in-rubber length gauges[8], and sonomicrometers[9-11], revealed conflicting results concerning the significance of papillary muscle dynamics in the mechanics of atrioventricular valve function. Different concepts of papillary muscle function were postulated ranging from a purely isometric contraction[3, 12, 13] to a regular systolic shortening[4, 6, 7, 9-11]. The significance of ischaemic papillary muscle dysfunction as a cause of mitral incompetence is still not clearly defined[14-20]. The discrepancy of the results may be, in part, explained by the limitations of the method used.

It is the purpose of this chapter to characterize the contractile behaviour of the papillary muscle of the intact left ventricle under different physiological and pathophysiological conditions. Special interest was focused on the following questions:

1. How do the papillary muscles behave during phasic changes of pressure and geometry in the left ventricle?
2. Does a direct relationship exist between papillary muscle dynamics and wall motion with respect to amplitude and velocity?
3. How does acute ischaemia affect papillary muscle function?
4. Does mitral incompetence result from acute ischaemic dysfunction of the papillary muscle?

Material and methods

Studies were performed in a total of 20 anaesthetized open-chest mongrel dogs. Animals of either sex weighing from 20 to 25 kg were initially anaesthetized with sodium pentobarbital (20 mg/kg body weight; Nembutal, Deutsche Abbot GmbH, Ingelheim, Germany). Anaesthesia was maintained by continuous infusion of piritramide (1.5 mg/kg/h; Dipidolor, Janssen Pharmaceutica, Duesseldorf, Germany) and ventilation with a mixture of 50% nitrous oxide and 50% oxygen (Servoventricular 900, Elema-Schönander, Stockholm, Sweden). A left thoracotomy was performed in the 5th intercostal space and the heart was then exposed and suspended in a pericardial cradle.

The left anterior descending coronary artery (LAD) and the circumflex branch (LCC) were dissected free near its origin for placement of electromagnetic flow probes (Statham SP 2202; Statham Instruments Inc., Oxnard, USA). A micrometer-driven snare was placed 10 mm distal to the flow tansducer to produce temporary coronary stenosis or occlusion. Cardiac output was measured by an electromagnetic flow probe placed around the ascending aorta. Left ventricular pressure (LVP, LVedP) and aortic pressure (AoP) were monitored by high-fidelity micromanometers (Millar Microtip PC 470, 7F; Millar Instruments Inc., Houston, USA) introduced via the carotid and the femoral artery, respectively. Right and left atrial pressures were recorded with Statham P23Db (Statham Instruments Inc., Hato Rey, Puerto Rico) pressure transducers. *dP/dt* was registered on-line by differentiating the LVP signal (Brush Differentiator Model 13–4214–01; Gould Brush Inc., Cleveland, USA).

The animals underwent total cardiopulmonary bypass. Ventricular fibrillation was produced, the left atrium opened, and the mitral leaflets retracted. Two modified miniature ultrasonic crystals (1.5–2.0 mm in diameter) were implanted through a small endocardial incision by means of a slitted Teflon tube. The crystals were inserted into the tip of both the anterior (APM) and posterior papillary muscle (PPM) under visual control[9, 21]. The leads of the transducers, which formed a free loop within the ventricle to prevent any tension, were led out through a tiny needle wound through the free wall of the ventricle. The inferior sonomicrometer transducers were inserted through the ventricular wall into the root of both papillary muscles using the same technique. The proper placement was controlled from inside the ventricle (*see Figure 32.1*).

The distance between the transducers ranged between 16 and 25 mm. Circumferential and longitudinal motion of the corresponding left ventricular wall were recorded by cylindrical gauges (2.0 mm outer diameter)[20] implanted into the subendocardial muscle layer. By continuous measurement of ultrasonic transit time between two piezoelectric crystals, acting as emitter and receiver, the phasic changes in papillary muscle (PM) and wall segment length (L–WS) were recorded. Details on this method have been published elsewhere[21, 23].

Measurements were performed during steady state conditions 40–60 minutes after cardiopulmonary bypass was terminated.

Changes in myocardial pump and muscle functins were induced by changing preload, afterload, and contractility. Preload was increased by rapid intravenous infusion of blood; afterload was augmented by intermittant cross-clamping of the descending aorta; and the contractile state was altered by infusion of calcium and isoproterenol (Isuprel). Papillary muscle function during ischaemia was studied after graded stenosis or occlusion of the LAD and LCC, respectively.

To detect mitral incompetence during ischaemic papillary muscle dysfunction, a careful analysis of left atrial pressure patterns was performed. In order to unveil even a small reflux into the left atrium, an indicator technique was used. A high frequency response thermistor was placed in the left atrium and a small catheter

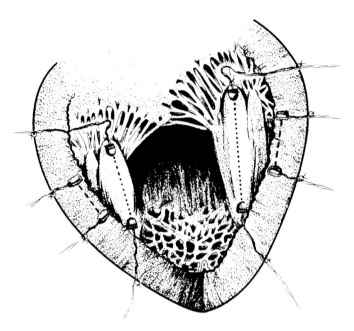

Figure 32.1 Placement of pairs of ultrasonic transducers in the anterior and posterior papillary muscle of the left ventricle.

was introduced into the left ventricle from the apex. During papillary muscle ischaemia cold saline (5 ml, 4°C) was injected into the ventricle and temperature recorded within left atrium.

All data collected are expressed as the mean ± SE.

Results

Normal pattern of *in-situ* papillary muscle motion

Figure 32.2 shows schematically the pattern of PM and ventricular wall motion. Under physiological conditions the length of a wall segment increases sharply during early diastole, reaching a maximum with atrial contraction. Small changes in length occur during the isovolumic period reflecting changes in ventricular geometry. During this phase length increases slightly parallel to the minor heart axis but decreases along the longitudinal axis. Throughout ventricular ejection segments shorten with almost constant velocity. The minimal length of the longitudinal segment is most often reached at the time of aortic valve closure whereas the circumferential segment continues to shorten until the end of ventricular systole. These changes in length during the isovolumic phases reflect changes in ventricular geometry, i.e. the transition from an ellipsoid to a more spherical shape during pressure development and the reverse during ventricular relaxation.

In contrast, the pattern of the papillary muscle shows a very moderate changes in length throughout diastole. As shown in *Figure 32.3* about 40% of lengthening occurs during the short isovolumic phase. In some experiments the increase in length during isovolumic systole reached up to 65% of the total amplitude

The P–L loop of the papillary muscle reflects the altered time course of contraction during ischaemia (*see Figure 32.7*). The PM was extensively stretched during both the isovolumic contraction and ventricular ejection phases as indicated by an increased right slant of the loop. During ventricular ejection, the force developed by the intact wall muscle cannot be overcome by the ischaemic papillary muscle. Shortening is delayed until the pressure falls to about 50% of peak value. Under these conditions the loop will be generated paradoxically in a clockwise direction.

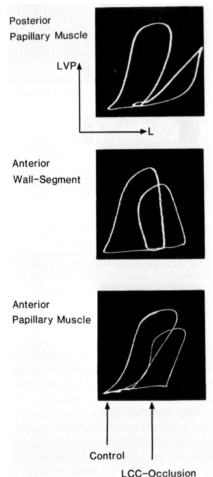

Figure 32.7 Changes in the morphology of pressure length loops in response to acute left circumflex coronary artery occulusion.

The loop area is no longer an expression of active work but now reflects the energy dissipated by the passive stretching of the ischaemic muscle. The P–L loops of the intact wall segment and the anterior papillary muscle are shifted to the right to reflect greater enddiastolic and maximal lengths. Despite the maintained extent of shortening, peak LVP was reduced indicating severe depression of overall left ventricular performance.

Discussion

The ultrasonic transit time method was found to be an adequate and reliable tool in studying the *in-situ* papillary muscle function. The main advantage of this method lies in the use of two separate low-mass transducers without any mechanical inter-connection. This configuration eliminates strain on the crystals during ventricular contraction. Implantation of transducers during cardiopulmonary bypass is a relatively atraumatic method, which ensures an accurate placement of the transducers along the major papillary muscle axis. In only 1 out of 21 experiments did autopsy reveal an improper placement of transducers in the papillary muscles.

Normal papillary muscle function

Under normal physiological conditions the pattern of *in-situ* papillary muscle dynamics is characterized by a slow increase in length during early and mid-diastole. A brief lengthening occurs associated with atrial contraction. With the onset of systolic pressure in the left ventricle, the length of the PM increases sharply reaching its maximum length at the opening of the aortic valve. This suggests that as long as the mitral valve is open, only moderate tangential forces act on the papillary muscles. As a result, pre-tension of the PM is low during diastole. After valve closure, which in respect to the PM appears as a passive mechanism, pressure in the LV rises sharply. This in turn stretches the papillary muscles, since the mitral leaflets now act as the second anchoring point for the PM.

This level of tension is thus directly transmitted to the papillary muscles and thereby determines the force of contraction. This, however, does not imply that the activation of the PM is delayed in relation to the contraction of the ventricular free wall[24]. The observed initial increase in length must be considered a mechanism which allows the leaflets to return into the atrioventricular plane. Further PM lengthening might reflect the functional correction of the position of the mitral leaflets during changes in ventricular geometry associated with displacement of PM axes.

This investigation on PM motion agrees precisely with the results of previous studies from our laboratory[9, 10]. Similar results were found by Cronin and co-workers[6,7] who used standard Walton–Brodie strain gauges. Fisher and associates[8], using mercury-in-rubber length gauges, also described a lengthening during the isovolumic systole. Discordant results were obtained by Hirakawa and colleagues[11]. In their study, sonomicrometers quite similar to those used in the present investigation were implanted into the *anterior* PM by penetration from the epicardial surface. They found a small decrease in the length of the anterior papillary muscle during the isovolumic period followed by a more extensive shortening during ventricular ejection. In three of the experiments, on the *posterior* PM, however, a lengthening was revealed during isovolumic systole. These contradictory results remain unclear. In a cineradiographic study Grimm *et al.*[4] calculated the distance between metal markers for successive frames. They found a phasic pattern of papillary muscle motion, which is characterized by a rapid increase in length during early diastole and a shortening during ventricular systole.

In contrast to these studies, which at least agree in that the papillary muscle shortens during ventricular ejection, other investigators postulated a purely isometric function of the papillary muscles[3, 12, 13]. This concept, however, could not be confirmed by recent experimental investigations[9, 11].

The onset of shortening of both papillary muscles coincides with the onset of shortening in subendocardial circumferential wall segments, which supports the studies on the anterior PM of Hirakawa *et al.*[11] Cronin *et al.*[7] assumed that other portions of the ventricle contract in advance of the papillary muscles. These findings do not agree with the sequence of contraction proposed by Rushmer[25], Burch and Depasquale[3], and Hider *et al.*[26] These authors have postulated an early activation of either the anterior or both papillary muscles preceding the mechanical contraction of the free left ventricular wall. The extent of shortening of each one of the papillary muscles averaged 20% of maximal length. Grimm *et al.*[4] found a 22.8% shortening of the papillary muscle. In contrast, Hirakawa *et al.*[11] reported only a 10% shortening of the anterior PM.

The characteristic pattern of PM motion can be influenced by a high LV filling pressure and/or an altered pressure–volume relation. If the pressure in the left ventricle rises sharply during early diastole, a parallel increase in PM length will be observed. Thereby the early diastolic pressure level determines the extent of early diastolic lengthening. At high diastolic pressure levels most of the PM elongation is moved up from the isovolumic systole to the diastole. The pattern of papillary muscle dynamics will thus be markedly altered and may closely resemble the pattern of a wall segment. Papillary muscle and ventricular functions are closely related. In response to changes in preload, afterload, and contractility, the papillary muscles behave like ventricular wall segments.

Papillary muscle function during ischaemia

The papillary muscles of the left ventricle are supplied by large branches of the epicardial coronary arteries[27]. They penetrate the ventricular wall radially and end in fine arborizations connected to the subendocardial plexus. The anterior papillary muscle is supplied by the left anterior descending coronary artery, the diagonal artery and the marginal branches. The posterior PM is supplied by the left circumflex branch and/or the right coronary artery. Because of this special vascular architecture, no adequate experimental method exists to produce reversible selective papillary muscle ischaemia. The placement of sutures around the base of the PM combined with the production of a patchy infarction of the adjacent ventricular wall as described by Mittal *et al.*[18] results in an irreversible infarction of the PM and is a very traumatic method which, in addition, may influence the functional architecture of the structures itself. Tsakiris *et al.*[20] injected formalin directly into the PM to produce infarction. By this irreversible procedure the muscle properties are changed and thus this method fails to resemble the situation of PM ischaemia in man. Lacking adequate techniques to produce selective papillary muscle ischaemia, temporary stenosis and occlusion of the LAD and LCC were used in this study. By this manoeuvre not only the PM but also large parts of the ventricular free wall and septum were rendered ischaemic.

A few beats after coronary occlusion, progressive dysfunction of both the depending PM and the adjacent ventricular wall developed in all experiments as shown previously[9, 10]. The morphology of the pressure–length loops of the PM and the wall segments changed progressively. When profound ischaemia has developed, the P–L loops will be generated in a clockwise direction indicating that no effective work is being performed by the ischaemic muscle. According to Tyberg *et al.*[28] the 'negative loop area' resulting from the lengthening during systole resembles the energy dissipated by the passive stretching of the ischaemic muscle. The response of the anterior and posterior PM to ischaemia did not differ functionally.

Despite severe ischaemic dysfunction of the papillary muscle, none of the animals in the entire series developed haemodynamic signs of mitral incompetence. There was also no evidence for indicator reflux into the left atrium during PM ischaemia. These findings confirm the results of a previous study from this laboratory. Tsakiris *et al.*[20] have shown that isolated PM infarction does not result in mitral incompetence. Similarly, Mittal and associates[18] could not produce mitral incompetence by infarction of the PM and the adjacent left ventricular wall. The authors concluded that mitral insufficiency is produced by papillary muscle dysfunction in combination with dyskinesia of the left ventricular free wall and ventricular dilatation. In contrast, Brazier *et al.*[16] suggested a 25% incidence of mitral incompetence when the entire subendocardium was rendered ischaemic. In this study the oxygen supply/demand ratio was changed by arteriovenous fistula, anaemia, and aortic stenosis. Hirakawa and co-workers[11] suggested that ischaemic PM dysfunction, following LAD or LCC occlusion, should result in a loss of proper apposition of the mitral valve leaflets and thereby may explain the occurrence of mitral incompetence.

The failure to produce acute mitral insufficiency by acute PM and adjacent ventricular wall ischaemia in the present series may be explained by several different mechanisms: we hypothesize that the effect of systolic PM elongation is counteracted to some degree by the systolic bulging of the adjacent ventricular wall, i.e. the point of anchorage of the papillary muscle moves in the opposite direction. As the ventricle dilates in response to ischaemia, the axis of the PM becomes more tangential. Both mechanisms taken together may reduce the net effect of the lengthening of the subvalvular apparatus on the position of the mitral leaflets.

The existence of excessive valvular tissue in relation to the mitral orifice area and systolic atrioventricular ring contraction[29] might still allow contact between the free margins of the mitral leaflets despite elongation of the subvalvular apparatus.

It is, however, conceivable that these mechanisms fail. Mitral incompetence might develop after papillary muscle infarction and later fibrosis. Associated substantial dilatation of the entire ventricle including the mitral annulus, reduction of atrioventricular ring contraction, and akinesia of the adjacent ventricular wall may be contributing factors to the pathogenesis of the clinical syndrome generally described as ischaemic papillary muscle dysfunction.

The proper PM function is only one of several components which, in a finely coordinated system, provide the functional integrity of the mitral valve.

Conclusion

The contractile behaviour of the papillary muscles reflect their task in controlling the proper positioning of the valve leaflets during phasic changes in ventricular geometry and pressure. The anterior and posterior papillary muscle did not differ functionally. According to the Frank–Starling mechanism and to changes in myocardial contractility, the papillary muscle behaves like ventricular wall segments. In response to ischaemia, identical changes of both papillary muscles and the wall segments were recorded. Acute ischaemic dysfunction of either the anterior or posterior papillary muscle does not result in acute mitral incompetence.

Acknowledgement

We acknowledge the skilful technical assistance of Mrs A. Bernhard-Abt, Mrs C. Schuelgen, and Mr S. Balteskonis.

References

1. BRUTSAERT, D.L. and SONNENBLICK, E.H. (1971). Early onset of maximum velocity of shortening in heart muscle of the cat. *Pfl. Arch.*, **324**, 91–99
2. EDMAN, K.A.P. and NILSSON, E. (1972). Relationships between force and velocity of shortening in rabbit papillary muscle. *Acta. Physiol. Scand.*, **85**, 483
3. BURCH, G.E. and DEPASQUALE, N.P. (1965). Time course of tension in papillary muscles of the heart. *J. Am. Med. Assoc.*, **192**, 701
4. GRIMM, A.F., LENDRUM, B.L. and LIN, HUN-LIN. (1975). Papillary muscle shortening in the intact dog: a cineradiographic study of tranquilized dogs in the upright position. *Circ. Res.*, **36**, 49
5. ARMOUR, J.A. and RANDALL, W.C. (1971). *In vivo* activity of the right ventricular papillary muscles. *Proc. Soc. Exp. Biol. Med.*, **136**, 534
6. CRONIN, R.E. and RANDALL, W.C. (1968). Direct examination of papillary muscle function in the canine left ventricle. *Texas Rep. Biol. Med.*, **26**, 419
7. CRONIN, R., ARMOUR, J.A. and RANDALL, W.C. (1969). Function of the in-situ papillary muscle in the canine left ventricle. *Circ. Res.*, **25**, 67
8. FISHER, V.J., STUCKEY, J.H., LEE, R.F. and KAVALER, F. (1965). Length changes of papillary muscles of the canine left ventricle during the cardiac cycle. *Fed. Proc.*, **24**, 278
9. HAGL, S., HEIMISCH, W., MEISNER, H. *et al.* (1976). Direkte Messung der Funktion der Papillarmuskeln des linken Ventrikels während akuter Koronarokklusion beim Hund. *Thoraxchirurgie*, **24**, 303
10. HAGL, S., HEIMISCH, W., MEISNER, H., BRAUN, E., MENDLER, N. and FRANKLIN, D. (1976). Function of normal and ischemic papillary muscles in the canine left ventricle. *Eur. Surg. Res.*, **8** (Suppl. I), 129
11. HIRAKAWA, S., SASAYAMA, S., TOMOIKE, H., *et al.* (1977). *In situ* measurement of papillary muscle dynamics in the dog left ventricle. *Am. J. Physiol.*, **233**, H384
12. BURCH, G.E., DEPASQUALE, N.P. and PHILLIPS, J.H. (1968). Syndromes of papillary muscle dysfunction. *Am. Heart J.*, **75**, 399
13. KARAS, S. and ELKINS, R.C. (1970). Mechanism of function of the mitral valve leaflets, chordae tendineae and left ventricular papillary muscle in dogs. *Circ. Res.*, **26**, 689
14. ANDERSEN, J.A. and FISCHER–HANSEN, B. (1973). Isolated acute myocardial infarction in papillary muscles of the heart: Clinicopathological study of 9 cases. *Br. Heart J.*, **35**, 781
15. ARANDA, J.M., BEFELER, B., LAZZARA, R., EMBI, A. and MACHADO, H. (1975). Mitral valve prolapse and coronary artery disease. Clinical, hemodynamic and angiographic correlations. *Circulation*, **52**, 245
16. BRAZIER, J.R., MALONEY, J.V. and BUCKBERG, G.D. (1975). Papillary muscle ischemia with patent coronary arteries. *Surgery*, **78**, 430
17. EDWARDS, J.E. (1971). Clinicopathologic correlations: Mitral insufficiency resulting from 'overshooting' of leaflets. *Circulation*, **43**, 606
18. MITTAL, A.K., LANGSTON, M., COHN, E.E., SELZER, A. and KERTH, W.J. (1971). Combined papillary muscle and left ventricular wall dysfunction as a cause of mitral regurgitation: An experimental study. *Circulation*, **44**, 174
19. SHELBURNE, J.O., RUBINSTEIN, D. and GORLIN, R. (1969). A reappraisal of papillary muscle dysfunction. *Am. J. Med.*, **46**, 862
20. TSAKIRIS, A.G., RASTELLI, G.C., DES AMORIM, D., TITUS, J.L. and WOOD, E. (1970). Effect of experimental papillary muscle damage on mitral valve closure in intact anaesthetized dogs. *Mayo Clinic Proc.*, **45**, 275
21. HAGL, S., HEIMISCH, W., MEISNER, H., ERBEN, R., FRANKLIN, D. and SEBENING, F. (1975). Ultraschallverfahren zur direkten Erfassung der regionalen Myokardfunktion. *Thoraxchir.*, **23**, 291
22. HEIMISCH, W., HAGL, S., GEBHARDT, K., MEISNER, H., MENDLER. N. and SEBENING, F. (1981). Direct measurement of cyclic changes in regional wall geometry in the left ventricle of the dog. *Innov. Tech. Biol. Med.*, **2**, 487

23. FRANKLIN, D.L., KEMPER, W.S., PATRICK, T. and MCKOWN, D. (1973). Technique for continuous measurement of regional myocardial segment dimensions in chronic animal preparations. *Fed. Proc.*, **32,** 343

24. SALISBURY, P.F., CROSS, C.E. and RIEBEN, P.A. (1963). Chorda tendinea tension. *Am. J. Physiol.*, **205,** 385

25. RUSHMER, R.F. (1956). Initial phase of ventricular systole: Asynchronous contraction. *Am. J. Physiol.*, **184,** 188

26. HIDER, C.F., TAYLOR, D.E.M. and WADE, J.D. (1965). The sequence of mechanical contraction of the left ventricle of the dog. *Proc. Physiol. Soc.*, 34P

27. ESTES, E.H., DALTON, F.M., ENTMAN, M.L., DIXON, H.B. and HACKEL, D.B. (1966). The anatomy and blood supply of the papillary muscles of the left ventricle. *Am. Heart J.*, **71,** 356

28. TYBERG, J.V., FORRESTER, J.S., WYATT, H.L., GOLDNER, S.J., PARMLEY, W.W. and SWAN, H.J.C. (1974). An analysis of segmental ischemic dysfunction utilizing the pressure-length loop. *Circulation*, **49,** 748

29. CHIECHI, M.A., LEES, W.M. and THOMPSON, R. (1956). Functional anatomy of the normal mitral valve. *J. Thoracic. Surg.*, **32,** 378

33

Preservation and restoration of the mitral mechanism during inferior wall aneursymectomy

W. D. Johnson, P. M. Pedraza and Kenneth L. Kayser

Inferior ventricular aneurysm is infrequently encountered in a coronary bypass population. In our experience, inferior aneurysms have been present in only 1% of patients operated on for coronary disease, and 10% of all patients with ventricular aneurysm. Various authors[1-8], reporting on surgical treatment of ventricular aneurysm, have observed an incidence of 0–17% in the inferior position. Autopsy series, however, have shown an incidence of 15–36%[9-12].

Clinical material

The subject study group of this report consists of 41 patients with aneurysm of the inferior wall of the left ventricle. To qualify for inclusion, the aneurysm had to be located primarily in the inferior (diaphragmatic) wall of the left ventricle and, furthermore, the aneurysm closure must have required a suture line at least 6 cm long. All aneurysms were of the 'true' type where the myocardium was completely replaced by a thin wall of scar. In all patients, the posterior papillary muscle was solid scar with no contractile capability whatever. The papillary chordae mechanism was invariably lengthened, and the valve proper was frequently damaged. Preoperative mitral insufficiency wsa present in 11 of 41 patients (27%), with V waves in the left atrium ranging up to 85 mm Hg. All patients had extensive coronary disease in other parts of the heart and required an average of 3.6 bypass grafts to revascularize the remaining myocardium. Many of the patients had been declined for surgery elsewhere, either due to fear of injury to the mitral mechanism, diffuse coronary disease, or poor ventricular function.

Surgical technique

In the earlier years of this series, we developed a technique that allows resection of the aneurysm and restoration of mitral valve function without replacement of the valve. The same technique, when used for inferior aneurysmectomy without preoperative mitral incompetence, prevents the development of mitral insufficiency.

The technique involves two basic maneuvers:

1. Plication of the mitral annulus.
2. Suspension of the scarred posterior papillary muscle distally.

Once on heart–lung bypass, the heart is elevated, exposing the inferior wall. A long incision is made parallel to the posterior descending artery almost to the mitral annulus (*see Figure 33.1*). The incision must be close to the posterior descending. An incision only 2–3 cm lateral to the posterior descending artery will usually divide the posterior papillary muscle and greatly complicate the repair.

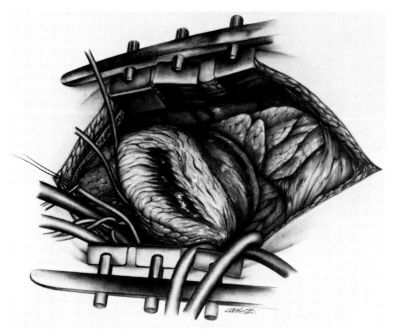

Figure 33.1 Incision for inferior aneurysm is made close to the posterior descending artery. Incision further laterally must be avoided to prevent injury to posterior papillary muscle.

Once the ventricle is open, the posterior papillary muscle (always solid scar) is easily identified (*see Figure 33.2*). The papillary muscle and chordae tendineae structure is always elongated, but intact. Mural thrombus has been seen only once. The scarred base of the septum can be easily identified on the other side of the ventriculotomy. Closure of the ventriculotomy is initiated by placing the first suture well laterally. It is inserted below the coronary sinus and passed through the mitral annulus. As it comes through the ventricular wall, it should come out just below the mitral leaflet, 3–4 cm lateral of the incision (*see Figure 33.2*). The suture is carefully passed behind the chordae tendineae and exited through the scar at the base of the septum. The other end of this mattress suture is passed through the scar a centimeter or so towards the apex. This sutre is also carefully passed behind the chordae tendineae and exited through the scar at the base of the septum. As the sutures progress toward the apex, wider and wider bites are taken on the septal side (*see Figure 33.3*).

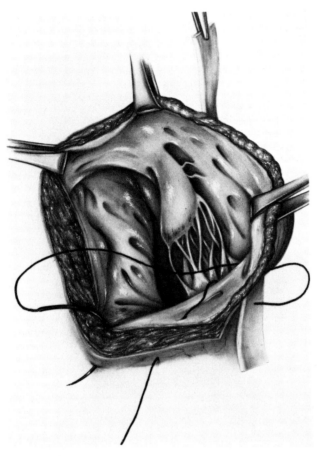

Figure 33.2 Inferior aneurysm open. The posterior papillary muscle, always solid scar, is easily identified. The chordae tendineae are elongated. The first suture is placed from outside through the mitral
annulus and enters the ventricle at the inferior edge of the mitral leaflet. It is usually 3–4 cm lateral to the
ventriculotomy. The suture then goes through the scar at the base of the septum adjacent to the annulus.

When the posterior papillary muscle is reached (solid scar), the sutures are
passed directly though the scarred muscle and angled at 45 degress or more towards
the apex. After all of the sutures are in place, the ventriculotomy is tied shut.
Excess scar is removed and a second layer of reinforcing sutures is placed in
standard fashion (*see Figure 33.4*). This method of closure has two purposes:

1. The first stitch placed at the mitral annulus plicates the annulus and reduces the
    circumference by several centimeters.
2. The sutures through the scarred papillary muscle pull distally and help reduce
    or prevent prolapse of the mitral valve.

We do not know which maneuver is more important, but the combination nearly
always eliminates mitral insufficiency when present, or prevents its occurrence. All
other coronary arteries that need bypass grafts and/or endarterectomy are taken
care of after the aneurysmectomy closure and valve reconstruction are completed.

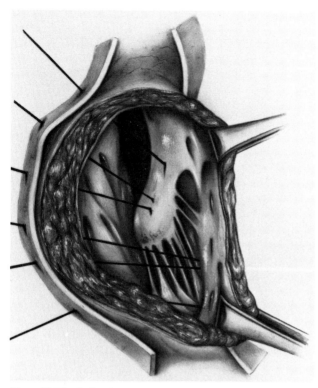

Figure 33.3 In closing the aneurysm, wider and wider bites are taken on the septal side. Sutures are passed directly through the scarred posterior papillary muscle and angled 45 degrees or more towards the apex. When closed this pulls the papillary mechanism distally and reduces prolapse.

Results

Eleven of the 41 patients presented with mitral insufficiency. Of these, three required mitral valve replacement and one had a ring annuloplasty. Of the 30 patients without significant mitral insufficiency preoperatively, one patient had a valve replacement. In none of the other patients was a significant mitral insufficiency present following the operative procedure. Three of the five patients requiring valve replacement had clear evidence of rheumatic involvement. Two patients (5%) died within 30 days of surgery. Of 23 hospital survivors operated before 1980, there were five (22%) late deaths over an average follow-up time of 33 months.

Discussion

The pathogenesis of inferior (diaphragmetic) wall aneurysm formation has been thoroughly reviewed by Buehler *et al.*[1] These authors devote much of their discussion to the distinction between true and false aneurysm. They describe a false aneurysm as one separated from the ventricular cavity by 'a circumscribed

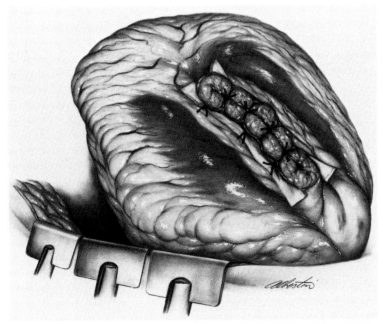

Figure 33.4 After all of the sutures are in place, the ventriculotomy is tied shut. Excess scar is removed and a second layer of reinforcing sutures is placed.

fenestration or elongated cleft'. Some, if not all, of these 'false' aneurysms are thought to be formed by a healed ventricular rupture. In general it is believed that false aneurysms represent a smaller loss of myocardium than true aneurysms[1]. This is undoubtedly true because large ventricular rupture is totally incompatible with life, whereas large myocardial infarction is frequently not fatal.

We have found only two other reports on surgical treatment of inferior wall aneurysm[1, 4]. Loop *et al.* report on 11 patients, without mitral involvement, operated on from 1966 to 1972. There were no coronary bypasses, but two patients received a Vineberg implant. One of the ten aneurysms was of the false type and six of 11 had mural thrombus. It is not clear whether patients with mitral involvement were excluded from the series, or not seen. They report no surgical mortality and only one late death. Buehler *et al.*[1] report on ten patients operated on in 1975 and before. They classified six aneurysms as false and four as true. Four patients had single bypass and five mitral replacement. Three of the four patients with true aneurysm required valve replacement. There was one surgical and one late death.

In our series of 41 patients there were no false aneurysms and only one mural thrombus. Patients received an average of 3.6 bypass grafts. The mitral mechanism was extensively involved in all, but valve replacement was required in only four (plus one mitral ring). There were two 30 day and five late deaths. These results indicate that inferior aneurysm combined with extensive coronary artery disease can be treated surgically. Even when the mitral mechanism is involved, valve replacement is usually not necessary. Surgical and late mortality are acceptable in view of the extent of disease.

Summary

Forty-one patients with aneurysm primarily in the inferior wall were operated. Eleven of the 41 presented with mitral insufficiency; only four required a valve prosthesis. Of the 30 without preoperative mitral insufficiency, only one required valve replacement. The patients received an average of 3.6 bypass grafts per patient. There were two (5%) 30 day deaths and five (22%) later deaths over an average follow-up of 33 months.

Inferior ventricular aneurysms, with or without mitral insufficiency, can usually be resected successfully without replacement of the mitral valve. Plication of the mitral annulus and suspension of the posterior papillary muscle distally to reduce prolapse are the two basic maneuvers used to eliminate or prevent mitral insufficiency. Needed bypass grafts are always constructed at the time of surgery.

References

1. BUEHLER, D.L., STINSON, E.B., OYER, P.E. and SHUMWAY, N.E. (1979). Surgical treatment of aneurysms of the inferior left ventricular wall. *J. Thorac. Cardiovasc. Surg.*, **78**, 74
2. RAO, G., ZIKRIA, E.A., MILLER, W.H., SAMADANI, S.R. and FORD, W.B. (1974). Experience with sixty consecutive ventricular aneurysm resections. *Circulation*, **49**, Suppl. 2, 149
3. FAVALORO, R.G., EFFLER, D.B., GROVES, L.K., WESTCOTT, R.N., SUAREZ, E. and LOZADA, J. (1968). Ventricular aneurysm. Clinical experience. *Ann. Thorac. Surg.*, **6**, 227
4. LOOP, F.D., EFFLER, D.B., WEBSTER, J.S. and GROVES, L.K. (1973). Posterior ventricular aneurysms. *N. Engl. J. Med.*, **288**, 237
5. LOOP, F.D., EFFLER, D.B., NAVIA, J.A., SHELDON, W.C. and GROVES, L.K. (1973). Aneurysms of the left ventricle. Survival and results of a ten-year surgical experience. *Ann. Surg.*, **178**, 399
6. IBARRA–PEREZ, C. and LILLEHEI, C.W. (1969). Resection of postinfarction ventricular aneurysms and simultaneous myocardial revascularization. *J. Cardiovasc. Surg.*, **10**, 419
7. CASTANY, R., CERENE, A., PUEL, P. and ENJALBERT, A. (1974). Left ventricular aneurysm resulting from myocardial infarction. *J. Cardiovasc. Surg.*, **15**, 74
8. NAJAFI, H., DYE, W.S., JAVID, H., HUNTER, J.A., GOLDIN, M.D. and SERRY, C. (1975). Current surgical management of left ventricular aneurysm. *Arch. Surg.*, **110**, 1027
9. DUBNOW, M.H., BURCHELL, H.B. and TITUS, J.L. (1965). Postinfarction ventricular aneurysm: a clinicomorphologic and electrocardiographic study of 80 cases. *Am. Heart J.*, **70**, 753
10. SCHLICHTER, J., HELLERSTEIN, H.K. and KATZ, L.N. (1954). Aneurysm of the heart: a correlative study of one hundred and two proved cases. *Medicine (Baltimore)*, **33**, 43
11. TODD, T.C. and MOSCOVITZ. (1969). Ventricular aneurysms in the aged. *Can. Med. Assoc. J.*, **100**, 162
12. WANG, C.H., BLAND, E.F. and WHITE, P.D. (1948). A note on coronary occlusion and myocardial infarction found post mortem at the Massachusetts General Hospital during the twenty year period from 1926 to 1945 inclusive. *Ann. Intern. Med.*, **29**, 601

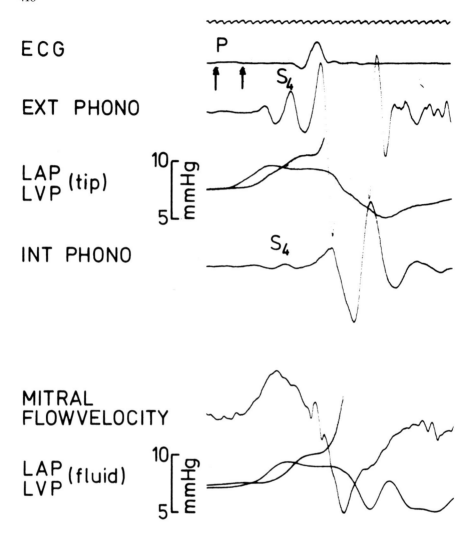

Figure 34.2 Pressure–flow–sound relationship during and after atrial contraction.

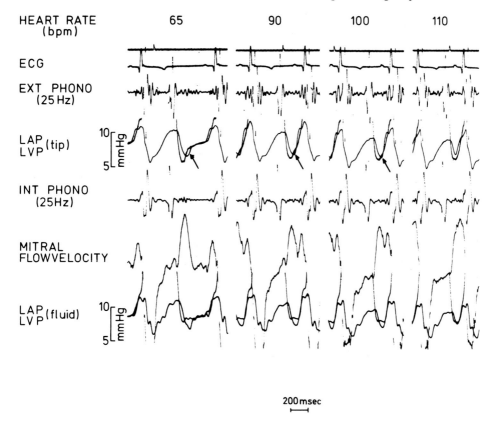

Figure 34.3 Continuous changes of mitral flow and transmitral pressure gradient after administration of atropine. Arrows indicate negative gradient.

Inflation of the balloon resulted in a fall of all diastolic pressures, a fading out of the rapid filling wave and the A wave, a much slower deceleration of diastolic flow and the disappearance of the gallop sounds. In nine dogs where gallop sounds could be recorded from the chest wall, the microphone was placed in direct contact with the epicardial surface of the freely exposed left ventricle, carefully avoiding contact with the chest wall. With the microphone on the epicardium, comparable low-frequency vibrations could be recorded. These findings strongly suggest that impact of the heart against the chest wall is not essential for the genesis of gallop sounds. We conclude that LV pressure rise in response to filling (so-called rapid filling wave and A wave) reverses the transmitral pressure gradient and decelerates flow. During this process of deceleration, the cardiohemic system will be set into vibrations which may become audible and recordable from the chest if they are transmitted with sufficient intensity.

By this mechanism both LV filling rate (dependent on cardiac output, relaxation and atrial contraction strength) and the height and speed of LV pressure in early and late diastole (dependent on viscoelastic properties of the myocardium) will determine the amount of deceleration and hence the occurrence and the intensity of gallop sounds.

420

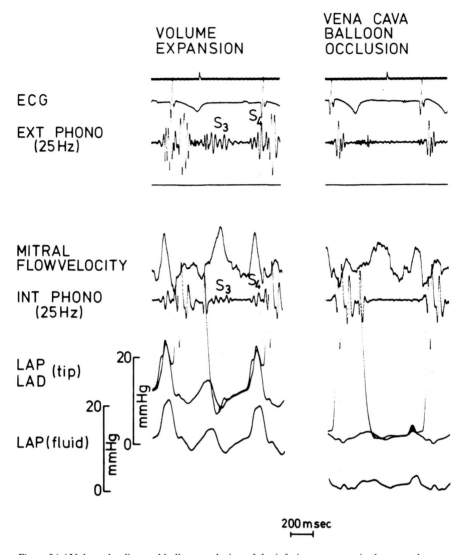

VOLUME
EXPANSION

VENA CAVA
BALLOON
OCCLUSION

ECG

EXT PHONO
(25 Hz)

S₃ S₄

MITRAL
FLOWVELOCITY

INT PHONO
(25 Hz)

S₃ S₄

LAP (tip)
LAD

20

mmHg

20

LAP(fluid)

mmHg

0

0

200 m sec

Figure 34.4 Volume loading and balloon occlusion of the inferior vena cava in the same dog.

Reference

1. RUSHMER, R.F. (1976). *Cardiovascular Dynamics*, 4th edn., p. 421. Philadelphia: W.B. Saunders Company

35

Pulmonary function 8 years after mitral valve replacement

Kim Böök and Alf Holmgren

Mitral valve replacement will in most instances result in marked improvement of central haemodynamics in patients with severe mitral valve disease. This has been shown in several reports of both early and late follow-up results[1-4]. The fate of the lungs is more controversial and not so well documented, especially regarding long-term findings. Mitral valve disease may indeed be regarded as a disease affecting both central haemodynamics and lungs; follow-up studies must take into consideration both these factors and relate each of them to the degree of improvement in patients who have undergone mitral valve replacement. We have focused our interest on haemodynamic studies after mitral valve replacement; our earlier reports[5-7] are in agreement with other publications on similar patients. It is generally accepted that mitral valve replacement results in improved physical work capacity, reduces the incidence of atrial fibrillation, increases cardiac output, reduces pulmonary arterial and left atrial pressures and decreases pulmonary vascular resistance. The patients experience less distressing symptoms and can be referred to a better functional capacity group according to NYHA classification.

The improved pulmonary circulation prompted a study regarding the reversibility of the deterioration of lung function and mechanics in patients who had had their mitral valve replaced[8]. In this chapter we present determinations of static and dynamic lung volumes, ventilation and alveolar gas exchange including diffusing capacity as well as pressure–flow relationship in the lung circulation, before and 1 year after mitral valve replacement. The improvement in lung function was slight in comparison with the significant haemodynamic improvement, indicating that the lung changes in mitral valve disease were less reversible. It was concluded that either the lung function impairment was more irreversible than haemodynamic changes or that the observation period of 1 year was too short, i.e. lung function might improve further with time. To clarify this, the present study was undertaken and the same patients were re-investigated 8–9 years after mitral valve replacement with identical methods regarding lung function and haemodynamic evaluation.

Materials

Fourteen patients were re-investigated 8–9 (mean 8.4) years after mitral valve replacement. The same patients had also been evaluated 7–13 (mean 9.5) months after surgery. There were eight women and six men and the age at operation ranged from 35 to 63 with a mean age of 51 years. The patients were accepted for mitral valve replacement due to clinical and haemodynamic signs of advanced mitral valve heart disease. The standard preoperative evaluation was performed in every patient and included bicycle ergometer work test, determination of total haemoglobin and total blood volume, determination of heart volume in the supine position, static and dynamic spirometry, analyses of central circulation with left and right heart catheterization and left ventricular angiography. In these patients determinations of ventilatory function and alveolar gas exchange including diffusing capacity and blood gases were added to the standard preoperative evaluation.

Isolated mitral stenosis was present in no patient, isolated mitral incompetence in six patients and combined mitral lesion in eight patients. Before surgery, five patients were in Group II and nine in Group III (NYHA). The patients generally had a low work capacity, heart volume and total haemoglobin were large, and mean pressures in the pulmonary artery and left atrium as well as the pulmonary vascular resistance were elevated.

Surgery with excision of the diseased mitral valve and replacement with Bjork–Shiley tilting disc mitral valve prosthesis was performed 1970–1972. A first postoperative follow-up study was performed 7–13 (mean 9.5) months following operation. The same protocol as in the preoperative evaluation was followed and included lung function studies. A new re-investigation was then repeated 8–9 (mean 8.4) years after surgery again using identical methods as in the preoperative evaluation.

Methods

Right and left heart catheterization was performed in the standard way in all patients. Pulmonary function was analyzed with conventional methods. Functional residual capacity was determined with helium dilution in a closed system with simultaneous measurement of total lung capacity. Dynamic spirometry was performed with a computerized Bernstein sprimeter. Normal values were computed from the regression equation published by Berglund et al.[9] Alveolar gas exchange and ventilation was analyzed with Douglas bag technique as was the steady state diffusing capacity for carbon monoxide during exercise. All calculations were performed off line on an IBM 1800 computer.

Results

Inherent in a retrospective study of this type is the high degree of selection. At the time of surgery it may be stated that only patients with moderate to severe mitral valve disease were accepted for valve replacement. They all showed signs of pulmonary circulatory changes of varying degree. Ventilatory function was far from normal. We must point out, though, that patients with severe tricuspid incompetence, needing surgical intervention, are not included in the series. At the early follow-up, a little less than a year following surgery, a certain selection had already occurred since the most seriously ill patients had already died or were in too bad a clinical state to undergo a re-investigation. At late follow-up a further selection has taken place, in part mirrored by the smaller number of patients taking part in this evaluation. Only the patients with the best myocardial and pulmonary functional reserve are left for study. It might be added that very few of the patients asked to join the study refused to do so. Apart from this, it must be pointed out that the patients are more than 8 years older than when they were operated on. Bearing the selection and the age factor heavily in mind, we may now proceed to present our results.

There were no changes in Functional Class (NYHA) when comparison was made between the early and the late follow-up. The increase in functional ability seen 1 year after surgery was maintained after 8 years. In *Table 35.1* some relevant preoperative data are compared with the late follow-up. In a similar comparison between preoperative data and the early follow-up highly significant improvement was observed but in this table only minor changes are seen. Thus, the central circulation has somewhat deteriorated 8 years after surgery in comparison with the situation 1 year after surgery.

TABLE 35.1 Some anthropometric data, circulatory data and intracardiac pressures before and 8.4 years after mitral valve replacement

Variable	W_{max} (kpm/min)	HV (ml)	THb (g)	$\bar{P}_{PA}$ (mm Hg)		$\bar{P}_{LA}$ or $\bar{P}_{PCV}$ (mm Hg)		PVR (units)		AVD (ml/l)	
				R	E	R	E	R	E	R	E
Pre x̄	417	1421	673	25.9	42.8	18.7	31.9	3.30	3.86	62.7	117.7
SD	257	648	180	6.0	11.7	4.2	7.9	1.46	1.86	7.1	17.7
Post x̄ (II)	544	1294	623	21.4	38.3	15.0	30.3	2.68	2.58	52.5	104.6
SD	168	601	141	4.2	8.8	5.0	8.7	1.14	1.28	7.6	14.3
d̄	−127	127	50	4.5	4.4	3.7	1.6	0.62	1.28	10.2	13.1
n	14	13	14	13	12	14	12	13	12	14	9
p	<0.05	>0.3	<0.05	<0.05	>0.02	>0.05	>0.4	>0.1	<0.05	<0.01	<0.01
Sign	x		x	x					x	xx	xx

W_{max} = Maximum working capacity; HV = heart volume; THb = total haemoglobin; $\bar{P}_{PA}$ = pulmonary arterial mean pressure; $\bar{P}_{LA}$ = left atrial mean pressure; $\bar{P}_{PCV}$ = pulmonary capillary venous pressure; PVR = pulmonary vascular resistance; AVD = arterio-venous oxygen difference; Pre x̄ = mean value of variable pre-operatively; Post x̄ = mean valve of variable post-operatively; d̄ = mean difference; sign = significance; R = rest; E = exercise.

Working capacity before operation and at the two postoperative evaluations is depicted for the individual patients in *Figure 35.1* and the majority of patients are able to perform at a greater work load at the late follow-up. The pulmonary artery mean pressure increase at rest and during exercise is shown in *Figure 35.2* and the same general pattern may be observed regarding the mean left atrial pressure in *Figure 35.3*. Without doubt, an impairment of the central haemodynamic situation is seen after 8 years compared with after 1 year but it is rather slight.

Regarding pulmonary function it seems logical to first look at the state of pulmonary vascular bed. *Figure 35.4* shows the pulmonary vascular resistance at 1 year plotted against the 8-year figures at rest and during exercise. As might be expected, most patients show a slight but definite increase. In *Figure 35.5*, where the preoperative findings are compared with both of the postoperative studies, a net decrease of the pulmonary vascular resistance is demonstrated.

Vital capacity, expressed as per cent of predicted value, is increased already at the early follow-up and even more so at the 8-year evaluation (*see Figure 35.6*)

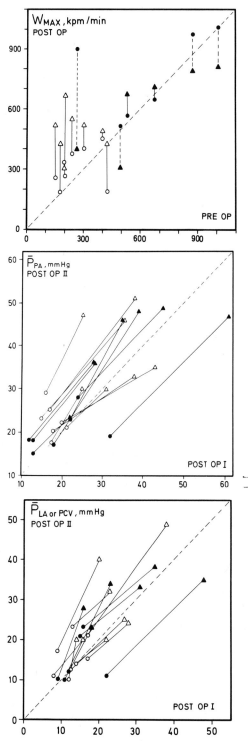

Figure 35.1 Maxium working capacity (W_{max} (kpm/min)) before 1 year and 8 years after mitral valve replacement in 14 patients.
o = Females at 1 year after operation;
● = males at 1 year after operation;
△ = females at 8 years after operation;
▲ = males at 8 years after operation. Observations in patients increasing their W_{max} at 8 years are joined by unbroken line; those in patients decreasing their W_{max} at 8 years are joined by broken line.

Figures 35.2 Pulmonary arterial mean pressure, $\bar{P}_{PA}$ (mm Hg) at 1 year and 8 years after mitral valve replacement at rest and during exercise in 13 patients. o = Females at rest; ● = males at rest; △ = females during exercise; ▲ = males during exercise.

Figure 35.3 Left atrial, ($\bar{P}_{LA}$ (mm Hg)) or pulmonary capillary venous pressure, (P_{PCV} (mm Hg)) at rest and during exercise 1 year and 8 years following mitral valve replacement in 14 patients. Symbols as in *Figure 35.2*.

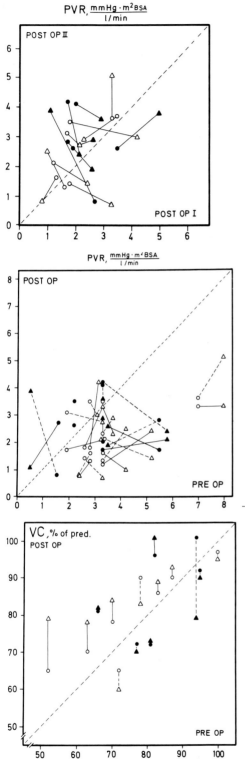

Figure 35.4 Pulmonary vascular resistance (PVR (mm Hg/*l*/min/m² BSA)) at rest and during exercise 1 year and 8 years after mitral valve replacement in 13 patients. Symbols as in *Figure 35.2*.

Figure 35.5 Pulmonary vascular resistance (PVR (mm Hg/*l*/min/m² BSA)) at rest and during exercise before, 1 year and 8 years following mitral valve replacement in 13 patients. o = Females at rest; ● = males at rest; △ = females during exercise; ▲ = males during exercise; —— = observations at 1 year; – – – = observations at 8 years.

Figure 35.6 Vital capacity (VC), expressed as per cent of predicted value, before, 1 year and 8 years after mitral valve replacement in 14 patients. Symbols as in *Figure 35.1*.

indicating an improved ventilatory function of the lungs. An even more marked improvement of gas exchange, expressed as diffusing capacity for carbon monoxide (*see Figure 35.7*), is seen in all but two patients and the increase is significantly greater at 8 years compared with the 1-year follow-up. When alveolo-arterial oxygen difference is related to oxygen consumption there is a significant increase preoperatively in comparison with normals (*see Figure 35.8*), but a tendency toward normal values is found 1 year after operation. Eight years after operation, however, a return to preoperative levels is demonstrated.

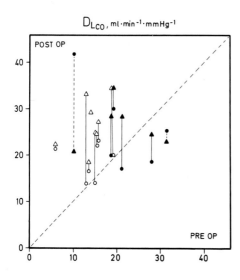

Figure 35.7 Diffusing capacity for carbon monoxide (D_{LCO} (ml/min/mm Hg)) before, 1 year and 8 years following mitral valve replacement in 13 patients. Symbols as in *Figure 35.1*.

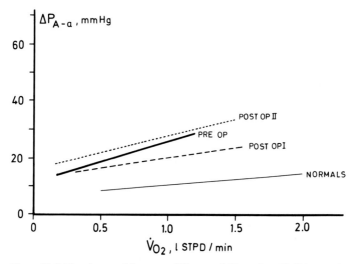

Figure 35.8 Alveolo–arterial oxygen difference (ΔP_{A-a} (mm Hg)) in relation to oxygen consumption ($\dot{V}_{O2}$ (*l* STPD/min)) in normals and before, 1 year and 8 years after mitral valve replacement.

Discussion

In summary, the central circulatory state has slightly deteriorated during the 7 years elapsing between the early and late follow-up, and is believed to be due mainly to the age factor. The same pattern is demonstrated regarding pulmonary circulation. Working capacity is, however, for the majority of patients, increased at 8 years in comparison with the 1-year evaluation. Ventilatory function is clearly improved—only a very slight improvement is demonstrated 1 year following surgery but after 8 years this improvement is much more prominent. Since the vascular resistance in the lung has increased, this improvement must be due to a better bellows function resulting in a more effective diffusion capacity. In contrast to this the alveolo-arterial oxygen difference increased at late follow-up. This alveolo-arterial oxygen difference increase may be caused by the presence of a shunt, by changes in the ventilation–perfusion ratio or by poor diffusion. There is no reason to believe that major shunts are present in this group of patients and the diffusion capacity is shown to increase. Changes in the ventilation–perfusion ratio due to aging is a possible explanation but remains to be proven, and is planned to be undertaken using the inert gas technique.

In conclusion, this chapter shows that despite haemodynamic improvement, lung function remains poor at an evaluation performed 1 year after mitral valve replacement but after 8 years the ventilatory function is somewhat restored due mainly to a better bellows function. The impaired lung function caused by long-standing mitral valve disease takes many years to recover.

References

1. BRAUNWALD, E., BRAUNWALD, N., ROSS, J. and MORROW, A. (1965). Effects of mitral valve replacement on the pulmonary valvular dynamics of patients with pulmonary hypertension. *N. Engl. J. Med.*, **273**, 509

2. RAMSEY, H., WILLIAMS, C., JR., VERNON, C., WHEAT, M., DAICOFF, G. and BARTLEY, T. (1971). Hemodynamic findings following replacement of the mitral valve with the Ball valve prothesis. *J. Thor. Cardiovasc. Surg.*, **62**, 624

3. LEE, S., ZARAGOZA, A., CALLAGHAN, J., ROSSAL, R. and FRAZER, R. (1971). Hemodynamic changes following mitral valve replacement with the Starr–Edwards and Cutter–Smeloff protheses. *J. Thor. Cardiovasc. Surg.*, **61**, 688

4. HOLLINRAKE, K., BAIDYA, M. and YACOUB, M. (1973). Haemodynamic changes in patients with high pulmonary vascular resistance after mitral valve replacement. *Brit. Heart J.*, **35**, 1047

5. BJÖRK, V.O., BÖÖK, K., CERNIGLIARO, C. and HOLMGREN, A. (1973). The Björk–Shiley tilting disc valve in isolated mitral lesions. *Scand. J. Thor. Cardiovasc. Surg.*, **7**, 131

6. BJÖRK, V.O., BÖÖK, K. and HOLMGREN, A. (1973). Significance of position and opening angle of the Björk–Shiley tilting disc valve in mitral surgery. *Scand. J. Thor. Cardiovasc. Surg.*, **7**, 187

7. BÖÖK, K. (1974). Mitral valve replacement with the Björk–Shiley tilting disc valve. *Scand. J. Thor. Cardiovasc. Surg.*, Suppl. 12

8. BÖÖK, K. and HOLMGREN, A. (1979). Long term changes of pulmonary function following cardiac surgery. *Cardiac Lung*, p. 433. Italy: Piccin Medical Books.

9. BERGLUND, E., BIRATH, B., BJURE, J., *et al.* (1963). Spirometric studies in normal subjects. *Acta Med. Scand.*, **173**, 185

36

Chordal rupture: Repair or replacement?

Keith Dawkins, David Oliveira, Philip Kay and Matthias Paneth

Introduction

With the introduction of open-heart surgery in the 1950s, effective surgical treatment for mitral regurgitation became available for the first time[1-3]. In many cases of mitral regurgitation secondary to ruptured chordae tendineae (RCT) there is no shortage of relatively normal valve tissue. This fact, together with the known problems associated with prosthethic valves, has stimulated the development of conservative procedures in this condition.

McGoon[4] in 1958 was the first to describe a specific technique for the repair of RCT although the condition had been treated prior to this with annuloplasty[5, 6]. Since then there have been a substantial number of reports dealing with a variety of repair techniques and the results obtained with them[7-27]. Others, in view of the initially rather variable outcome following repair, have preferred mitral valve replacement[28-31].

In recent years the advantages of repair over replacement in selected cases of mitral regurgitation have become clear, but there are no large series comparing the two operations in cases due solely to RCT. The purpose of this chapter is to review all cases of surgically treated RCT seen recently at the Brompton Hospital and to carry out such a comparison.

Patients and methods

The case records of all 211 patients found to have RCT at open-heart surgery for mitral regurgitation in the years 1970–1980 inclusive were reviewed. Patients with non-rheumatic mitral regurgitation due to 'floppy valves' caused by a dilated annulus (without RCT) were excluded from the study. In patients where there had been extensive destruction or retraction of valve tissue secondary to previous rheumatic heart disease, surgery or bacterial endocarditis, repair was clearly not feasible, and these patients were also excluded. No patients with ruptured papillary muscle have been included, nor have patients who underwent additional surgery (e.g. aortic valve replacement, tricuspid plication, CABG etc.). The remaining 183 patients represent a population that might reasonably have been treated with repair or replacement, and form the basis of this chapter. The mean age at the time of surgery was 57 years (range 4–78 years), 87 of whom were males and 96 females (1:1.1). Of the 183 patients, 82(45%) underwent mitral valve repair, and 101(55%) mitral valve replacement. In 11 patients mitral repair was technically unsatisfactory, and mitral replacement was carried out at the same operation. Five further patients required late mitral valve replacement (mean 1.4 years after repair), for significant mitral regurgitation.

Results

Mitral valve repair

82 patients underwent mitral valves repair, with a mean (±SD) age of 59±12 years. In 75(91%) no clear aetiology for the chordal rupture could be defined, and these patients are subsequently referred to as having 'spontaneous' rupture. In 7(9%) documented subacute bacterial endocarditis had occurred on a previously normal valve. 59(72%) of patients were in sinus rhythm, 22(27%) in atrial fibrillation, and 1 in complete atrioventricular block. 70(85%) of patients had rupture of the posterior chordae, 10(12%) rupture of the anterior chordae, and 2 rupture of the chordae to both mitral valve cusps. Of the 11 patients in whom mitral repair was unsuccessful, and mitral replacement had to be undertaken at the same operation, 7 had posterior rupture, 2 had anterior rupture, and 2 rupture of the chordae to both cusps. Four of the 5 patients requiring late mitral replacement had anterior rupture, and the remaining patient posterior rupture (*see Figure 36.1*).

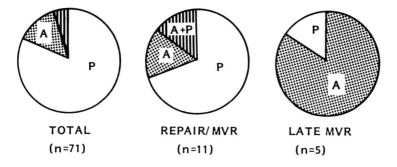

A = ANTERIOR, P = POSTERIOR, A + P = BOTH CUSPS

Figure 36.1 Mitral valve repair: cusps involved. MVR = Mitral valve replacement.

SURGICAL TECHNIQUE

Mitral valve repair was based on the method of Carpentier[25], in which a triangular section of the anterior mitral valve leaflet, and/or a trapezoid section of the posterior leaflet was resected as appropriate to restore valve competence. In addition, two circumferential 2–0 Ethilon sutures were used to reinforce the annulus. The repair technique used has evolved during the time course of the series, and descriptions of the earlier[21], and more recent[22, 26] methods have been published. Patients were not routinely anticoagulated following surgery.

EARLY MORTALITY

The in-hosptial early mortality in this group was 4/82(4.9%). Three of these patients had undergone simple mitral repair. One died of pump failure, one of haemorrhage, and one of an acute myocardial infarct. One further patient died following attempted mitral repair followed by mitral replacement, from valve dehiscence caused by prosthetic endocarditis.

LATE MORTALITY

During the follow-up period (mean 3.6 years, range 0.08–12.2 years), 4 further patients died: 2 of pump failure, 1 fom SBE, and 1 died suddenly (possibly as a result of an arrhythmia).

Mitral valve replacement

101 patients (mean age 56±15 years) underwent mitral valve replacement. In 79(78%) chordal rupture was 'spontaneous'. 16(16%) had documented SBE, 11(11%) on a normal valve, and 5(5%) on a valve previously affected by rheumatic carditis, 5(5%) had ischaemic heart disease, and 1(1%) had RCT complicating acute rheumatic fever. 58(57%) were in sinus rhythm, and the remaining 43(43%) in atrial fibrillation. RCT were found in the posterior cusp in 31(31%), anterior cusp in 58(57%), and involving both mitral cusps in 12(12%).

SURGICAL TECHNIQUE

Mitral valve replacement was undertaken using standard techniques with a variety of prostheses. 46(46%) had a Starr–Edwards 6120 prosthesis, 27(27%) a Bjork–Shiley tilting disc valve, 18(18%) a Carpentier–Edwards porcine xenograft, 9(9%) an aortic homograft, and in one patient on Omniscience tilting disc valve was implanted. Following surgery, patients were anticoagulated with warfarin to maintain the British Standard Prothrombin Ratio at 2.0–2.5.

EARLY MORTALITY

In the valve replacement group the hospital mortality was 5/101 (5%). Four patients died of pump failure, and 1(1%) of prosthetic endocarditis.

LATE MORTALITY

During the follow-up period a further 23 patients died. The causes of death are listed in *Table 36.1*. In one patient (*see Table 36.1*) death was due to pulmonary edema caused by thrombosis of a Bjork–Shiley valve as a result of discontinuing oral anticoagulants. Details of the 8/23(35%) of patients dying from cerebrovascular events are listed in *Table 36.2*. Mean age of this subgroup was 55 years (range 40–71 years). Five out of eight were males, and six out of eight were in sinus rhythm. Five out of eight sustained cerebral emboli, and two of these patients suffered a previous embolism, prior to the event that caused death. In two out of eight the cause of death was cerebral haemorrhage. In the remaining patient the cause of the cerebrovascular event was unknown. Post-mortem confirmation was

TABLE 36.1 Mitral valve replacement: Causes of late mortality

Cerebrovascular events	8 (35%)
Pump failure	6
Sepsis	3
SBE	2
Sudden death	1
Hepatic failure	1
Haemorrhage	1
Prosthetic thrombosis*	1

*See text.

TABLE 36.2 Mitral valve replacement: Cerebrovascular events causing late mortality

Age (years)	Sex	Valve	Rhythm	Pathology
71	M	SE	SR	Embolism
67	F	SE	AF	Haemorrhage
61	F	SE	SR	Embolism
40	F	SE	SR	Embolism
47	M	BS	SR	?
52	M	BS	AF	Embolism (×2)
65	M	BS	SR	Haemorrhage
40	M	HOMO	SR	Embolism (×2)

SE = Starr–Edwards; BS = Bjork–Shiley; HOMO = aortic homograft; SR = sinus rhythm; AF = atrial fibrillation.

available in five out of eight patients. There was no statistical difference in the incidence of thromboembolism with the various types of prosthesis. The lack of complications with the Carpentier–Edwards xenograft is probably related to the fact that these valves were only implanted in 18% of patients, mainly in the last few years, resulting in a shorter period of follow-up in this subgroup.

ACTUARIAL SURVIVAL

Actuarial survival curves (32) predict a 6-year survival of 88(±6.9)% for those patients who underwent mitral valve repair, compared with a 6-year survival of 68(±5.7)% for mitral valve replacement (p < 0.01) (*see Figure 36.2*). Patients who had attempted repair followed by mitral valve replacement have been included in the valve replacement group for the purposes of actuarial analysis.

FUNCTIONAL CLASS

Preoperatively, 56% of the valve replacement group and 51% of the repair group were in New York Heart Association functional class III or IV. Postoperatively, 82% of the replacement group and 83% of the repair group were in NYHA class I.

CARDIAC CATHETERIZATION

It is not the policy at the Brompton Hospital to catheterize routinely all patients with valvular heart disease[33]. In this series 30 out of 82(37%) of the repair group, and 47 out of 101(47%) of the replacement group underwent cardiac catheterization. Actuarial survival at 6 years was not influenced by cardiac catheterization (catheter group, 80±6.1%; no catheter group, 80±7.7%; difference not significant) (*see Figure 36.3*).

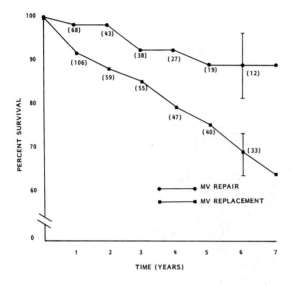

Figure 36.2 Actuarial survival curves in patients undergoing mitral valve repair or replacement.

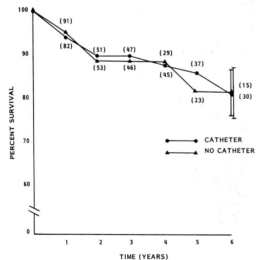

Figure 36.3 Actuarial survival curves in patients with chordal rupture receiving a catheter and in those not receiving a catheter.

Discussion

Not all cases of RCT will require surgery. In the eight cases reported by Ronan *et al.*[34] three improved and were maintained on medical treatment 6, 12 and 36 months after their initial symptoms. However, these cases represent the minority and for most the choice lies between mitral valve replacement and repair.

The decision as to when to operate in mitral regurgitation may not be straightforward. Kay et al.[23] state that the criteria should be solely symptomatic, but a recent study[35] of prognostic factors in surgery for non-rheumatic mitral regurgitation found that variables such as short history (< 1 year) and a normal left ventricular end-diastolic volume index($< 100 \, ml/m^2$) were favourable prognostic factors. An ejection fraction of under 0.5 was uniformly associated with a poor outcome. These results suggest that operative intervention should be considered earlier rather than later before irreversible myocardial damage occurs.

Having decided to operate the choice of surgery lies between repair and replacement. This decision is best made after inspection of the valve, and Carpentier et al.[25] have published detailed indications for and against repair depending upon the precise cause of the regurgitation. Other factors to be considered include the experience of the surgeon in the repair technique and the results from previously published series. This present series is not strictly comparable with earlier reports as there are no other large series dealing exclusively with cases of mitral regurgitation secondary to RCT.

Comparison between the repair and replacement groups is only meaningful if there are no significant differences in the incidence of risk factors between the two groups. The two groups were comparable for age and preoperative functional status. Early mortality for mitral repair or replacement was very similar at 4.9% and 5.0%, respectively, which compares favourably with other series. The differences in late mortality between the two groups are striking. There were no cerebrovascular episodes in the repair group, but 10 episodes occurred in the replacement group, resulting in eight deaths. Of interest is the low incidence of atrial fibrillation in these patients (2 out of 8), despite the higher incidence of atrial fibrillation in the replacement group as a whole (43 vs. 27%). In five out of eight patients death was due to thromboembolism, a complication of the prosthesis, in two out of eight it was due to cerebral haemorrhage complicating anticoagulant therapy, and in the remaining patient the cause of the cerebrovascular event was unknown. The results in the replacement group were not biased by one particular prosthesis performing badly (see Table 36.2).

The results of this series, therefore, are in agreement with those of Yacoub et al.[27], which is the only other sizeable series comparing the two operations in a relatively uniform population, in demonstrating the significantly greater survival with repair. In the survivors, both operations produced a similar improvement in functional status. However, in Yacoub's series only a proportion of patients had mitral regurgitation secondary to chordal rupture; furthermore mitral repair was compared with mitral replacement using a free aortic homograft in all patients, and not a mechanical prosthesis.

The influence of which leaflet is affected on the success or otherwise of the repair is shown in Figure 36.1. Thus anterior leaflet chordal rupture is associated with a disproportionately high incidence of both intra-operative and late failure of repair. This conforms with the experience of Carpentier et al.[24] who found that if resection of one fourth or more of the anterior leaflet was required to control regurgitation, the repair was contraindicated. Similarly, Gerbode et al.[19] treated four cases of anterior leaflet RCT and two out of the three with RCT to both leaflets in their series with mitral valve replacement. Other authors, although not commenting on the actual incidence of anterior leaflet RCT, do not seem to have had an excess of failed repairs in this group[23, 26].

The surgical management of valvular heart disease without prior cardiac

37

The reconstruction of the mitral valve with stabilized biological tissue in 33 clinical cases

R. Deac, D. Bratu, M. Liebhart, S. Bradisteanu, M. Poliac, E. Fagarasan and V. Bilca

The complex structure of the mitral valve and its interrelated function with other components of the mitral apparatus and left ventricle make duplication with an artificial substitute difficult.

Clinical application of heart valve replacement and the search for an ideal valvular substitute has entered the third decade. While the search continues, conservative surgery of the mitral valve is still indicated in cases with anatomically correctable lesions. Although the literature contains much information about mitral valve reconstruction procedures for mitral incompetence[1-8], there are few reports on the conservative surgery with leaflet advancement for mitral stenosis. We are not aware of the utilization of a stabilized biological tissue for mitral valve reconstruction in cases with isolated or predominant mitral stenosis.

Dissatisfaction with the long-term results, the hemodynamic performance, the need for anticoagulant treatment, the high cost of available valvular substitutes and improved surgical techniques with myocardial protection offered by the hypothermic cardioplegia has renewed interest in the reconstruction of the mitral valve.

Previous works of Sauvage et al.[9], Selmonosky et al.[10], Bailey et al.[11, 12], Marion et al.[12] and Frater et al.[13] have described reconstruction of the mitral valve by leaflet advancement using autologous biological tissue (pericardium, fascia lata). The long-term fate of these tissues in the mitral area has not been reported, and there is concern that shrinkage of autologous fresh pericardium and fascia lata will cause stricture of the valve repair. Stabilized biologic tissue of human or animal origin do not have this tendency, thus prompting us to evaluate its use for leaflet advancement. In this sense, it is used in combination with complete valvotomy for mitral valve reconstruction for mitral stenosis.

Material and methods

Between February 1980 and July 1983, 33 patients with predominant mitral stenosis of rheumatic origin underwent surgery. In this group, 29 were females (87%) and four males (12.2%). The mean age was 35 (age range 22–56 years). Eighteen patients had isolated mitral stenosis, six had predominant stenosis associated with mitral incompetence and nine cases had mitral stenosis associated with other valvular lesions. Twenty-two patients were in sinus rhythm and 12 in atrial fibrillation. At the time of operation, two patients were in New York Heart Association Functional Class II, 29 in Class III and one in Class IV. Two patients had previous closed mitral valvotomy. Left atrial thrombus was found intraoperatively in five patients and two patients had previous cerebral embolism. Only eight patients, mainly those with associated anomalies, had hemodynamic studies performed before the operation.

Complete mitral valvotomy combined with mitral valvuloplasty by patch advancement of the mural leaflet were performed in 27 cases of mitral stenosis as an isolated lesion or associated with minor to moderate mitral incompetence. In three cases, the above-mentioned procedures were combined with aortic valvuloplasty for lesions not requiring valve replacement and in two cases were additional procedures for aortic valve replacement. In one case, two other conservative procedures were necessary for tricuspid and aortic valve lesions, combined with the mitral procedures.

Operative technique

The patients were operated on through median sternotomy under cardiopulmonary bypass with moderate body hypothermia (25–30°C) combined with cardioplegic arrest and local cooling for myocardial protection. Left ventricular (LV) vent was introduced via LV apex. Wide exposure of the mitral valve was obtained through an incision in the left atrium (LA), posterior to the interatrial groove, and facilitated by the flaccid heart under cardioplegia.

Intraoperative findings

The mitral orifice was estimated by the operating surgeon as being between 1 and 1.5 cm^2 in 18 cases and below 1 cm^2 in nine cases. Twenty-four cases showed alterations at the papillary muscle level. There were six patients with one papillary muscle in contact with the free margin of the leaflet and seven patients with both papillary muscles at the level of the leaflet. In 12 cases, incision of one papillary muscle was performed and in the other 12 cases both papillary muscles were incised. In this group of 24 patients, five valves were fenestrated. In 24 cases, there were changes at the chordae level with thickening, fusion and shortening. In all 33 cases, the mural leaflet was thickened and shortened. Both commissures were fused and fibrotic.

Complete mitral valvotomy was performed by bilateral commissurotomy, splitting of the papillary muscles and mobilization of leaflets and subvalvular structures. The shortened mural leaflets was incised at its insertion for most of the circumference up to 5–10 mm to the commissural area. Few third-degree chordae were sectioned. Through this incision, the subvalvular structures are examined from the ventricular aspect and further mobilization of the chordae, papillary muscles and leaflets is performed. Commissurotomy is carried further from this approach. The decision to reconstruct or to replace the valve is made only after the examination of the mitral apparatus from above and below through the described incision.

After the complete valvotomy which produced an adequate mitral orifice, a stabilized biological tissue patch was inserted in the incision at the base of the mural leaflet by a continuous single 3/0 Ethibond suture. The stabilized biological tissue patch was tailored according to the size of the orifice in the mural leaflet and to the desired shape of the leaflet to allow efficient coaptation with the anterior leaflet. One important technical detail is to suture from the annulus to the patch to avoid a close contact between the tissue and the LV wall. The position and the shape of the reconstructed leaflet will be determined by this suture.

In 29 cases, the biological tissue patch used was human dura mater stabilized with Glutharaldehyde and in four cases the patch was heterologous pericardium. The competence of the mitral valve was assessed intraoperatively by known procedures:

1. Visual examination of the mobility and passive coaptation by simple approximation of the two leaflets.
2. Testing the valve closure in relaxed state of the LV with fluid under pressure introduced via left ventricular vent at the apex (aorta cross clamped).
3. Filling of the LV cavity with blood from aortic incompetence (aorta unclamped).
4. Inspection of the valve in the beating heart with protective measures taken against air embolism.
5. Inspection of the mitral valve with the finger through the left atrial appendage and extracardiac palpation of the LA to detect thrill of mitral incompetence.
6. Use of a sterile stethoscope to detect murmurs.
7. Pressure measurements.

The cardiopulmonary bypass time varied from 65 to 116 minutes with a mean of 81 minutes for isolated procedures and from 105 to 173 minutes (mean 134 minutes) in the group with associated procedures. Two cases were operated upon with a beating heart with a mean perfusion time of 100 minutes. Thirty-one cases were operated upon under cardioplegia with a mean aortic cross-clamped time of 47 minutes for isolated procedures and 68 minutes for the group with associated procedures.

The first patients were anticoagulated with prothrombin depressant for 6 weeks. Three patients were on continuous anticoagulation treatment, two for aortic valve replacement with Bjork–Shiley valves and one for left atrial thrombus removed at the operation (patient in atrial fibrillation).

Intraoperative assessment of mitral valve competence showed mild mitral regurgitation in four cases. In two cases, the incompetence at the commissural area was corrected by sutures with Teflon pledgets, and in the other two cases it was left uncorrected.

Results

There was no operative or hospital death in the present series. Thirty-three patients left the hospital and 32 (97%) were followed up between 4 and 32 months after the operation (mean 13.8 months). One 32-year-old patient, operated upon in April 1982 for mitral stenosis and left atrial thrombus, left the hospital in good clinical condition, but did not answer our call for follow-up. We received no information about complications or death in this case.

All the patients examined recently have improved after operation except two of them. Twenty-one patients are now in NYHA Class I, eight in Class II, one in Class

II and one in Class IV. One patient, although improved after the operation, is still in Class III. She has a 3/VI systolic murmur in the mitral area since the operation due to a mild regurgitation at posteromedial commissure. The second patient with other valvular-associated lesions did not improve after the operation. She is now in the hospital 30 months after the operation with tricuspid incompetence and chronic renal failure. She has a 1/VI systolic murmur at the apex.

At clinical examination, two patients have systolic murmurs, grade 3/VI in the mitral area (one with mitral incompetence before the operation). Five patients have a 1–2/VI systolic murmur at the apex (three had mitral incompetence before the operation). Twenty-two patients have competent mitral valves. Eight patients with previous mitral incompetence have no systolic murmur in the mitral area. To summarize, 23 patients had no systolic murmur, six had a 1–2/VI murmur and three had a 3/VI murmur.

The cardiothoracic ratio could be calculated in 30 patients: in three cases it did not change in comparison with before the operation, in 19 cases decreased and in seven cases increased (five with systolic murmurs).

The LA size measured in 26 cases decreased in 16, did not change in five and increased in five cases.

Three patients have a diastolic rumble at 6, 6 and 7 months after the operation, respectively. In another eight patients, a short diastolic rumble could be detected after exercise at 10–32 months after the operation. Eleven patients have normal heart sounds.

Discussion

In the surgical treatment of predominant stenotic lesions of the mitral valve, we have preferred the open-heart approach since 1975. The safety of open valvotomy and better control of the operative technique[14], was proved in our first series of 100 cases without operative or hospital death.

In spite of adequate valvotomy some of the mitral valves which were competent on the operative table had systolic murmurs of mitral incompetence shortly after surgery.

In up to 20% of patients, the residual mitral incompetence was due to impaired coaptation related to the thickened and shortened mural leaflet.

Correction of the mitral incompetence at the commissural area could be performed by annuloplasty sutures at the price of rendering the mitral orifice smaller than optimal.

The literature suggests that the mitral leaflet is involved in the physiological and pathological mitral valve closure. The ratio of rough zone to clear zone in the middle scallop of the posterior leaflet is 1.4, while in the anterior leaflet it is 0.6. This implies that a greater portion of the posterior leaflet comes into contact with the anterior leaflet during valve closure[15]. The mobility of the posterior leaflet was restricted by disease more frequently than the anterior leaflet[1]. A good hinge movement is required for the posterior leaflet and the subvalvular apparatus must be explored and freed if indicated[6]. In other cases, the posterior leaflet is tethered down and has no full excursion to meet the anterior leaflet[6]. Carpentier[3] has shown that this frequent finding is due to the retraction of secondary chordae at that point and therefore must be sectioned selectively[6].

In cases with advanced lesions of the subvalvular structure and anterior leaflet or calcification of the valve, we performed mitral valve replacement. In other patients, we found lesions with marginal indications for valve replacement, in whom the valve could be salvaged by a reconstructive procedure. We judged that some of the explored mitral valves had components too good to be replaced in spite of lesions at different levels of the subvalvular apparatus.

The refined reconstructive techniques developed by Carpentier[2-4] and Duran[6, 7], have opened the era of modern conservative surgery of the mitral valve. Previous works of Lillehei, Merendino, Kay, Wooler, Reed, McGoon, Gerbode, and many others, described various techniques to correct mitral incompetence[8]. On the basis of these well-known techniques[9-12, 15], 33 patients had mitral valve reconstruction with complete valvotomy and patch extension of the mural leaflet with stabilized biological tissue. In an effort to preserve an adequate mitral orifice and a competent valve, we elected the insertion of a pliable tissue patch to the mural leaflet in order to provide a larger area for coaptation with the anterior leaflet and a mobile hinge for movement of the thickened mural leaflet.

Because autologous tissue (pericardium, fascia lata) used in the technique described by Sauvage[9], Bailey[11], Marion[12], Selmonosky[10] and Frater[13] has the disadvantage of fibrotic thickening in valvular area, we felt that human dura mater stabilized with glutaraldehyde would be the ideal tissue because it is readily available, sterile, pliable, less antigenic and durable, without calcification. Also, the similarity to aortic leaflet structure, with bundles of collagen crossing each other in opposite directions was felt to be an advantage. Obtained from young donors 12 hours after death, it is washed and preserved for 14 days in purified 0.5% glutaraldehyde buffered at pH 7.4. For storage, a solution of formaldehyde 5.4% is used. The thin dura mater tissue from young donors retains its pliable structure after fixation and cross-linking with glutaraldehyde. Experimental studies in dogs showed good preservation of dura mater structure and good thrombo-resistance up to 14 months after the insertion of a conduit with a valve between the right ventricle and pulmonary artery. The tissue has been also used in 15 clinical cases for closure of atrial septal defects and for right ventricular outflow tract reconstruction in tetralogy of Fallot since 1976. There is no evidence of shrinkage, calcification or aneurysmal dilatation. As an allograft, it is hoped to be less antigenic than a xenograft.

The pericardial xenograft tissue was selected for use in four cases based on large experience of various centers with pericardial xenograft valves.

The indications for mitral valve reconstruction with stabilized biological tissues were:

1. Predominant rheumatic mitral stenotic lesions with short and thickened mural leaflet in adult patients.
2. Without significant pathology of the anterior leaflet.
3. No calcification.
4. Small LV inadequate for a large biologic or prosthetic valve to match the surface area of a given patient.
5. Less than severe pathology of subvalvular structures.

Cases of pure mitral incompetence with alteration of the valvular collagen are an indication for valve replacement, in our experience. Until further clarification of tissue valve calcification in children, we would not recommend the use of leaflet extension with biological stabilized tissue.

The operative procedure to be performed for a stenotic lesion of the mitral valve is decided only intraoperatively after careful assessment of every component of the mitral apparatus. Every effort should be made to attempt the reconstruction before the decision to replace the valve was taken.

Cases with pericardial adhesions due to previous operations with distortion of the LV dynamics would not be considered for reconstruction.

In cases with an unsatisfactory reconstructive procedure valve replacement is indicated. In the present series, no valve replacement was felt indicated after the reconstruction. In three cases, the reconstructive procedure was considered 'aggressive', as there were significant lesions in the subvalve mechanism.

Associated anomalies are not a contraindication to reconstructive procedure with leaflet advancement, although the operative time will be longer for multiple valve procedures. The isolated procedure was performed in our series in less than one hour of cardioplegic arrest and 1 hour and 30 minutes perfusion time. When associated with other valvular procedures, the cross-clamping time of the aorta was over 1 hour and perfusion time 2 hours.

The advantages of the procedure are preservation of the patient's own valve, absence of thromboembolic complications and freedom from anticoagulant treatment. The reconstructive procedure was done with no mortality.

Conclusions are somewhat in question due to the small number of patients in this series and the very short follow-up. The procedure is a palliative operation. The more severe the deformity of the leaflets and subvalvular apparatus at the time of the operation, the greater the likelihood that the patient will require valve replacement in the future[14, 16]. As a more aggressive approach, it seems possible to resect and replace larger parts of the leaflet with stabilized biological tissue if the free margin of the original leaflet and its chordal attachment can be preserved.

The long-term fate of the stabilized biological tissue in the functioning leaflet of the mitral valve is important as regards the future of biological valves. The reconstructive procedure, as described, offers the possibility to explore and correct subvalvular lesions not obvious through the mitral orifice and from the atrium. The procedure may be combined with other reconstructive procedures of the mitral valve.

In this era of better valvular substitutes, there is ongoing need for comparison between improved procedures of reconstruction and valve replacement.

Conclusions

1. Mitral valve reconstruction with stabilized biological tissue is possible in predominant stenotic lesions with favorable anatomy.
2. Complete mitral valvotomy combined with extension of posterior leaflet produced an adequate mitral orifice and a competent valve.
3. In cases with short posterior leaflet, the decision for replacement or reconstruction is facilitated by an incision at its base, which allows exploration of the mitral apparatus.
4. Satisfactory results have been obtained with low mortality and morbidity. Valve replacement was avoided or delayed in this group of patients.
5. The long-term fate of stabilized biological tissue is not known, but satisfactory function of the mitral valve is proven up to 2½ years after the operation.

References

1. BURR, L.H., KRAYENBUHL, C., SUTTON, M.S.I. and PANETH, M. (1977). The mitral plication suture. A new technique of mitral valve repair. *Journal of Thoracic and Cardiovascular Surgery*, **73**, 589
2. CARPENTIER, A. (1969). La valvuloplastie reconstitutive. Une nouvelle technique de valvuloplastie mitrale. *La Presse Medicale*, **77**, 251
3. CARPENTIER, A. (1976). Plastic and reconstructive mitral valve surgery. In *The Mitral Valve* (ed. D. Kalmason), p. 527. London: Acton
4. CARPENTIER, A., DELSCHE, A., DAUPTAIN, I., SOYER, R., BLONDEAU, P., PIWNICA, A. and DUBOST, Ch. (1971). A new reconstructive operation for correction of mitral and tricuspid insufficiency. *Journal of Thoracic and Cardiovascular Surgery*, **61**, 1
5. CARPENTIER, A., CHAUVAUD, S., FALIANI, I.N., *et al.* (1980). Reconstructive surgery of mitral valve incompetence. Ten year appraisal. *Journal of Thoracic and Cardiovascular Surgery*, **79**, 330
6. DURAN, C.G. and UBAGO, I.L.M. (1976). Conservative mitral valve surgery: problems and developments in the technique of prosthetic ring annuloplasty in *The Mitral Valve* (ed. D. Kalmason), p. 549. London: Acton
7. DURAN, C.G., POMAR, J.L., REVUELTA, I.M., *et al.* (1980). Conservative operation for mitral insufficiency. *Journal of Thoracic and Cardiovascular Surgery*, **73**, 825
8. OURY, I.M., PETERSON, R.L., FOLKERT, H.T.L. and DAILY P.O. (1977). Mitral valve replacement versus reconstruction. *Journal of Thoracic and Cardiovascular Surgery*, **73**, 825
9. SAUVAGE, L.R., WOOD, S.I., BERGER, K.E. and CAMPBELL, A.A. (1966). Autologous pericardium for mitral leaflet advancement finding in the human after 56 months. *Journal of Thoracic and Cardiovascular Surgery*, **52**, 849
10. SELMONOSKY, C.A. and EHRENHAFT, I.L. (1969). The technique of open mitral reconstruction in the treatment of acquired and congenital mitral incompetence. *Journal of Thoracic and Cardiovascular Surgery*, **10**, 426
11. BAILEY, C.P., ZIMMERMAN, I., HIROSE, T. and FOLK, F.S. (1970). Use of autologous tissues in mitral valve reconstruction. *Geriatrics*, **25**, 119
12. MARION, P., CHAPSAUR, S., ESTANOVE, S. and GEORGE, M. (1970). L'allongement valvulaire dans la chirurgie conservative de la valvule mitral. *Annales des Chirurgie Thoracic et Cardiovasculaire*, **9**, 417
13. FRATER, R.W.M., BERGHIUS, I., BROWN, A.L. and ELLIS, F.H., JR. (1965). The experimental and clinical use of autogenous pericardium for the replacement and extension of mitral and tricuspid valve cusp and cordae. *Journal of Cardiovascular Surgery*, **6**, 214
14. HOUSMAN, L.B., BONCHEK, L., LAMBERT, L., GRUNKEMEIER, G. and STARR, A. (1977). Prognosis of patients after open mitral commissurotomy. *Journal of Thoracic and Cardiovascular Surgery*, **73**, 5
15. RANGANATHAN, N., SILVER, M.D. and WIGLE, E.D. (1976). Recent advances in the knowledge of the anatomy of the mitral valve. In *The Mitral Valve* (ed. D. Kalmason), p. 7. London: Acton
16. BYRNE, I., KIRSCH, M.M., MORRIS, J.D. and SLOAN, H. (1980). Long term results of open mitral valvuloplasty. *Annals of Thoracic Surgery*, **29**, 142

38

The 'dynamic' mitral ring: A new concept in treating mitral insufficiency

F. Alonso–Lej

Basic studies in dogs[1, 2] have demonstrated that during systole the mitral annulus experiences two modifications: the mural portion contracts, shortening its length, while the aortic portion is displaced upwards towards the aorta.

The contraction of the annulus reduces the area of the mitral orifice by as much as 36%[1] and even up to 40%[2]. This contraction and shortening of the annulus takes place only in the portion that supports the mural or posterior leaflet (*see Figure 38.1*). This part of the annulus does not contract uniformly. A segment between the center of the leaflet and the posterior commissure shortens by as much as half its length. Laterally it shortens gradually less until the level of the posterior commissure and a point near the anterior one where the length remains unchanged. At the same time that the mural annulus contracts, the aortic annulus moves upward, displaced by the jet of blood, propelled by the ventricular diastole. This displacement is maximal at the center. All these movements change somewhat the valvular plane.

The utilization of mitral rings[3, 4] opened an important field in the reconstruction of the mitral valve, avoiding in many cases its replacement by a prosthesis. On the

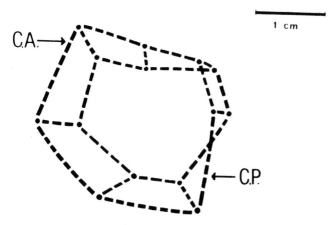

1 cm

C.A.

C.P.

Figure 38.1 Diastolic and systolic sizes of the annulus. CA = Anterior commissure; CP = posterior commissure.

other hand the annuloplasties that reduced the annulus by different suture techniques[5–7] have the disadvantage of narrowing the orifice and not avoiding a possible relapse of insufficiency. The use of bioprosthesis does not solve all the problems related to tromboembolic phenomena and its durability is limited. Therefore, the obvious trend in mitral surgery is to reconstruct the valve, provided that the tissues are preserved. Some type of ring is mandatory in those cases in which mitral insufficiency is a component of valvular pathology. In the market there have been until now two types of rings: rigid and 'flexible'.

The rigid types[4, 8] approximate the leaflets to the center of the orifice, remodelling the architecture of the valve. Their main disadvantages are concerned with two different aspects. First, they do not allow the selective adjustment of the ring to the specific type of regurgitation. Second, they avoid the physiological shortening and displacement of the annulus during the cardiac cycle. Therefore, if the surgeon inserts a large ring (diastole size) some regurgitation will occur during systole because the annulus attached to it cannot contract, and the leaflets will not meet each other, not leaving the orifice tightly closed. Consequently, the surgeon has to use a smaller ring (systolic size) to obtain the approximation of the leaflets during systole, sacrificing some area during diastole (in fact producing some stenosis).

Most of the flexible rings—all of them developed by Spanish surgeons[9–11]—allow the physiological modification of the annulus during the cardiac cycle (shortening and displacement) but do not provide it with the necessary support to maintain the remodelling of the valve. This is particularly noted as the peripheral ends of the leaflets near the commissures. In certain cases, due to this reason, the commissures do not close tightly during diastole. On the other hand, they do not always permit its selective readjustments to the specific type of influx.

The 'dynamic' ring developed by us comprises the advantages of both types, eliminating the disadvantages. The selective features of the ring are (*see Figure 38.2*):

1. Two rigid components of malleable stainless steel 1 mm in diameter, to achieve the remodelling of the annulus where it is especially needed, that is, at the level of the commissures.
2. A soft component in a selected portion of the ring, corresponding to the mural leaflet, to allow the maximal contraction of this part of the annulus during systole. For this reason the rigid components are not symmetrical, because the segment of maximal contraction is nearer the posterior than the anterior commissures. This soft component is of Dacron velour, which also covers as a sleeve the entire ring constituting its only visible part.
3. To permit the shortening of the soft portion of the ring accompanying the contraction of the annulus, the rigid part should be discontinued by a spring, (acting as a hinge) to allow the rigid 'mural' ends to approximate to each other. The spring is of stainless steel, 0.28 mm in diameter. The rigid components are screwed to the spring. This flexible component of the ring is inserted at a point that corresponds to the middle of the annulus of the aortic leaflet. At the same time this spring permits the physiological cephald displacement of the annulus of the aortic leaflet during systole.
4. A thread of 000 monofilament travels twice along the inside of the ring to allow when necessary the narrowing of the ring, shortening the soft components.

The insertion of the ring requires a careful technique and an adequate exposure.

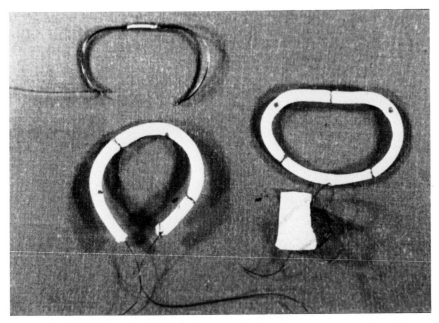

Figure 38.2 Components of the dynamic ring.

Two marks are placed in the atrial side to facilitate the orientation of the ring. These marks correspond to the prolongation of the commissures. In the first place two mattress sutures are placed in the annulus opposing both commissures. These sutures are utilized, similarly to the technique described by Dr Carpentier, to decide the proper size of the ring, although the special dynamic characteristics of our ring allowed the use of a 'diastole' size instead of the 'systolic' size necessary when a rigid ring is utilized. Between these sutures and all along the aortic annulus three or four wider mattress sutures are placed. Both needles of these mattress sutures spear the interior border of the rigid part of the ring to allow better approximation of the leaflets. Then the ring goes down over the annulus and the sutures are knotted. This part of the insertion is similar to the technique used to place a Carpentier ring. With the ring in position a running suture is utilized to complete the insertion using both distal sutures including the ends of the rigid components first and later the soft part. The fact that this part of the ring is not rigid permits its separation from the tissues, facilitating an adequate placement of the stitches.

It is very important that the stitches facing the mural leaflets are placed just outside the annulus, because if any small portion of the leaflet is included in the stitch the leaflet can be deformed. Once the ring is sutured in place a bolus of fluid under pressure is injected into the left ventricle, to estimate the accuracy of the repair. If the leaflets contact tightly protruding into the auricle, and a jet of fluid escapes when we push them into the ventricle we conclude that the regurgitation has been corrected. Otherwise, the heart is allowed to beat and the left ventricle filled with blood following any of the methods described in the literature[12–16]. To adjust the ring to each particular case, two different manoeuvers may be necessary depending on the different situations encountered.

First, if there is a 'leak' through one of the commissures (*see Figure 38.3*) the corresponding rigid component is narrowed (reducing its curvature) compressing both ends with a clamp, and approximating the commissural ends of the leaflets obliterating the reflux (*see Figure 38.4*). To facilitate this manoeuver the rigid ends present a small notch, where the tip of the clamp is applied to avoid slipping.

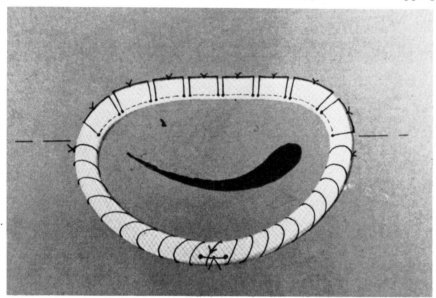

Figure 38.3 'Leak' through a posterior commissure.

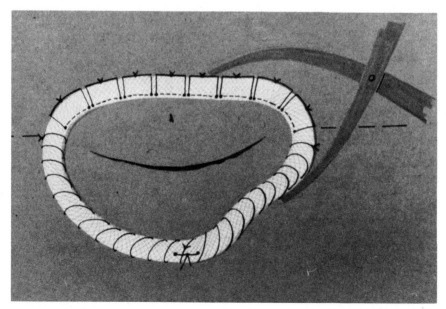

Figure 38.4 Correction of the leak shown in *Figure 38.3*, narrowing the corresponding rigid component.

Secondly, if the 'leak' is extended along the free ends of the leaflets (*see Figure 38.5*), because they do not reach each other, we can approximate them and reduce the size of the ring by pulling gradually on both ends of the thread that travels doubly inside the ring until the regurgitation disappears (*see Figure 38.6*). When the leak is controlled, the suture is tightened, maintaining the ring in its new

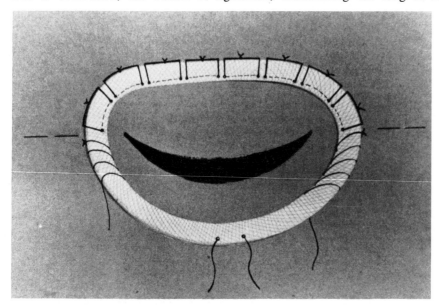

Figure 38.5 'Leak' through the entire orifice.

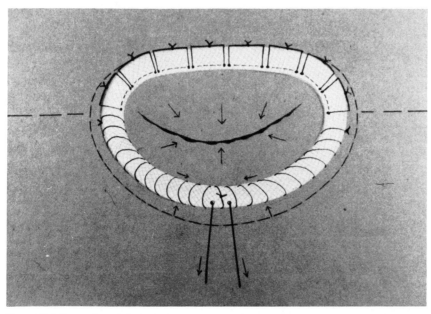

Figure 38.6 Correction of the leak shown in *Figure 38.5*, narrowing the ring shortening of the soft component by pulling the thread.

dimensions. In certain cases both manoeuvers may be necessary. The dynamic features of the ring can be observed during the operation and later on radiologically. During the operation we have seen sometimes how the blood escapes from the ventricle through the valve during diastole. These leaks disappeared during systole when the annulus mitralis and the ring contracted, reducing their sizes.

The first prototype dates from 1977. There was a 35-year-old female patient who suffered from a mitral valvulopathy with stenosis and insufficiency. A complete valvulotomy and insertion of a 'dynamic' ring was carried out. The ventriculography showed complete closure of the valve during systole. In diastole one can see the lateral separation of the mural ends of the rigid components (increasing the area to the mitral orifice) and the cephaled displacement of the aortic ends, therefore following the physiological modifications of the mitral annulus during the cardiac cycle and obtaining the maximal mitral area in diastole without regurgitation during systole. The same radiological findings have been encountered in the other cases operated upon (*see Figure 38.7*).

In conclusion, we have presented a mitral ring that offers the possibility of adapting itself to the special characteristics of each specific case. A ring that maintains the remodelling of the mitral valve and allows at the same time the physiological changes, narrowing and displacement of the mitral annulus during the cardiac cycle, therefore permitting the use of diastole sizes. We have placed this ring in over 20 cases with excellent results. In due time we will publish our results.

References

1. TSAKIRIS, A.G., VON BERNUTH, G., RASTELLI, G.C., BURGOIS, M.J., TITUS, J.J. and WOOD, E.H. (1971). Size and motion of the mitral valve annulus in anaesthetized intact dogs. *J. Appl. Physiol.*, **30**, 611
2. POMAR, J.L., CUCCHIARA, G. and DURAN, C.M.G. (1978). Tratamiento quirúrgico conservador de las valvulopatías auriculoventriculares, I. Anuloplastias mitrales. *Cirug. Es.*, **32**, 1
3. CARPENTIER, A. (1969). La valvuloplastie réconstitutive. Une nouvelle technique de valvuloplastie mitrale. *Presse Med.*, **77**, 251
4. CARPENTIER, A., DELOCHE, A., DAUPATAIN, J., *et al.* (1971). A new reconstructive operation for correction of mitral and tricuspid insufficiency. *J. Thoracic. Cardiovasc. Surg.*, **61**, 1
5. MARENDINO, K.A. and BRUCE, R.A. (1957). One hundred seventeen surgically treated cases of valvular rheumatic heart disease. Preliminary report of two cases of mitral regurgitation treated under direct vision with the aid of a pump oxigenator. *JAMA*, **1964**, 749
6. KAY, E.B., NOGUEIRA, C. and ZIMMERMAN, H.A. (1968). Correction of mitral insufficiency under direct vision. *Circulation*, **21**, 568
7. WOOLER, G.H., NIXON, P.G., GRIMSHAW, A. and WATSON, D.A. (1962). Experiences with mitral valve repair in mitral incompetence. *Thorax*, **17**, 49
8. COOLEY, D.A., FRAZIER, O.H. and NORMAN, J.C. (1976). Mitral leaflet prolapse: surgical treatment using a posterior annular collar prosthesis. *Cardiovasc. Dis. Bull. Texas Heart Inst.*, **3**, 381
9. ARCAS, R. (1976). Tesis doctoral. *Annuloplastia Mitral con Soporte Flexible Circular*. Faculted de Medicina, Universidad de Navarra
10. POMAR, J.L., FIGUEROA, A., OCHOTECO, A., UBAGO, J.L.M. and DURAN, C.G. (1978). Clinic hemodynamic evaluation of 118 patients undergoing mitral flexible ring annuloplasty. *Amer. J. Cardiology*, **41**, 422
11. SAURA, E., VALLE, J.M. and PUIG MASSANA, M. (1980). Anillo flexible y ajustable en cirugía conservadora de la válvula mitral. I congreso Nacional de la Asociación Española de Cirugía Cardiovascular, Sevilla
12. MULLIN, M., ENGELMEN, R., ISOM, D., BOYD, A., GALSSMAN, E. and SPENCER, F. (1974). Experience with open mitral comissurotomy in 100 consecutive patients. *Surgery*, **76**, 974
13. POMAR, J.L., CUCCHIARA, G., GALLOW, J.I. and DURAN, C.G.M. (1978). Intraoperative assessment of mitral valve function. *Ann. Thorac. Surg.*, **25**, 354
14. KING, H., CCSCKI, J. and LESHNOWER, A. (1980). Intraoperative assessment of the mitral valve following reconstructive procedures. *Ann. Thorac. Surg.*, **29**, 81

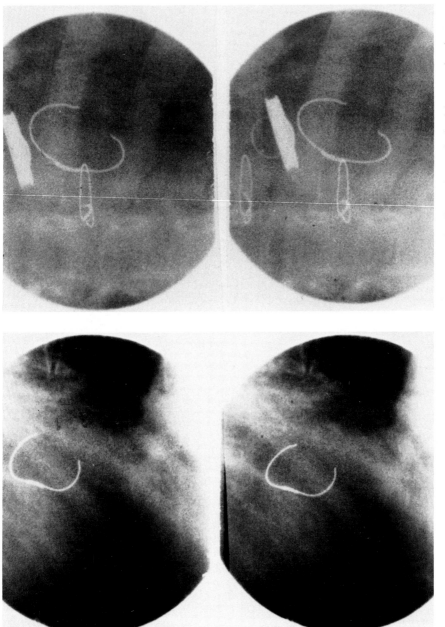

Figure 38. 7 Two patients with a dynamic ring, showing reduction of the ring during systole. The aortic prosthesis of the second patient (right half of figure) shows that the systole occurs by an opening of the obturator disc.

15. NAIR, K.K. and YATES (1977). Direct evaluation of mitral valve function during surgery following conservative procedures. *J. Thor. Cardiovasc. Surg.*, **73,** 684
16. HALSET, W.L., ELLIOT, D.P. and WALKER, L.L. (1980). Simplified intraoperative technique to test mitral valve repair. *J. Thor. Cardiovasc. Surg.*, **80,** 792

39

Valve replacement for chronic mitral insufficiency: Long-term follow-up using technetium–99m–pertechnetate scintigraphy

E. Kreuzer, B. Reichart, N. Schad and G. Bougkioukas

Summary

An average of 19.8 ± 11 months after valve replacement for chronic mitral insufficiency left and right ventricular global function was assessed non-invasively in 12 patients. Preoperative deterioration in contractility influenced the long-term outcome after surgical intervention. Preoperative ventriculography of the nine men and three women (age at operation 48 ± 13 years), revealed increased end-diastolic volumes (EDV) (239.9 ± 66 ml) and end-systolic (ESV) volumes (73.5 ± 26 ml).

$49.4 \pm 9\%$ of the stroke volume (175.5 ± 47 ml) regurgitated into the left atrium. The ejection fraction (EF) was normal in all cases ($67.7 \pm 6\%$). Postoperatively, end-diastolic and end-systolic volumes of the left ventricle were normal at rest ($121.8 \pm 3\%$ and 52.8 ± 35 ml, respectively) and after peak exercise (122.0 ± 29 and 37.6 ± 22 ml, respectively). The ejection fraction responded physiologically to exercise by increasing from 57.7 ± 12 to $69.7 \pm 10\%$ ($p < 0.05$). Volumes and ejection fraction of the right ventricle were within normal ranges both at rest and after exercise.

The mean rapid filling rate increased after peak exercise from 211.9 ± 50 to 433.4 ± 178.1 ml/sec. The pulmonary transit time measured 7.3 ± 1.2 s at rest and 4.4 ± 1.2 s after exercise. Both parameters revealed a physiological function of the implanted valve prosthesis (10 Bjork–Shiley and two Carpentier–Edwards).

In this series, valve replacement for chronic mitral insufficiency was able to normalize left ventricular function. At present, radionuclide ventriculography (technetium-99m–pertechnetate scintigraphy, first-past technique) is probably the most promising technique for evaluating the function of both ventricles after mitral valve replacement.

Introduction

Obtaining an accurate long-term prognosis in patients with valve replacement for chronic mitral incompetence continues to pose problems. Usually, judgement is based on clinical examination and additional information is drawn from the ECG and chest X-ray. Exact data of right and left ventricular performance may be obtained by cardiac catheterization. This invasive method is inconvenient for the patient and not without risk. Grading according to criteria of the New York Heart Association depends on the patient's subjective report. Non-invasive methods, like echocardiography and scintigraphy, are being employed. This study deals with 12 patients who underwent valve replacement for chronic mitral incompetence and were periodically examined using the first-pass of a technetium-99m–pertechnetate bolus as a non-invasive procedure which is easy to carry out and yields objective information of the left and right ventricular performance and the function of the implanted mitral valve prosthesis.

Patients

The study covers nine males and three females who were operated on between January 1977 and December 1980. The age of the patients at the operation varied between 23 and 70 years (mean age 48.3 ± 13 years).

The left ventricular end-diastolic (EDV) and end-systolic volumes (ESV) calculated from preoperative contrast angiograms according to the formula of Sandler and Dodge[1] were increased (230.9 ± 66 ml and 73.5 ± 26 ml). 49.4 ± 9% of the total stroke volume (157.5 ± 47 ml) regurgitated into the left atrium. The left ventricular ejection fraction (EF) proved normal in all patients (67.6 ± 6%).

In two patients, the right heart catheterization revealed normal mean pulmonary pressures (< 20 mm Hg). Seven patients had slightly (20–35 mm Hg) and three moderately (35–60 mm Hg) elevated pulmonary pressures.

According to history, intra-operative findings and histological examination of the resected mitral valve tissue, mitral insufficiency was due to bacterial endocarditis in five cases, of rheumatic origin in four; degenerative changes were observed in three patients.

Operative technique

Surgery was performed using a Bentley bubble oxygenator and general hypothermia of 28°C. During the intracardiac procedure, the aorta was cross-clamped and 4°C cold cardioplegic solution (Bretschneider) was infused into the aortic root for myocardial protection; in addition, the pericardial well technique (Shumway) was applied. Ten Bjork–Shiley and two Carpentier–Edwards prostheses were implanted with diameters of 27 mm (2 patients), 29 mm (9 patients) and 31 mm (1 patient).

Assessment of postoperative right and left ventricular function using technetium-99m–pertechnetate scintigraphy (first-pass technique)

The patients were studied 19.8 ± 8 months (range 9–42 months) postoperatively both at rest and after age-related maximum exercise during which heart rate doubled from 78 ± 14 to 149 (23/s). During both parts of the study (15–20 mCi technetium-99m–pertechnetate were used each) the patients were sitting on a bicycle ergometer in the RAO position. An automatic injector was applied to secure an intravenous, ECG triggered, injection of the radioactivity as a bolus which arrived at the tricuspid valve during systole. The distribution of the radioactivity was recorded applying a fast multicrystal camera (System 77, Baird–Atomic Corporation) in connection with a computer which stored all scintigraphic pictures (*see Plate 39.1*).

The end-diastolic volume (EDV) was calculated by a formula experimentally derived in a balloon model by Nikel[2]:

$$EDV \text{ (ml)} = CV (K_1 . NTC - K_2 (1 + K_3z)^2)$$

Where NTC = normalized total count rate, calculated as the count integral of the ventricle divided by the maximum count density; z = distance from collimator to ventricle; and K_1, K_2, K_3, CF are constants ($K_1 = 11.5 \text{ ml/cm}^2$; $K_2 = 6.8 \text{ ml}$; $K_3 = 0.051 \text{/cm}$; CV = 0.81 (for position of the heart in RAO 30 degrees without dimension)).

ESV and EF (*see Plates 39.2 and 3*) were estimated as follows:

$$ESV \text{ (ml)} = \frac{\text{end-systolic counts}}{\text{end-diastolic counts}} . EDV$$

$$EF \text{ (\%)} = \frac{\text{end-diastolic counts} - \text{end-systolic counts}}{\text{end-diastolic counts}} . 100$$

Function of the prosthesis implanted in the mitral position was assessed by the mean pulmonary transit time (PTT) and the rapid diastolic filling rate of the left ventricle (RFR). PTT was defined as the time a radionuclide bolus needed to travel from the pulmonary artery to the left atrium. According to Upton and co-workers[3] 5.8 ± 1 s is normal at rest and 2.5 ± 0.4 s after exercise.

RFR was calculated as the volume of the rapid diastolic filling divided by its duration (normal: 207 ± 54 ml/s at rest and 411 ± 119 ml/s after exercise).

Results

Figure 39.1 shows the postoperative functional classification according to the New York Heart Association in comparison with the preoperative grades. On an average, the patients improved from preoperative class 2.6 to postoperative 1.8.

Postoperative left and right ventricle function (Technetium-99m–pertechnetate scintigraphy (*see Table 39.1*))

During peak exercise, heart rate increased from 78 ± 14 to 149 ± 23/s. At the same time EDV of the left ventricle measured 121.8 ± 38 ml at rest and 122 ± 29 ml during exercise. The ESV decreased during exercise from 52.8 ± 35 ml to 37.6 ± 22 ml ($p < 0.05$). Exercising EF increased from 57.7 ± 12 to $69.7 \pm 10\%$ ($p < 0.05$). With heart rate cardiac output nearly doubled, from 6.4 ± 2 to 10.3 ± 2.8 l/min ($p < 0.05$).

The volumes and the EF for the right ventricle were within normal ranges both at rest and during exercise.

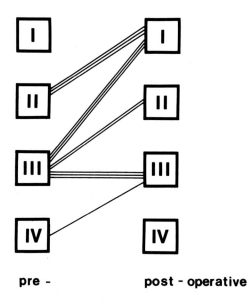

N.Y.H.A.

pre -   post - operative

Figure 39.1 Clinical staging according to the New York Heart Association (NYHA) classification; pre- and postoperative grades of 12 patients receiving valve replacement for chronic mitral insufficiency.

Function of the implanted valve prosthesis

The mean pulmonary transit time—though elevated in comparison with normal subjects, was reduced in all cases during exercise. The average was 7.3 ± 1.2 to 4.4 ± 1 s ($p < 0.05$). The rapid diastolic filling rate of the left ventricle averaged postoperatively 211.9 ± 50 ml/s at rest and doubled under maximum exercising conditions to 433.4 ± 118 ml/s ($p < 0.05$). Again an increase was obtained in every single case.

Discussion

While grading of the patients clinical condition (NYHA classification), ECG and chest X-ray are all useful in assessing right and left ventricular hemoydnamics, but give only an indirect evauation of the dynamics as they really are. Evidence that classification relies to a high degree on the patient's subjective report (*see Figure 39.1*) is supported by the scatter throughout our groups when compared with

---

Plate 39.1 12-image view, depicting the travel of a compact 15–20 mCi technetium-99m–pertechnetate bolus from the vena cava, the right atrium (views 1 and 2) to the right ventricle (views 3 and 4) through the lungs (views 5–8) to the left atrium and ventricle (views 9–12).

Plate 39.2 Left ventricular ejection fraction (RAO-position) at rest (upper panel) and during exercise (lower panel). The global ejection fraction is divided into 10 fractions; each fraction is symbolized by a different tint. The marginal bright tint stands for 100% ejection fraction; the lowest ejection fraction is measured around the left ventricular base.

Plate 39.3 Right ventricular ejection fraction (RAO—position at peak exercise). (For explanation, *see* Plate 39.2.)

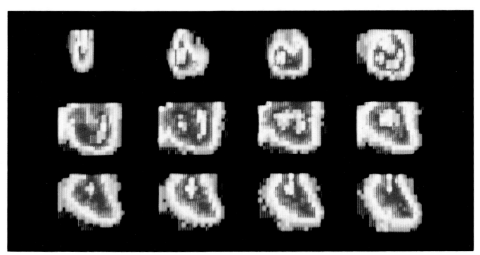

Plate 39.1

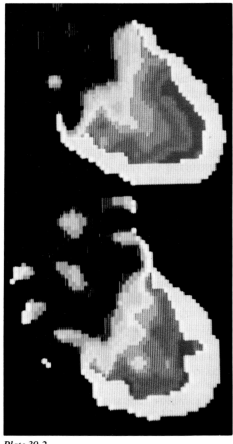

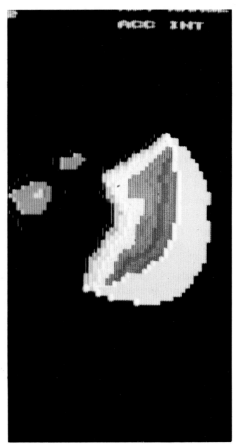

Plate 39.2

Plate 39.3

Our data are in conflict with the results of the Durham group[11], which also studied patients with valve replacement for chronic mitral insufficiency using similar scintigraphic methods: this group were unable to find any postoperative unchanged high EDV and ESV, causing wide standard deviations of the means. According to Schuler and co-workers[12], those ventricles obviously had become dependent on the preoperatively systolic afterload reduction due to chronic mitral insufficiency.

Both the rapid diastolic filling rate of the left ventricle and the mean pulmonary transit time aided in evaluating the function of the prosthesis in the mitral position. A significant increase of the rapid diastolic filling rate of the left ventricle due to exercise is more meaningful as a demonstration of adequate function than the values shown at rest. In our 12 cases, without any exception, the RFR of the left ventricle increased, and on an average, doubled. The PTT may be modified by diseases of the lungs or right ventricular dysfunction.

None of our patients showed markedly elevated pulmonary mean pressure preoperatively. Additionally, normal right heart function was proved by postoperative scintigraphic measurements (see Table 39.1). Under exercise condition the PTT decreased from 7.3 ± 1.2 s to 4.4 ± 1 s ($p<0.05$). These values are in agreement with numbers issued by Scholz[10] and Reyrich[13] obtained in healthy volunteers.

Conclusion

Technetium-99m–pertechnetate scintigraphy of the heart is a non-invasive method which may be applied repeatedly in sequential studies without introducing substantial or systematical errors. This technique is ideal in obtaining right and left ventricle performance both at rest and during exercise. The effect of surgical intervention and the function of implanted mitral valve prosthesis may be evaluated on a long-term basis. This group of patients with mitral regurgitation with minimally elevated PA pressure had consistent improvent in ventricular diameter 19 months postoperatively.

References

1. SANDLER, H. and DODGE, H.T. (1968). The use of single plane angiography for the calculation of left ventricular volume in man. *Amer. Heart J.*, **75**, 325
2. NICKEL, O. and SCHAD, N. (1978). Image analysis of the heart action recorded with a high speed multicrystal gamma camera. *Med. Prog. Technol.*, **5**, 1
3. UPTON, M.T., RERYCH, S.K., NEWMAN, G.F., BOUNOUS, E.P. and JONES, R.H. (1980). The reproducibility of radionuclide angiographic measurements of left ventricular function in normal subjects at rest and during exercise. *Circulation*, **62**, 126
4. SCHAD, N. (1977). Non-traumatic assessment of left ventricular wall motion and regional stroke volume after myocardial infarction. *J. Nucl. Med.*, **18**, 333
5. SCHAD, N. and NICKEL, O. (1978). Radionuclide angiography in coronary heart disease: Where do we stand? *Cardiovasc. Radiol.*, **1**, 27
6. SCHAD, N. and NICKEL, O. (1979). Assessment of ventricular function with first-pass angiocardiography. *Cardiovasc. Radiol.*, **2**, 149
7. SCHAD, N. and NICKEL, O. (1980). Nichtinvasive Beurteilung der regionalen Funktion des linken Ventrikels; erste Tracer Passage. *Radiologie*, **20**, 56
8. SCHAD, N. and NICKEL, O. (1981). Noninvasive assessment of left ventricular function. In *Radiology Today* (eds M.W. Donner and F.H.W. Henck), Vol. **1**

9. NICKEL, O., SCHAD, N., ANDREWS, E.J., FLEMING, J.W. and MELLO, M. (1982). Scintigraphic measurements of left ventricular volumes from the count density distribution. *J. Nucl. Med.*, **23,** 404

10. SCHOLZ, P.N., RERYCH, S.K., MORAN, J.F., *et al.* (1980). Quantitative radionuclide angiography. *Catherization and Cardiovascular Diagnosis*, **6,** 265

11. PETER, C.A., AUSTIN, E.H. and JONES, R.H. (1981). Effect of valve replacement for chronic mitral insufficiency on left ventricular function during rest and exercise. *J. Thorac. Cardiovasc. Surg.*, **82,** 127

12. SCHULER, G., PETERSON, K.L., JOHNSEN, A., *et al.* (1979). Temporal response of left ventricular performance to mitral valve surgery. *Circulation*, **59,** 1218

13. RERYCH, S.K., SCHOLZ, P.M., NEWMAN, G.E., SABISTON, D.C. and JONES, R.H. (1978). Cardiac function at rest and during exercise in normals and in patients with coronary heart disease. *Ann. Surg.*, **187,** 449

Section 11

40

Summary and overview

William W. Angell

The Surgery Panel at the International Mitral Valve Symposium (San Diego, California, 1982) was comprised of cardiovascular surgeons with unusually extensive experience and expertise. Cogent issues pertaining to mitral valve replacement were addressed in a unique manner.

Mitral valve replacement devices

By way of introduction, the following list describes five valve types:

1. Prosthesis:
   (a) Ball—Starr and Sutter.
   (b) Disc—Bjork and Medtronic–Hall.
   (c) Leaflet—St. Jude.
2. Tissue:
   (a) Porcine—Carpentier and Hancock.
   (b) Pericardial—Ionescu.

As reported by the manufacturers, the frequency of use of tissue versus mechanical valves for mitral valve replacement was approximately equal in 1982. However, in some centers prosthetic valves are used exclusively where in others only tissue valves are used. *Table 40.1* depicts an attempt to rate the valve types according to their critical characteristics or by the complications associated with them.

The *caged ball valve* has been used the longest, but it accounts for only about 10% of the valves implanted. The *pericardial valve,* while having the best *in-vitro* hemodynamic characteristics along with the lowest reported incidence of thromboembolism, also accounts for less than 10% of valves utilized. Thus, 80% of mitral valves implanted are either *disk prostheses* or *porcine bioprostheses*. The tilting disk valve used in the mitral position has *in-vitro* hemodynamic characteristics which are not substantially different from any other valve type, and it has a higher reported incidence of thromboembolism and thrombosis. Its *in-vitro* hemodynamics are not as good as the bileaflet or pericardial valve. Yet this device continues to be the most popular type for valve replacement.

One might draw the conclusion from this comparative analysis that selection of valve type is based on factors other than hemodynamic characteristics, clinical

TABLE 40.1 Rating of types of valve according to critical characteristics or complications

Variable	Valve				
	Ball	Disc	Leaflet	Porcine	Pericardial
Hemodynamics:	1	3	3	1	3
In vitro	1	3	3	1	3
In vivo	2	2	3	2	2
Clinical	2	2	2	2	2
Thrombosis and/					
or embolism:	1	1	1	3	3
Without anticoagulant	0	0	0	3	3
No significant embolism or residual	1	1	1	2	2
Durability:	3	2	1	1	1
Immediate	3	2	2	2	2
Short term	3	2	2	2	2
Long term	3	2	0	1	1
	20 (5)	20 (6)	18 (5)	20 (5)	24 (7)

Normal = 4; Optimal = 3; Standard = 2; Adequate = 1; Unknown or Inadequate = 0.

efficacy, or longevity of experience. Hence this assessment of mitral valve replacement devices shows that:

1. The valve with the best score was amongst the least popular.
2. The valve with the longest experience was among the least popular.
3. The most popular valve was suboptional by all criteria.

Valve selection is on the basis of criteria other than those analysed.
    Some of the factors affecting valve selection are:

1. Anticoagulation.
2. Spontaneous valve failure.
3. Thromboembolism risk.
4. Hemodynamics, *in vivo* and *in vitro*.
5. Other—physicians–surgeons–patients bias, valve profile, ease of insertion.

Probably the most significant of these is the personal preference of the surgeon or the surgical team that is using a given valve type. As noted in many reported series, the selection of a valve is often based on a group's developmental work with a particular valve or on a traditionally stated preference or interest in the evaluation of a particular valve type. Choice of a valve replacement device may be made through preference of patient, surgeon or cardiologist, all of which are influenced by product marketing. Emphasis is on the name of the valve or name associated with the valve, its appearance, the data that's presented by the manufacturer, the time at which the product is brought into the market, the climate of that market at that time, the personality of the individuals associated with the company and their local representatives.

In many instances, the commercial valve manufacturing companies exert a strong influence in the market place based on service, availability, personality of the contacting representatives or the general salesmanship of the company. The literature in general has had little influence on the selection of valve type because it is scant, biased, selected with short duration of follow-up and of greatest accuracy and validity. As *Tables 40.2* and *40.3* illustrate, there are relatively few completely reported series of valve replacement patients, with (1) a substantial and chronological period of follow-up time; (2) inclusion of all patients operated so that the series is not selected; (3) reporting of all complications; and (4) an adequate percentage of patient follow-up.

While it has been stated by Dr Duran that reporting methods have greatly improved, there is still a striking paucity of good comparable surgical results in series of patients meeting the above criteria for statistical significance. We are particularly indebted to Stanford for consistently reporting their data in this manner. While they do have a bias toward the tissue valve they, unlike many reporting groups, have no vested interest in a particular valve replacement device.

TABLE 40.2 Analysis of series of patients receiving mitral valve replacement with mechanical prosthesis

Valve type	No. of patients	Years follow-up			% operative mortality	Late mortality		% 4-year actuarial survival
		Max.	Mean	Pt-yrs		Total	%/Pt-yr	
Bjork–Shiley	230	6.5	3.7		4.7	10.5		89*
	203	9.0	2.5	482	4.0	18.5	7.5	72*
Starr–Edwards 6120	515	11.0	4.3	2159	9.7	36.8	7.9	68
	134	12.0	5.4	639	11.9	28.0	5.1	80
Starr–Edwards 6300	362	8.2			10.8	15.8		74†
Starr–Edwards 6400	205	4.3	1.8	353	4.0	6.1	3.4	85*

*Excludes operative mortality.
†Excludes non-cardiac deaths.
A/C = Anticoagulated patients; Other = irregularly anticoagulated; Pt-yr = patient-year.

TABLE 40.3 Analysis of series of patients receiving mitral valve replacement with porcine xenograft

Valve type	No. of patients	Years follow-up			% operative mortality	Late mortality		% 4-year actuarial survival
		Max.	Mean	Pt-yrs		Total	%/pt-yr	
Hancock	561	7.3	2.5	1302	8.9	14.3	5.5	72
	381	4.5	2.0	714	10.5	14.2	2.0	82.5
	335	6.2			6.9	8.3		70
	147	6.3	4.5	558	15.0	26.5	2.0	78.5
	131	6.3	2.8	357	6.0	11.5	4.2	85
	120	4.1	1.5	170	8.3	13.6	8.8	70
	111	4.0	1.8	172	11.7	13.3	7.6	
Carpentier oxidized	15	6.0	3.6	48	13.0	23.0	6.3	80
Angell–Shiley	94	8.3	2.6	221	10.0	21.0	8.1	69
	60	1.7	0.8	47	1.6	3.4	4.3	

Pt-yr = Patient-year.

Mitral valve repair

As the incidence of rheumatic mitral valve disease has progressively declined, other types of mitral valve pathology have emerged. The International Mitral Valve Symposium participants were strongly in favor of expanding the techniques for mitral valve reconstruction over mitral valve replacement because of the differences in surgical results.

To this end, it was felt that *diagnostic methods* for evaluating valve pathology should be directed towards defining those lesions which are amenable to repair. The criteria for referral of patients for surgery in cases where valve repair is a certainty or a high probability may be different from the criteria for those patients who require valve replacement. Surgical techniques are more complicated, and the repair may not result in a perfectly competent valve. In spite of residual stenosis or insufficiency, the required valve may still have a better long-term prognosis for the patient than a perfectly competent prosthesis. Also, in most series, repair carries a lower operative risk than replacement.

Earlier referral of patients for repair of mitral valve regurgitation was recommended by all panelists. There is good evidence that early correction of mitral valve regurgitation will insure better postoperative myocardial function with less left ventricular dilatation and failure. In the later stages of mitral regurgitation, the downhill clinical course due to congestive failure can occur in spite of total repair of the mitral valve lesion. In an attempt to make an earlier diagnosis of patients with deteriorating left ventricular function, the use of indices that are load-dependent is good in concept but not yet well defined. Ejection fraction is still the best standarized method for the evaluation of left ventricular function. Different levels should be set for normal inpatients with mitral valve regurgitation. Even with this consideration, ejection fraction is still the best predictor of postoperative left ventricular contractility.

Preservation of left ventricular contractility is enhanced little by medical management. Patients with mitral regurgitation must be continually evaluated for changes in ventricular function. In the presence of adequate diuretic and unloading therapy, symptoms and signs may not determine when the patient is the best candidate for invasive diagnostic evaluation and surgery. Chronic atrial fibrillation results in a significantly poorer long-term prognosis with either mitral valve repair or replacement, and optimally patients should be considered surgical candidates prior to the time they develop atrial fibrillation.

While enthusiasm for valve repair is shown by all cardiologists, it must be noted that if valves are badly damaged, long-term function is not substantially better than with a replaced valve. *Pathology* therefore should be clearly delineated and valves separated into those that are otherwise of good character and quality anatomically, but have specific defects. Localized segmental prolapse of the posterior leaflet with disrupted chordal mechanism is an entirely different form of mitral valve regurgitation from the thickened, fibrotic, generally deteriorated valve secondary to extensive pathology in leaflet and subvalvular mechanism. One should therefore divide mitral pathology into categories based on the long-term prognosis with repair as contrasted to the requirement for valve replacement, both being profoundly influenced by left ventricular performance. On the one hand is the presence of very localized segmental posterior leaflet prolapse with an otherwise normal mitral valve apparatus, and the spectrum then progresses through generalized valve prolapse with the stretching of leaflets and chordae in the so-called 'floppy valve' syndrome. These may well be repairable but do not have the same excellent long-term results as localized posterior leaflet defects. The rheumatic valves with generalized fibrosis and calcification resulting in mixed mitral stenosis and insufficiency are sometimes repairable but may carry no better prognosis than the long-term results with mitral valve replacement. The objective is to separate the types of pathology preoperatively and to allow, and even encourage, the surgeons to make the appropriate choice between repair and replacement based upon the valvular anatomy.

Toward this end, there has been striking improvement in ultrasonic diagnostic techniques and interpretation. Both Drs Kalmanson and Duran emphasized, however, that a full invasive cardiac catheterization is still necessary for patients who are candidates for mitral valve surgery. The combination of echo and Doppler flow techniques is permitting a more precise evaluation of regurgitant flow and localization of the anatomic lesion. Future methods will add substantially to our preoperative assessment of the mitral valve mechanism, the state of ventricular function and the appropriate timing of invasive catheterization and surgery. Preoperative definition of the anatomy, with characterization of specific pathology and functional derangement, greatly enhances the surgeon's ability to perform reconstruction of the valve and to have that reconstruction properly evaluated following surgery. Dr Duran re-emphasized that the earlier surgery can be justified, the better the postoperative result will be, particularly if that interval is prior to the time chronic atrial fibrillation has occurred. He also expressed the opinion that clinical results from changes in valve design and manufacture techniques have not had a significant interval to allow accurate reporting. If there is consistency and standardization of reporting techniques, data will be comparable coming from various groups all over the world.

Mitral valve replacement

Dr Allen Johnson voiced the opinion of several cardiologists which suggests that there has been little or no progress in prosthetic valve replacement devices in the 7 years since the previous Mitral Valve Symposium. While we surgeons would disagree, it must be admitted that the clinical evidence for substantial improvement in either tissue valves or prosthetic valves has not been convincing. If there has been improvement in the basic preparation and construction methods of the valves or in valve design, it has not been borne out by published clinical data.

Dr Bjork had discussed previously the problem of strut fracture with the Bjork–Shiley valve. During the panel discussion, two patients from Australia were presented who died with strut fracture and release of the disk. Dr Bjork re-emphasized that struts should be of unit construction in the 60- and 70-degree tilting disk valve and that the mechanical failure has occurred only in the 20-mm size. He feels confident that the problem has been proven to be solved by the pulse duplicator and stress testing at Shiley Laboratories. Welded valves are no longer being made and should be removed from the inventory. Dr Starr answered that no matter how the tilting disk is constructed, it requires a bending or distortion of the monostrut to get the poppit in position. None of the mechanical components of the caged ball valve require distortion in order to insert the poppit. This is one of the greatest theoretical advantages of the caged ball type of mechanism versus the tilted disk. As far as he was aware, none of the data in the literature shows a statistically significant difference between any of the valve types in clinical complications or follow-up. The one exception is the personal series of Marion Ionescu with the pericardial valve. Dr Starr questioned whether this personal series could be reproduced in other hands.

Combined tricuspid and mitral disease

The question of tricuspid involvement with mitral valve disease was raised. It was noted that if the tricuspid valve is involved, then there is a 10% increase in the operative mortality for that patient group. Both Drs Carpentier and Duran agreed that the increased risk is expected with tricuspid involvement. In general, these patients have had long-standing mitral disease and represent a patient group who is at the end of the spectrum in the time course of their disease process. As has been stated earlier, surgical results are going to be related more to the timing of surgery than to any other single aspect of the patient's status. The point was also reiterated that tricuspid regurgitation should be corrected and that repair will improve the short- and long-term clinical result and decrease the operative mortality rate. It was also suggested that if tricuspid involvement is not secondary to mitral replacement, but is anatomically organic and relative to primary tricuspid disease process, there is no change in the morbidity and mortality associated with the combined tricuspid and mitral valve repair or replacement. The tricuspid valve, in all surgeons' opinion, should not be replaced and is virtually always amenable to repair. Ideally, mitral surgery should be done before there is tricuspid involvement. In Dr Bjork's experience, at 5 years, 60% of incompetent tricuspid valves were competent after mitral valve replacement.

Tissue valve deterioration

The significance of morphologic changes in tissue valves and their use as a predictor of valve durability was addressed. Dr Ionescu stated that he had no electron-microscopic data on the pericardial valve correlating with valve durability. Dr Oyer expressed the opinion that morphologic changes in the porcine valve would have predicted a much earlier deterioration rate than actually occurred clinically. While the morphology may be a predictor of deterioration, the time sequence and the percentage of valves that will deteriorate may be substantially different from what is seen microscopically. Conversely, it may be that we do not understand which kind of microscopic alteration will predict clinical deterioration. It is clear that the vast majority of tissue valves that have deteriorated have undergone calcification, and calcium may well be the causative agent in most, if not all, of the clinical porcine valve deterioration that has been seen during the first 10 years of experience. Doctor Carpentier's data indicates that there is no difference in the early morphologic changes of pericardial or porcine valves. One would expect that any biological valve that is created with a fixative agent and is then implanted and subsequently examined will show morphologic changes. This is in contrast to—and is a disadvantage of—the tissue valve compared with the prosthetic valve. Improved tissue preservation techniques by the manufacturers will hopefully increase the *in-vivo* durability of valves. In addition, many aspects of valve preparation are better controlled at the present time, particularly the condition of the tissue from the time it leaves the slaughter house until it arrives for fixation in the laboratory.

A representative from the Albert Einstein Medical Center showed tears in pericardial valves with the rest of the leaflets appearing grossly normal. He described *in-vitro* fatigue testing in which pericardial valves lasted approximately twice as long as porcine valves. Dr Carpentier suggested that tissue valves are biological and are in a biological environment before and after implantation. Using mechanical high-speed fatigue testing for this biological valve is less appropriate than using those devices for testing mechanical valves. One might speculate that the mechanical pulse duplicator is no more a compatible environment for a biological valve than is the human heart for a mechanical valve!

Dr Starr emphasized that the effect of changes in valve manufacturing and design takes a long time to become clinically evident. We will not know the effect of those changes for many years after they have been conceived, executed and then implanted in patients. These changes are not criteria for selection of a particular valve. Along this same line, valve changes must eventually be deleterious if enough changes are made. For example, certainly the desire is that durability of the tissue valves will increase. If increased durability could be proven in the tissue valve, it would then offer us a more viable alternative to the prosthetic valve. At present, however, we must wait 5–10 more years to prove that present methods will in fact prove to increase durability. In general, present changes in manufacturing, even if good in theory, should not be an argument for selection of a given valve type.

The experts' choice of valve

After addressing these issues and eliciting opinions on the eight valve types available, the experts on the panel were asked their preference and the reasons for choosing a specific valve type over another—but excluding their first choice. The rationale behind this question is that these experts have extensive experience and knowledge regarding valves, valve types, valve implantation techniques and the problems and causes associated with valve replacment. While their first choice may be biased, the second choice is commonly not, and yet is still based on their extensive experience. Dr Starr's second choice was the Carpentier–Edwards valve. His feeling was that more information is available about that valve type than the others. He conceded that there is no conclusive data at the present time, but felt that the Carpentier–Edwards valve may be better than the Hancock valve. The stent has theoretical advantages and has not been associated with some of the complications reported with the early Hancock valves. His objection to the pericardial valve is that there is no well-reported clinical data except in Dr Ionescu's hands, and those data were felt to be biased. He emphasized the point that if a surgeon wishes to avoid problems with implanting valves that may eventually turn out to be bad in design or construction, one should not use a valve that does not have a substantial clinical record, an example being the Braunwald–Cutter valve. The new valve types (e.g. the St. Jude valve) are wildcat valves of speculative nature. The surgeon who selects a new valve type without a clinical record will eventually be burned by the speculative nature of these devices.

This opinion was re-emphasized by Dr Matloff who suggested that although he used the St. Jude valve he anticipated that in using the new valve he must accept new problems. He also emphasized that it will take at least 15 years of experience to determine durability. When one considers the functional life span of a surgeon and the length of time required for individual evaluation, one cannot logically make more than one change in a career. Dr Bjork stated that he rarely used a second-choice valve but when he does he believes that one should go with a valve type that has the best clinical record. Dr Ionescu suggested that he found a rare indication for using a prosthetic valve. Some of these indications were: reoperation of a Jehovah's Witness, the presence of fungal endocarditis, and patients who have had four or five reoperations. When selecting a valve other than his own, he uses the Bjork–Shiley valve because of the substantial clinical record.

Dr Carpentier expressed the opinion that there was no absolute valve of choice because there is no perfect valve. In his experience, valve failure rate was the lowest for reconstruction and no statistical difference was noted for any of the other three valve replacement devices. Thromboembolism was substantially less with the bioprosthesis. Surgical mortality was lowest with reconstruction, followed by replacement with the bioprosthesis and the highest using prosthetic valves. Therefore, in his own individual experience, Dr Carpentier used reconstruction techniques wherever possible. The bioprosthesis is his first choice for replacement, and the Starr–Edwards valve is the preferred prosthesis. Dr Carpentier stressed that this is not because he has a long-standing friendly relationship with Dr Starr but is based on hard data from his own center.

Doctor ——— from St Thomas Hospital purported that their surgeons selected the valve type from the clinical data that is published and that they used the Starr–Edwards valve, the Carpentier–Edwards valve and the Bjork–Shiley valve in equal frequency. However, he also felt that the type of valve chosen is commonly due to the sales representative's personality and attractiveness and has little to do with the scientific data available on a particular valve product.

The question was raised to Dr Oyer as to whether the comparative studies between valve types in the same institution truly generated comparable data. He stated that they had not used a prosthetic valve since 1974 but that with the recent evidence of increasing failure rate with the bioprosthesis, they may consider a change in valve type sometime in the future. The Stanford experience with the original Starr–Edwards valve was good. In his opinion, that would be a reasonable consideration for an alternative valve type.

Dr Kalmason expressed an opinion that individual institutions have different results with different valve types. He believed that the cardiologist should decide which valve type is appropriate and send the patient to that center where the particular valve type is being used. The valve that a surgeon selects is due to an individual impression or opinion. Each center, particularly one doing a substantial volume of valve replacement surgery, should adopt a policy. The center's policy should, in Dr Carpentier's opinion, be determined by its own experience and not by the experience of other reported people. This emphasizes the fact that there are statistical differences in reports between groups using the same valve replacement device. Dr Starr is more likely to get better results with the Starr–Edwards valve than surgeons at Stanford using the same valve type. There are individual and acceptable reasons for this. It makes sense, therefore, for Dr Starr to come to the conclusion that for the patients he sees it is better for him to use the Starr–Edwards valve. For patients that are seen at Stanford, it is better for them to receive the porcine valve. This opinion was met with disagreement from Dr Matloff, who felt that for any individual patient there is a preferred valve type and that should be the basis of selection. The experience and expertise of the surgical group is most important in selection of a given valve type. Where cardiologists are experts in diagnosis, surgeons probably have a better knowledge and understanding of results associated with a given valve type. Therefore, the surgeon more appropriately makes the choice based on his experience and his understanding and interpretation of the experience of others.

From the audience, the Caster–Hall valve was described as having been released by Medtronic, and this valve has an extensive pre-release experience of nearly 5 years with excellent data collection. The manufacturers are to be complimented for the thoroughness, responsibility and maturity with which this device was introduced.

The moderator and panelists were polled for their choice of valves. Dr Starr's opinion was that one can address the issue with the patient in such a way that the patient's response is predetermined. He discusses the choice with patients but accepts the fact that the patient will take his recommendation for a Starr–Edwards valve. Dr Angell used porcine valves 90% of the time, and the preference for a porcine valve was expressed to the patient preoperatively. In virtually all instances, the patient takes this recommendation regarding selection. Dr Ionescu indicated that the patient leaves the choice to the surgeon, and that in his unit the pericardial valve was used exclusively. At Cedars–Sinai in Los Angels, Dr Matloff said that they were very careful to explain to the patient his choices. Selection is definitely left to the patient to avoid problems or complications relative to the choice of a particular valve type later in the patient's course. Dr Bjork indicated that in Sweden the surgeon makes the choice for the patient. At Stanford the porcine xenograft is used exclusively.

Thromboembolism and anticoagulation

A technical question of anticoagulation and the relationship of the atrial appendage obliteration to thromboembolism was addressed. There was a divergence of opinion on this point. Both Dr Bjork and Starr did not feel that the obliteration of the appendage was important and was perhaps a disadvantage. The experience of Drs Barratt–Boyes, Kirklin and Angell were quoted, suggesting that obliteration of the atrial appendage was a simple technique which eliminated a significant anatomical site for thrombosis. Early heparinization is not deleterious and has a low complication rate and is followed by an interval of 1–3 months coumadin therapy. In the experience of many, chronic coumadin therapy for all patients in atrial fibrillation was appropriate. There was not, however, a universal agreement on this point. Substantial numbers of patients with bioprosthetic mitral valve replacements are being managed without anticoagulation even in the face of atrial fibrillation. The prosthetic valves all require anticoagulants. Drs Starr and Smeloff pointed to a substantial number of patients with ball valves who have had their anticoagulant stopped and who have done well without long-term coumadin therapy. In prosthetic valve patients, if coumadin therapy is possible, the incidence of complications is lower. It was emphasized that anticoagulants can be stopped intermittently for other surgical procedures without significant complications.

Mitral valve disease in children

Dr Carpentier expressed a strong preference for valve repair in 90% of children. In those cases where the valve could not be repaired, a bioprosthesis was used. With this comes an understanding that the patient will need a reoperation for a larger valve. The accelerated deterioration in the younger age group was accepted. In patients 10–20 years of age, a Starr–Edwards prosthetic valve was used. The group in Hanover, Germany, reported an experience of 15 children with the St. Jude valve using only aspirin as an anticoagulant. Dr Starr had a preference for the use of ball valves in children except where it is essential that a low-profile valve be used. In that case, he selected the Bjork–Shiley valve. His experience after 14 years is that the thromboembolism incidence in children is the same as with adults or even less. In India, where there is a large problem with rheumatic fever, and where prosthetic valve replacement is required often in children, the thromboembolism incidence is 1½–2% per year. Dr Ionescu indicated that his experience with children was small and the results with valve replacement poor.

Concluding remarks by Dr Carpentier—mitral valve symposium II

It is urged that as physicians dealing with patient care, we should not be disappointed or discouraged with the 'State of the Art' of mitral valve surgery. Over the past 7 years since the previous Mitral Valve Symposium, all of the techniques have substantially improved, including valve repair, the techniques of cardiopulmonary bypass, valve design and cardiac preservation. This in turn has improved the results with valvular surgery. Twenty years ago, all patients with the diagnosis of serious valvular heart disease died, and now we are looking at a 90% survival rate at 5 years. The physicians involved and the commercial companies have combined and contributed to provide a very impressive level of expertise in the care of patients who require surgery for valvular heart disease.

Appendix

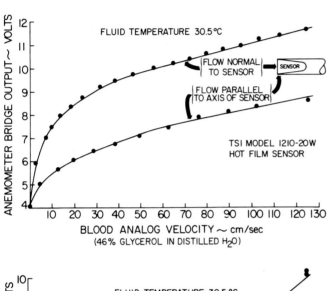

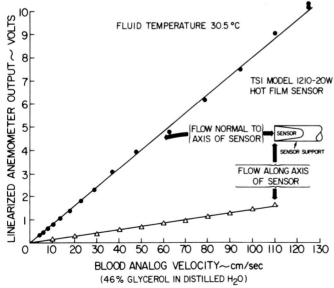

Figures 3.A1 and *3.A2* Calibration curves for TSI Model 1210–20W hot-film probe (*see text* p. 20).

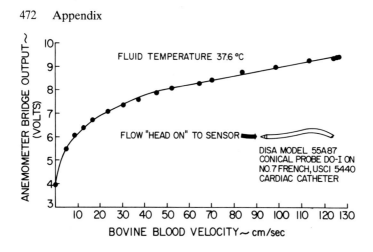

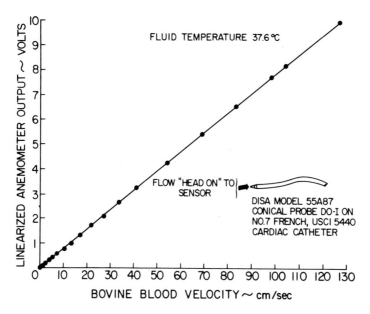

Figures 3.A3 and *3.A4* Calibration curves for DISA Model 55A87 Conical probe (*see text* p. 31)

Index